Oral Pathology

Color Atlas of Dental Medicine

Editors: Klaus H. Rateitschak and Herbert F. Wolf

Oral Pathology

Peter A. Reichart and Hans Peter Philipsen

Translated by
Thomas Hassell, D.D.S., Ph.D.
Bellevue, USA

1072 Illustrations

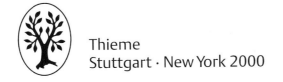

Thieme
Stuttgart · New York 2000

Authors' Addresses

Peter A. Reichart, D.D.S.
Professor
Zentrum für Zahnmedizin
Charité
Augustenburger Platz 1
13353 Berlin
Germany

Hans Peter Philipsen, D.D.S.
Professor
Edif. El Cóndor, Apt. 30
Guadalmina Alta
29670 San Pedro de Álcantara
Spain

Editors' Addresses

Klaus H. Rateitschak, D.D.S., Ph.D.
Dental Institute, Center for Dental Medicine
University of Basle
Hebelstr. 3,
4056 Basle,
Switzerland

Herbert F. Wolf, D.D.S.
Private Practitioner
Specialist of Periodontics SSO/SSP
Löwenstrasse 55,
8001 Zurich,
Switzerland

Library of Congress Cataloging-in-Publication Data

Reichart, P. (Peter) [Oralpathologie. English] Oral pathology/Peter A. Reichart and Hans Peter Philipsen; translated by Thomas Hassell. p.; cm. – (Color atlas of dental medicine) Includes bibliographical references and index.
ISBN 3131258810 (GTV : hardcover) –
ISBN 0-86577-932-5 (TNY)
1. Mouth–Diseases–Atlases. I. Philipsen, H. P. (Hans P.) II. Title. III. Series.
[DNLM: 1. Stomatognathic Diseases–pathology–Atlases.
WU 17 R348o 2000a]
RC815. R39513 2000
616.3'107–dc2l
00-055193

Illustrations by Joachim Hormann, Stuttgart

This book is an authorized translation of the German edition published and copyrighted 1999 by Georg Thieme Verlag, Stuttgart, Germany.
Title of the German edition: Oralpathologie

© 2000 Georg Thieme Verlag,
Rüdigerstraße 14,
D-70469 Stuttgart, Germany
Thieme New York, 333 Seventh Avenue,
New York, N.Y. 10001 USA

Typesetting by Müller, Heilbronn
Printed in Germany
by Grammlich, Pliezhausen

ISBN 3-13-125881-0 (GTV)
ISBN 0-86577-932-5 (TNY)   1 2 3

In the Series "Color Atlas of Dental Medicine"

K. H. & E. M. Rateitschak, H. F. Wolf, T. M. Hassell
- **Periodontology, 2nd edition**

A. H. Geering, M. Kundert, C. Kelsey
- **Complete Denture and Overdenture Prosthetics**

G. Graber
- **Removable Partial Dentures**

F. A. Pasler
- **Radiology**

T. Rakosi, I. Jonas, T. M. Graber
- **Orthodontic Diagnosis**

H. Spiekermann
- **Implantology**

H. F. Sailer, G. F. Pajarola
- **Oral Surgery for the General Dentist**

R. Beer, M. A. Baumann, S. Kim
- **Endodontology**

J. Schmidseder
- **Aesthetic Dentistry**

P. A. Reichart, H. P. Philipsen
- **Oral Pathology**

Foreword

Prof. Isaäc van der Waal

Oral and Maxillofacial Surgery/Pathology
University Hospital Vrije Universiteit / ACTA
Amsterdam, The Netherlands

The authors of *Color Atlas of Oral Pathology,* both world-renowned authorities in their field, have been able to write down and illustrate their vast knowledge and expertise in an extremely clear and didactic way. The enormous number, but above all the wide variety of oral diseases that are presented in this atlas offer a challenge to every dentist, who must be able to recognize and diagnose lesions of the oral cavity and the face at the earliest possible stage. The dentist must also recognize when the time is appropriate to refer the patient to a specialist if more experience, knowledge, and skills are required in the management of patients with more perilous maladies.

Indeed, the spectrum of the dentist's daily occupation has broadened tremendously in the past century, developing from a primarily technically oriented trade, repairing and replacing teeth, to a much more biologically oriented *pro-fession,* dealing with the diagnosis and often the treatment of numerous diseases and conditions that affect the oral cavity and its surrounding structures. This development in dentistry demands a comprehensive biological and medical education. Today's dentist and the dentists of the new millennium will benefit greatly from the contents of this atlas.

The authors have achieved a well-balanced structure in their chapters. Particularly their choice to focus on a number of specific anatomic oral subsites, such as lips, tongue, cheek, and palate, will be of great help in the everyday practice, when the dentist is confronted with an oral lesion whose pathogenesis and definition are not readily recognizable.

Dentists will embrace this atlas. And rightly so.

Preface

Oral pathology is an established scientific discipline in medicine and dentistry, whose goal is to describe and understand the anatomic and histopathologic aspects of human diseases.

Historically, oral pathology developed from two important sources: The first is to be found in the early decades of the 20th century and is based in oral medicine; the second is more recent, and finds its origin in the study of general pathology.

Morphologic studies of the dental hard tissues and the diseases of these tissues, primarily dental caries but also maladies within neighboring structures such as the periodontium, led to our earliest understanding of the histopathologic nature of these anatomic structures. Over the course of many decades, histologic examination of dental hard tissues was the primary pursuit in dental research; this led to its being called purely "*dental* pathology." Dental caries and its etiopathogenic aspects demanded the use of morphological methods and, increasingly, the development of novel sectioning and staining techniques. Dental caries research benefited early on from the use of the electron microscope.

At that time in history, histopathologic diagnosis of most oral diseases was relegated to general pathologists; there appeared to be no necessity for a specialized field of *oral* pathology. In retrospect, however, the classification of lesions such as odontogenic tumors and cysts was poorly detailed and also imprecise. For affected patients, this often meant unnecessary radical surgical therapy. This mind-set began to change in the early 1950s and throughout the 1960s. The specialty of "oral pathology" evolved into an accepted discipline with an active research agenda. In several areas of the world, such as the United States, Great Britain, Scandinavia, and the Netherlands, "oral pathology" evolved into an independent discipline with its own active research endeavors. Between 1950 and 1980, the literature provided many new descriptions of various oral diseases;

these were based upon improved histopathologic diagnosis and a more mature understanding of pathogenic mechanisms. This rapid development of the discipline of oral pathology can be closely linked with important pioneers such as Pindborg, Gorlin, Kramer, Lucas, and many others. The current World Health Organization (WHO) classification of the odontogenic tumors derives primarily from the original research work of these and other leaders in the dental medicine community.

The second innovative source for the development of oral pathology derived from general medical pathology. The introduction of advanced diagnostic techniques led, also in oral pathology, to critically important improvements for diagnostic precision and accuracy. For example, immunohistochemistry and cytochemical procedures have been established and accepted in oral pathology for many years. The use of numerous polyclonal and monoclonal antibodies has made it possible for the oral pathologist to differentiate between epithelial, mesenchymal, or neurogenic tissue components. Newer ultrastructural methods, on the other hand, have provided advances primarily in scientific investigations rather than in routine oral diagnosis. Most recently, molecular biological procedures such as the polymerase chain reaction (PCR) have also been utilized in the science of oral pathology. The goal of the contemporary methods of investigation is to obtain relevant information about various markers of tissue proliferation or oncogenes, ultimately providing insights concerning the risk of malignant transformation, for example, of an area of oral leukoplakia. These developments are extremely promising; however, so far there has been no real breakthrough. Routine examination of surgical biopsy specimens remains the basis for virtually all histopathologic diagnoses. Nevertheless, the diagnostic power that can be gleaned today from a simple oral biopsy has been greatly expanded.

At the present time, the discipline of oral pathology seems to be traversing a period of fundamental change. During the last ten years, it has become clear that pure "bench pathology" does not always provide the optimum diagnosis. Rather it is the combination of *clinical* oral pathology with histopathologic examination that leads to improved diagnosis and also to the quality control that has become more and more important.

The inclusion of oral medicine into the spectrum of knowledge of the oral pathologist would be a reasonable step in the right direction. The extent to which such combinations of disciplines might affect the structuring of university-based teaching of dentistry cannot yet be ascertained or even imagined. In this regard, one must also consider developments that may influence the entire future of dentistry as a profession. The worldwide reduction in the prevalence rate of dental caries has dramatically changed the nature and substance of dental practice over the past 30 years. Both the WHO and the Fédération Dentaire Internationale (FDI) have repeatedly emphasized this fact in recent reports. Dentistry's emphasis on restorative procedures, which has predominated in our profession since its very inception, must now yield to more medical activities by the dentist. This can also be seen in the FDI proposal for the term "oral physician." H. Löe (United States) recently outlined the major areas of emphasis within which such an "oral physician" would work:

- Diseases of the oral mucosa,
- TMJ disorders and diseases of the salivary glands, including the restoration of saliva production,
- Participation in the treatment of cancer patients and organ transplant patients,
- Diagnosis and treatment of facial pain,
- Psychosomatic oral diseases.

There exists today a clear trend for dentistry to position itself closer to medicine. This will be absolutely necessary if dentistry is to persist as a profession based upon academic principles.

This perspective for the future admonishes each dental practitioner to become more knowledgeable of and involved in oral pathology and oral medicine if our profession is to satisfy the inevitable demands. This *Atlas* is dedicated to a synthesis between clinical practice and oral pathology; it therefore pursues a wholly new concept, in order to simplify accurate and precise diagnosis. It will permit dental practitioners to better serve their patients; this is, after all, the most important and most noble goal.

Berlin, Germany, and   Peter A. Reichart
San Pedro, Spain   Hans P. Philipsen

Spring, 2000

Acknowledgements

This *Atlas* presents illustrations that have been collected over a period of more than 25 years. From our two extensive archives we have selected the most representative cases in order to offer the reader a spectrum of the most typical clinical, radiographic, and histopathologic findings. Our personal collections, however, were not always sufficient. So we asked colleagues for help in providing additional illustrative material from their own collections. We would like to express our sincere gratitude to all of these contributors.

The following individuals made available clinical, radiographic, and histologic illustrations or preparations, as well as electron photomicrographs:

Dr. Lis Andersen, Copenhagen, Denmark
Prof. T. Axéll, Oslo, Norway
Dr. Gudrun Bethke, Berlin, Germany
Prof. H. G. Gelderblom, Berlin, Germany
Prof. W. Golder, Berlin, Germany
Prof. Dr. U. Gross, Berlin, Germany
Prof. Dr. B. Hoffmeister, Berlin, Germany
Dr. K. Kalz, Berlin, Germany
Prof. J. Reibel, Copenhagen, Denmark
Prof. M. Shear, Simonstown, South Africa
Prof. K. Sugihara, Kagoshima, Japan
Prof. I. Thompson, Tygerberg/Stellenbosch, South Africa
Dr. H.-J. Tietz, Berlin, Germany
Prof. I. van der Waal, Amsterdam, The Netherlands

We thank Prof. J. Bier (Berlin) and Prof. B. Hoffmeister (Berlin) for providing biopsy materials.

The photographic documentation would not have been possible without the dedicated participation of photographers J. Eckert and R. Hoey, and graphic arts specialist W. Lorenz. We express our sincere gratitude to these three individuals.

We thank Dr. Christian Scheifele for preparing a computer program that significantly simplified our work with the layout and the text.

Ms. Christiane Schönberg, our secretary, deserves special thanks. During the long period of manuscript preparation, she was always patient and tireless in making corrections and additions.

We also thank Dr. Thomas M. Hassell (Seattle, USA) for turning our German sentences, phrases, and paragraphs into a coherent English-language text, and Ms. Debbie Sorensen (Seattle, USA) for preparing the English manuscript.

Our special thanks go to the editors of the *Color Atlas of Dental Medicine* series, Prof. K. H. Rateitschak and Dr. H. F. Wolf, for their knowledgeable guidance during preparation of the layout as well as for continuous motivation and collegial advice.

The employees at Thieme Publishers, especially Dr. Chr. Urbanowicz, Mr. K.-H. Fleischmann, and Mr. M. Pohlmann, deserve our gratitude for their valued assistance and support, and for their understanding cooperation.

We ask our spouses, Barbara Reichart and Kirsten Philipsen, to accept our heartfelt thanks for their understanding and support during the years that it required to produce this book.

Last but not least, we wish to recognize and thank the man who implanted in us the spark of enthusiasm for clinical and histologic oral pathology: Prof. Jens Jørgen Pindborg, Copenhagen (Denmark), who, unfortunately, died much too early.

Introduction

Many books about diseases of the oral mucosa, oral manifestations of AIDS, and other diseases of the oral cavity have been published in recent years. Several excellent textbooks of oral pathology have also appeared. In these works, one generally finds either clinical pictures and diagnoses alone, or—especially in oral pathology textbooks—histopathologic findings.

Why, then, another Atlas of Oral Pathology?

There were numerous reasons for compiling yet another atlas, the most important of them being:

● Our overriding desire to utilize exceptional illustrative materials to *forge a connection between clinical and histopathologic findings*. Only this combination will permit a successful search for the correct definitive diagnosis. This manner of presentation should also serve to improve understanding of the pathogenesis and etiology of various diseases.

● Most classical textbooks of oral pathology are arranged according to classifications of disease entities. Quite the contrary, the organization of this atlas is based upon the *sequence of steps generally followed during clinical examination of the oral cavity*.

What Do We Mean by That?

Every examination—including the examination of the oral cavity—must follow a systematic, recurring pattern. After documenting the patient's medical history, one proceeds to visual inspection and finally to palpation of any existing abnormality. Inspection generally begins by observing the patient's overall corporeal stature. Next, the face and especially the perioral region are considered. An intensive inspection of the lips is performed and then the patient is asked to open the mouth. Examination of the oral cavity is performed according to a systematic inspection of the various oral regions, such as the cheeks, the tongue, the floor of the mouth, the palate, etc. The organization and configuration of this *Atlas* follow the anatomic configuration of the oral region. However, for some diseases, such as odontogenic tumors, cysts, and salivary gland diseases, this principle is not applicable; in these cases, we have adhered to the more customary scheme of classification and presentation.

Within the various regions of the oral cavity, we have presented clinical and histopathologic information according to etiology: infections; mechanical, physical, chemical, or thermal causes; disturbances of keratinization; tumors etc. Because we have arranged the book in this way, the same disease process may be found in several chapters. For example, oral leukoplakia or carcinoma of the oral cavity as well as other diseases are presented several times according to their various localizations. We have taken care to reduce redundancy within the text whenever possible. In most instances, broader topics are distributed among the relevant chapters, so the reader can cross reference comprehensive information about each disease entity.

• To simplify the search for a diagnosis, we have included "*diagnostic keys*" in the index. These are collective terms under which the various disease processes are presented in the *Atlas*. For the mucosal lesions, color (white, black, blue, yellow) as well as surface structure (ulcerated, verrucous, etc.) are provided. The radiographic criteria include: radiolucent, radiopaque, sharply or poorly demarcated, circumscribed, homogeneous, non-homogeneous, etc.

• *Inspection of the face* and discovery of a possible lesion—for example, a black spot that has not previously been detected—should also be considered the responsibility of the dentist. This does not imply that the dentist should establish the definitive diagnosis, nor that treatment should be administered; rather, a patient who exhibits a suspicious lesion should be referred to an appropriate specialist.

• *HIV-infection* has dramatically expanded the spectrum of oral manifestations and their severity; it has also complicated oral diagnosis. For this reason, we have included a short chapter with some basic data and other information about the AIDS epidemic.

• It is obvious that the *literature* today in all areas of oral pathology and oral medicine has become practically impossible to master. We therefore have not cited case reports or older literature. Rather, we have concentrated primarily on comprehensive review articles and more recent publications.

Oral diagnosis is often difficult and challenging. It is our hope and desire that this *Atlas* will serve to sharpen practitioners' diagnostic skills and increase their joy in oral diagnosis.

Table of Contents

Oral Diagnosis

Oral diagnosis is an important, if not the *most* important, aspect of dental practice. The responsibility for oral diagnosis rests with the dental practitioner; unfortunately, this responsibility is too often neglected. Nevertheless, the onus is on the general dentist to recognize and detect orofacial abnormalities early on. If an oral lesion or condition is overlooked by the general practitioner, the best opportunity for timely and appropriate therapy will be missed.

What Is a Diagnosis?

Any dentist who examines a patient and formulates a diagnosis is assumed to have both detected and understood the type of disease suffered by the patient. During the course of the examination and the subsequent considerations, other disease processes will have been eliminated as probable diagnoses. Diagnosis, therefore, involves *recognition* and *differentiation.* These processes are crucial for establishing the definitive diagnosis.

The oral cavity of a human being may be affected by over 200 different diseases, some common and others less so; fortunately, only 3% are life threatening. The diagnosis of oral lesions is fundamentally an exercise in clinical pathology. In most instances, oral lesions are caused by pathogenic microorganisms or other disease-causing agents. In order for the clinician to recognize and describe the alterations, certain "references" must be present, which can be compared to the altered conditions.

It follows that a prerequisite for the detection of pathologic changes in the oral cavity is a thorough basic knowledge of the clinically normal appearance of the oral cavity and its adjacent structures. It is also important to recognize that the characteristics of a tissue cannot be satisfactorily evaluated without thorough knowledge of its microstructure. This is because the microanatomy of tissues correlates well with the clinical features, on which the clinical evaluation and ultimate diagnosis are based. For these reasons, the conscientious clinician cannot afford to ignore the importance of *normal* anatomy and histology of the various tissues of the oral cavity. The goal of this *Color Atlas of Oral Pathology* is to provide every dental practitioner with the basic histologic and clinical knowledge required to accurately arrive at a correct definitive diagnosis.

However, the diagnosis is not a goal *per se.* More importantly, it represents the basis for treatment and prognosis. Therefore, the clinician must follow a methodical diagnostic routine that identifies all of the clinical and histologic characteristics of a disease process.

The Diagnostic Sequence

The following diagnostic sequence has evolved from many years of clinical experience. It has proved to be both effective and practical:

1. Detection of a deviation from the normal
2. History (first appearance and clinical course)
3. Methodical examination of the oral cavity
4. Reexamination of the apparent change from the normal
5. Attempts to classify the lesion
6. Listing of possible diagnoses
7. Development of the differential diagnosis
8. Development of a working diagnosis (tentative diagnosis)
9. Formulation of the definitive diagnosis (supported by paraclinical findings, see below)
10. Paraclinical findings (radiograph, biopsy, microbiology, blood count, etc.)

It has been argued that an experienced diagnostician does not follow a cumbersome or formal process during the search for a diagnosis, but can diagnose any lesion after only a cursory examination. This is rarely true, however, because a diagnosis does not often result from an instant recognition of the pathologic process, but rather on the rapid and effective use of a diagnostic sequence, which must be perfected over many years. It is, of course, true that the astute diagnostician who has seen numerous intraoral lesions will more likely be able to rapidly anticipate the nature of a disorder.

The collection of information and data that serve as a basis for diagnosis derive in principle from three areas:

● From the specific medical and dental history,
● From the clinical examination, and
● From additional examinations, such as radiography, biopsy, microbiological evaluation or hematological analysis.

The first source, the patient's medical/dental history, will not be discussed further here. Readers interested in detailed information about this point are referred to the *Color Atlas of Oral Surgery for the General Dentist* (Sailer and Pajarola 1999), which provides an excellent and detailed description of anamnestic methodology.

In the following few pages, the individual steps of the diagnostic sequence are described in more detail.

1. Detection of a Lesion

It is important to remember that, in many cases, especially when pain or functional disturbance occur, the patient will be the first one to detect a problem.

2. History of the Primary Complaint, Its First Appearance and Clinical Course

This point of the diagnostic sequence is particularly important because valuable tips for the diagnosis can emerge. The most common primary complaints with diseases of the oral cavity are pain, soreness, a burning sensation in the mouth, bleeding, tooth mobility, delayed tooth eruption, dryness of the oral cavity, or swelling, to name but a few.

The patient should be encouraged to precisely describe the primary characteristics of the pain. Is it sharp or dull? What are its intensity, duration and localization, and what seems to trigger the pain? If the patient uses terms such as "soreness" or "burning" to describe the disorder, this provides a clue for mucosal inflammation or ulceration of varying origin. Burning of the tongue only occurs following atrophy or erosion of the lingual epithelium, often without any visible alteration. Numerous diseases can cause a burning sensation, ranging from geographic tongue through psychogenic disturbances. Intraoral bleeding may also result from various diseases, such as periodontitis, trauma, neoplasia, and diseases that are associated with disturbances of blood clotting.

Loss of alveolar bone or root resorption can lead to tooth mobility that may indicate various conditions, e.g., periodontal disease, trauma, normal resorption of the primary teeth, malignant tumors, or even rare conditions such as familial hypophosphatasia. Delayed eruption of teeth may be associated with cysts, odontomas, osseous sclerosis and tumors. In cases of generalized delayed tooth eruption, the clinician should consider the possibility of anodontia or cleidocranial dysostosis. A dry mouth (xerostomia) may be a consequence of the following disease processes: local infections such as candidiasis, infection of the major salivary glands, systemic dehydration or psychogenic disturbances. Xerostomia may also result as a side effect of numerous medications.

If the patient complains of a swelling, the following possibilities exist: inflammation or infection, cysts, benign and/or malignant tumors. When attempting to arrive at a diagnosis, it is helpful to determine the first appearance and the clinical course of any swelling:

● Swelling that increases in size before eating: salivary retention phenomenon.
● Swelling that increases in size slowly (over the course of months or years): reactive hyperplasia, chronic infections, cysts and benign tumors. If the duration encompasses weeks or months, malignant tumors must also be considered.
● Swelling that increases in size rapidly (hours to days): abscesses (painful), infected cysts (painful), salivary retention phenomenon (painless), and hematomas (painless, but uncomfortable when pressure is applied).

3. Methodical Examination of the Oral Cavity

For the examination of intraoral and extraoral structures, a careful and methodical sequence is very important; indeed, it is a prerequisite for a sound diagnosis. The sequence of the examination should never vary. It is extremely important to develop an examination routine. Only in this way will it be possible to avoid missing possibly important findings during the examination. The *extraoral* examination of the head and neck region is extensively described in the *Color Atlas of Oral Surgery for the General Dentist* (Sailer and Pajarola 1999); the interested reader will find helpful tips and additional details in that excellent book.

For the *intraoral* examination, one requires two mouth mirrors, sensitive fingertips for palpation, and two extremely attentive eyes. Even with rubber gloves, digital palpation provides the best and most reliable sense of the texture of any tissue alteration in the oral cavity. Dentures should be removed before the clinical examination begins. The following procedure is recommended for examination of the oral cavity:

The *lips* should be examined with the mouth closed and open. The color, texture and surface characteristics of the vermilion border and the adjacent skin must be carefully observed.

Mucosa of the lower lip and the vestibulum: The mandibular vestibulum should be examined with the mouth partially open. Any color changes or swelling in the area of the vestibulum and the gingiva must be documented.

Mucosa of the upper lip and the vestibulum: The examination of the maxillary vestibulum and the frenula should also be examined with the mouth partially open.

Commissures, buccal mucosa and vestibulum of the mandible and maxilla in the cheek region: Using two mouth mirrors serving as retractors and with the mouth wide open, the entire buccal mucosa extending from the commissure and to the anterior tonsillar pillar can be examined. Alterations of pigmentation, color, texture or mobility of the mucosa should be recorded. It is especially important to examine the commissures carefully, and to avoid covering them with the mouth mirrors during the examination.

Alveolar ridges (processes): These structures should be inspected from all aspects—buccal, palatal and lingual.

I	Lower lip (vermilion border and adjacent skin)
II	Upper lip (vermilion border and adjacent skin)
III	Mucosa of the lower lip and sulcus
IV	Mucosa of the upper lip and sulcus
V	Commissures, buccal mucosa and vestibula (maxillary and mandibular)
VI	Alveolar process, buccal (use two mirrors)
VII	Alveolar process, lingual (use two mirrors)
VIII	Alveolar process, anterior, with tongue in rest position
IX	Tongue protruded, held by the examiner
X	Lateral borders of the tongue, held by the examiner
XI	Tongue (ventral surfaces) and floor of the mouth
XII	Floor of the mouth with the mouth wide open
XIII	Hard and soft palate, mouth wide open, head tilted backward

1 Sequence of oral cavity examination
Step-wise course of the examination.

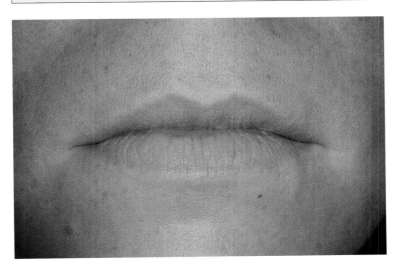

2 Steps I and II of the oral cavity examination
The vermilion border of the lips and the adjacent skin are carefully examined with the mouth closed.

Tongue: With the mouth partially open, the tongue is inspected in its normal *in situ* position; the dorsum of the tongue deserves special attention. Any changes, such as swelling, ulceration, coating, or variations in size, color or texture should be documented. In addition, any changes in the pattern of papillae on the lingual surface are recorded. The patient should then be asked to protrude the tongue, which permits evaluation of any abnormality in lingual mobility. Using the mouth mirror, the lateral borders and the ventral surface of the tongue are examined. The patient should be asked to move the tongue to the left, to the right, and upward. An excellent way to inspect the tongue is to carefully grasp the tip with a piece of gauze to assist full protrusion and to facilitate examination of the lateral borders.

Floor of the Mouth: While holding the tongue up, the floor of the mouth is examined for any swelling or other abnormalities.

Hard and Soft Palate: With the mouth wide open and the patient's head tilted backward, the base of the tongue is gently depressed with a mouth mirror. First the hard palate and subsequently the soft palate can than be thoroughly inspected.

3 Step I and step II of the examination of the oral cavity
With the mouth partially open, the vermilion border and adjacent skin are inspected.

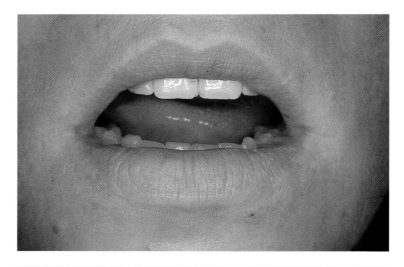

4 Step III of the examination of the oral cavity
After reflecting the lower lip, its mucosa and the vestibular sulcus are examined.

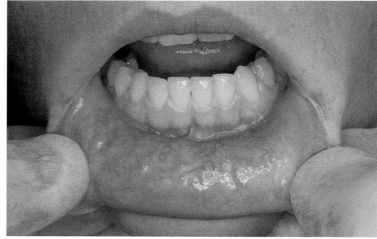

5 Steps IV and V of the examination of the oral cavity
After reflecting the upper lip, its mucosa and the vestibular sulcus are examined.

Right: The commissures of the mouth, buccal mucosa, and the vestibula of both maxilla and mandible are inspected. This is best performed with the mouth wide open. Two mouth mirrors can be used to reflect the cheeks and lips.

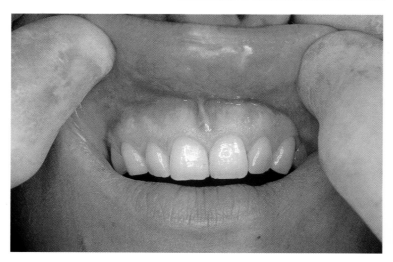
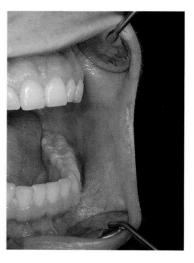

4. Further Examinations of Any Observed Abnormalities

At this point in the examination, new or previously unanswered questions frequently emerge. In many instances it is wise to re-examine any previously observed deviations from normal, in order to evaluate the original findings or to make more detailed clinical observations.

5. Attempt to Classify Any Observed Alterations

To classify diseases is to compile lists of the maladies suffered by humankind, and then to organize the lists in such a way that clinicians can more readily identify encountered abnormalities. Most formal classifications contain subgroups beneath major disease processes. In dentistry, one classifies cysts of the jaws, which are subclassified into odontogenic and nonodontogenic, inflammatory and developmental. There has been a tendency to construct classifications that are more detailed than is actually necessary for prognosis and patient treatment. Extremely detailed classifications may be more didactic than practical. Differentiation between a complex and a compound odontoma, for example, is unimportant in terms of prognosis and therapy. It stresses only the pathologic spectrum of odontoma. Differences of opinion during consideration of treatment principles usually revolve around the fact that too little attention

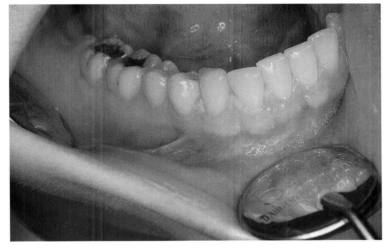

6   Step VI in the examination of the oral cavity
Buccal view of the alveolar process.

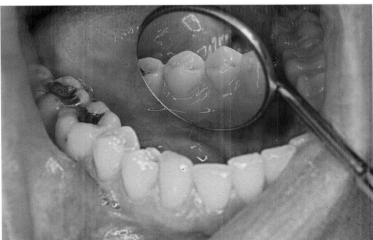

7   Step VII in the examination of the oral cavity
Lingual view of the alveolar process.

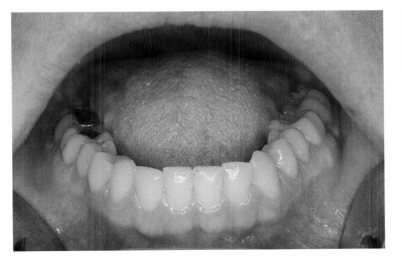

8   Step VIII in the examination of the oral cavity
Anterior view of the mandibular alveolar process.

has been paid to the clinical spectrum, or that various definitions exist for a certain disease entity. For example, many clinicians do not classify initial demineralization of the tooth surface as caries, but reserve this diagnosis for those cases where an actual defect (cavity) is present. Other clinicians speak of caries from the very onset of demineralization. Since incipient carious lesions are treated differently than frank cavity formation, it is likely that misunderstanding and differences of opinion may occur during a discussion of treatment.

6. Listing Possible Diagnoses

After all the diagnostic information has been assembled, a list of lesions should be formulated that corresponds to both the clinical and the radiographic findings. At this point, the order or sequence of the list is unimportant because the primary goal is to identify *all* possible pathologic processes that are similar to the observed alteration, either clinically or radiographically.

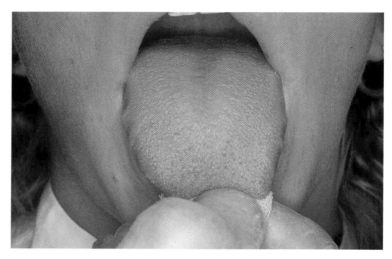

9   Step IX of the examination of the oral cavity
The tip of the tongue is held firmly by the examiner.

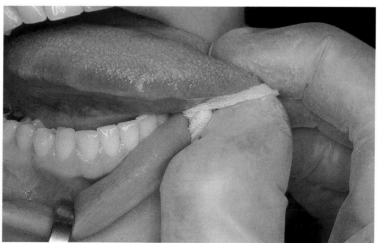

10   Step X of the examination of the oral cavity
Examination of the lateral borders of the tongue, whose tip is reflected by the examiner.

11   Steps XI through XIII of the examination of the oral cavity
Floor of the mouth, view from above.

Right: Hard and soft palate as viewed with the patient's head tilted back.

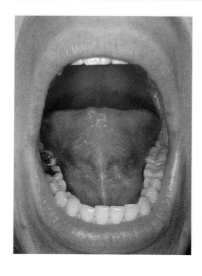

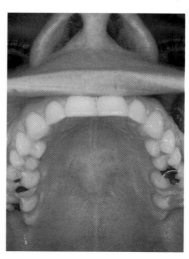

7. Formulating the Differential Diagnosis

Establishing the differential diagnosis consists essentially of *rearranging* the possible diagnoses listed under point 6 above. The most likely diagnosis ranks at the top of the list and the least likely diagnosis at the bottom. To become competent in the art and science of the differential diagnosis, the clinician must not only be cognizant of the signs and symptoms elicited by a great many oral diseases, but must also possess statistical knowledge of disease frequency (prevalence, incidence). Thus, it is especially important to know the *relative incidences* of various disorders; more common diseases will be near the top of the list while rarer disorders will rank near the bottom. When special circumstances are in evidence, the diagnostic list can be re-ordered. For this reason, during the formulation of the differential diagnosis, it is recommended that the more common diseases and disorders be listed first. It is also prudent to keep in mind that the frequency of many diseases can be influenced by factors such as age, gender, anatomic location and other factors.

8. Developing the Working Diagnosis (Preliminary Diagnosis)

The clinician now has a differential diagnosis, but this is not yet sufficient for proceeding with therapeutic measures. First it is necessary to re-check the credibility of the top choices:

- Through further examination of the lesion,
- Through renewed questioning of the patient, to broaden the medical/dental history,
- Through application of additional examination methods and, finally
- Through thorough re-evaluation of all the data and information collected thus far.

Once these tests of credibility have been performed, the much narrower spectrum of diagnoses (top choices) is referred to as the *working diagnosis.*

9. Formulating the Definitive Diagnosis

The definitive diagnosis of an oral lesion is often provided by the oral pathologist, who provides the biopsy report (see point 10, below). This report takes into consideration of all of the clinically relevant data in addition to any laboratory findings. Even in the absence of histopathologic findings, most oral lesions and conditions can be diagnosed on the basis of careful clinical observations and data (subjective symptoms and clinical findings).

There will be cases, however, where the diagnosis cannot be definitively made even by an experienced clinician. For this reason, the working diagnosis must not serve as the basis for initiating therapy. In such cases, the clinician must order additional (paraclinical) examinations (radiographs, cytologic smears, computed tomography, magnetic resonance imaging, biopsy, microbiologic or hematologic examinations). Of all of these tests, it is often the biopsy that provides the determining factor for securing of the definitive diagnosis.

General practitioners may be hesitant to perform a biopsy, because they are insecure or because they did not gain sufficient experience with biopsies during their training. In addition, uncertainty may be increased by inadequate knowledge of the indications for biopsy and for interpretation of the biopsy report. It is also important to realize that patients often associate the term biopsy, or tissue excision, with examination for malignancy. There are many reasons for de-dramatizing this attitude, since this diagnostic procedure in no way exclusively serves the detection of cancer. Patients should be given detailed information about the biopsy procedure and the reasons for performing it.

10. Biopsy

The biopsy can be defined as a diagnostic procedure, whereby tissue or cellular material is removed from the living organism in order to be microscopically examined and to prepare a description of the histological findings. Diagnostic biopsies are performed to confirm, to exclude or to make a definitive diagnosis at the earliest possible time, in order to institute curative therapy without delay.

The term biopsy is usually used to describe the surgical procedure, namely the harvesting of a sample of tissue. The bacteriologic examination of pus, bodily fluids, etc. is not normally included in the rubric biopsy; however, cytologic examination of smears (e.g., for detection of fungi) can be considered a special type of biopsy. Indications, contraindications and the procedures for various types of biopsy methods will be presented in the following chapter.

Biopsy

Indications for Biopsy

It is not necessary to biopsy every pathologic process that is discovered in the oral cavity. The following lesions serve as examples of situations where biopsy *is* indicated:

- Persisting white lesions of the oral mucosa. These are sometimes precancerous. The biopsy can establish whether the lesion is benign, precancerous or malignant.
- Ulcerations that persist for more than three weeks and fail to heal.
- Strong suspicion of malignancy. The dental practitioner should *not* perform the biopsy procedure but should refer the patient to a specialist.
- Persistent swelling without any clear diagnosis.
- Oral lesions that do not respond adequately to therapy.

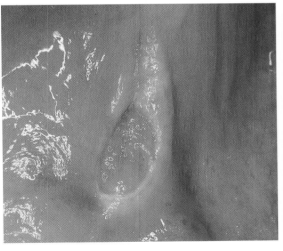
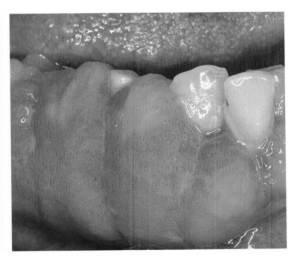

12 Indication for biopsy
Left: Chronic ulceration in the retromolar region. This lesion exhibited no tendency to heal over a 23-day period.

Right: This case of gingival hyperplasia persisted following conservative periodontal therapy, without significant improvement. This fact called into question the original diagnosis of plaque-induced gingivitis.

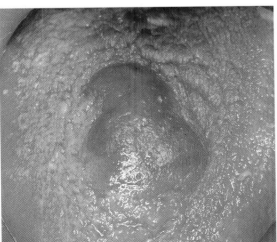
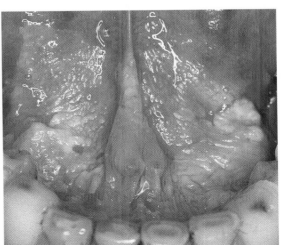

13 Indication for biopsy
Left: Persistent swelling on the dorsum of the tongue. It is not possible to achieve a definitive diagnosis from a clinical examination alone.

Right: Extensive leukoplakia of the floor of the mouth. In such cases, where the lesion is extensive and exhibits varying clinical appearances, two or three incisional biopsies should be performed.

Biopsy Procedures

When the decision is made to perform a biopsy, the *type* of biopsy must first be selected: either an *excisional* biopsy or an *incisional* biopsy. No attempt should be made to disinfect the biopsy site with a tinted disinfectant solution because this could influence the tissue preparation and lead to problems during interpretation of the histologic findings. If it is necessary to remove detritus from the biopsy site, the patient should rinse the mouth with chlorhexidine solution (0.2%). Biopsy instruments are usually the same instruments used for routine oral surgery. Electrosurgery or laser surgery are inappropriate.

It is important that the harvesting of the tissue specimen be performed meticulously. Pathologic alterations can only be properly interpreted if all tissue details are well preserved. Proper handling of the biopsy by the clinician, from surgical removal to fixation of the specimen, is of the utmost importance.

14   Biopsy instruments
Surgical instruments for a mucosa biopsy are kept in an appropriate container. The basic set includes: fine surgical forceps, vessel clamps, needle holder, Langenbeck retractors, suture scissors, atraumatic sutures, suction tip and gauze squares.

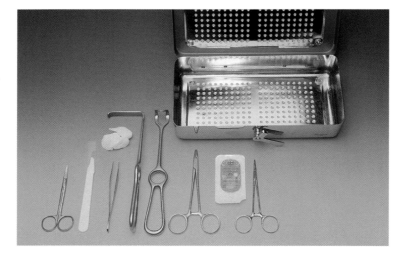

15   Excisional biopsy—schematic
Left: This procedure is indicated for mucosal lesions less than 10 mm in diameter.

Middle: The excision is performed by creating an elliptical incision, encompassing normal adjacent tissue.

Right: Vertical incision through the lesion, defining a wedge-shaped biopsy.

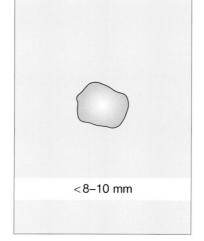

<8–10 mm

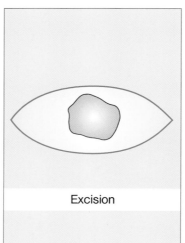

Excision

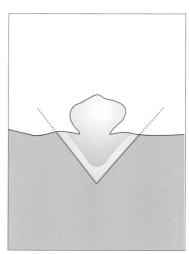

16   Excisional biopsy—"fibroma" of the buccal mucosa
The lines indicate the direction and the extent of the incision.

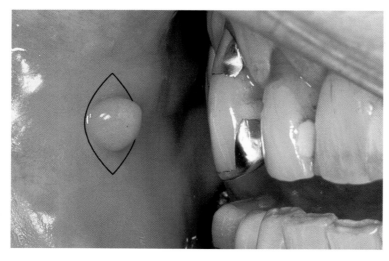

Excisional Biopsy

If the pathologically altered mucosa is small (0.8–1.0 cm in diameter or smaller), the entire lesion including a rim of adjacent normal tissue is removed *in toto.* This type of biopsy is referred to as an *excisional* biopsy.

Incisional Biopsy

If the diameter of the pathologic alteration is larger than ca. 1.0 cm, a representative sample of tissue from the boundary zone where normal and pathologically altered tissue adjoin should be harvested. This type of biopsy is referred to as an *incisional* biopsy. If the lesion is larger than 1.5–2.0 cm in diameter, and a single biopsy cannot encompass all of the characteristics of the change, two or more biopsies should be harvested. It is important to remove a representative normal tissue section in order to give the pathologist the best prerequisites to establish a proper diagnosis. Incisional biopsies must always contain adjacent normal tissue.

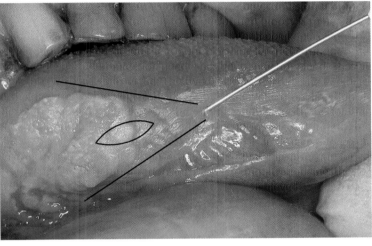

17 Incisional biopsy—injection
A biopsy is to be performed on the leukoplakia of the lateral border of the tongue. The anesthetic injection needle has been inserted. The two black lines depict the direction along which the anesthetic solution should be injected. Using this technique, it is only necessary to make a single needle insertion for adequate infiltration anesthesia to be achieved.

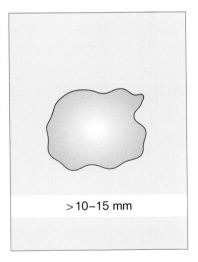

> 10–15 mm

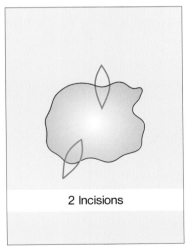

2 Incisions

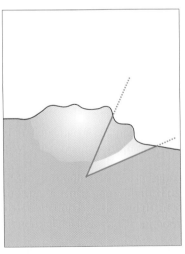

18 Incisional biopsy— schematic
Left: The example is a large mucosal lesion of 10–15 mm or larger, necessitating two biopsies to encompass all of the pathologic alterations.

Middle: Same lesion, depicting the possible biopsy sites.

Right: Vertical incision through the lesion with the creation of a wedge-shaped tissue section that includes adjacent normal tissue.

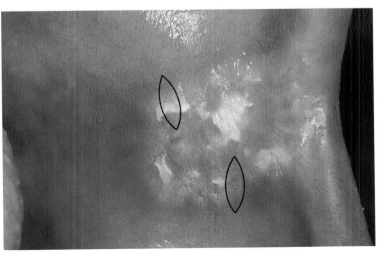

19 Incisional biopsy— erythroleukoplakia at the corner of the mouth
Two representative biopsies will be taken. The tissue specimens should include both the red and the white components of such lesions, including the normal adjacent mucosa.

Harvesting and Handling the Biopsy

Technical aspects of tissue removal follow the general rules applicable for all minor oral surgical procedures. It is important that the procedure be performed carefully to avoid tissue damage such as tears or crushing. Appropriate containers with fixative solution (formalin) and standard biopsy report forms from the cooperating pathology laboratory should always be available. It is also important to consider that the pathologist normally will not have the opportunity to examine the patient clinically. Thus, the pathologist is completely reliant on the clinical information provided by the dentist.

The instant the biopsy is removed from the oral cavity, the blood supply is severed and tissue autolysis immediately sets in. For this reason it is important that the tissue biopsy be immediately immersed in fixative solution to avoid any artifactual cellular changes. Any change in cytologic detail leads to problems during the histopathologic interpretation. The most common fixative is 10% buffered formalin solution. The amount of fixative used should be at least 10 to 15 times greater in volume than the tissue specimen.

20   Handling the biopsy
After removal of the mucosal biopsy, it should be placed on a piece of cardboard with the bleeding surface face down. This prevents the tissue piece from rolling up and ensures a good orientation of the tissue surface and the cut surfaces to each other. The biopsy, along with the preparation board, are then immersed in fixative solution.

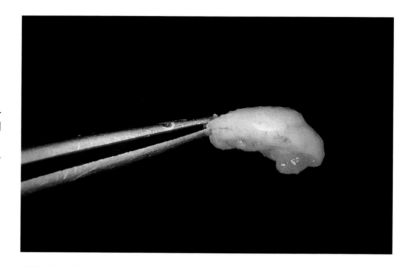

21   Containers for transporting the formalin-fixed biopsy
Plastic containers with screw caps are indicated for biopsy transport. Note that these containers have an inner and an outer vial.

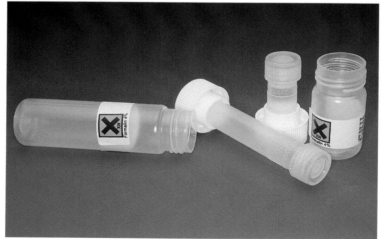

22   Punch biopsy instrument
The cutting end of this disposable instrument has a diameter of 6 mm. Using this circular scalpel, appropriate punch biopsies can be obtained.

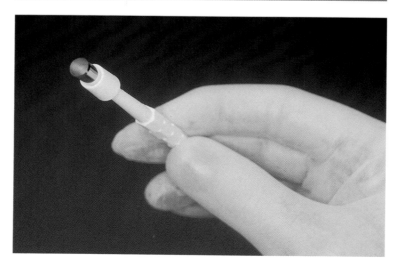

Local Anesthesia

It is impossible to harvest a biopsy without anesthesia. General anesthesia should only be used in patients with extreme dentophobia or mental disturbances. In almost every case the method of choice is local anesthesia. It is most important that the anesthetic solution *not* be injected into the biopsy site itself. In order to minimize hemorrhage, the anesthetic solution should contain a vasoconstrictor (epinephrine).

Punch Biopsy

In some cases, special biopsy instruments can be used when taking oral biopsies. For patients suspected of suffering from Sjögren's syndrome, a biopsy of the mucosa of the lip can provide a diagnostic evaluation of alterations in the minor salivary glands. The punch biopsy instrument, which is usually employed for skin biopsies, is particularly indicated in such cases. Using a 6 mm punch instrument, a cylinder of tissue can be removed that contains the labial mucosa as well as the submucosal salivary glands.

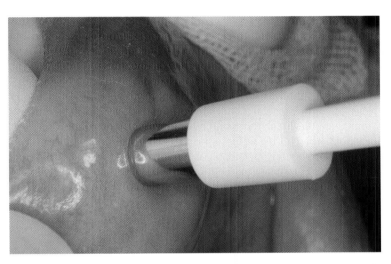

23 Punch biopsy
The punch biopsy instrument is applied to the mucosa of the lower lip with light pressure and a rotational movement. This creates a cylindrical block of tissue that can be removed using scissors. The resulting wound can be easily closed with a single suture. This is often not necessary, however, because the wound margins tend to collapse upon themselves.

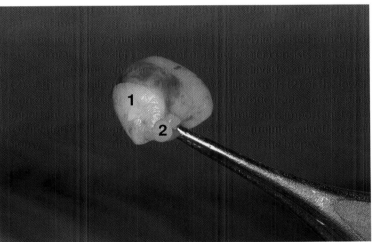

24 Tissue specimen resulting from a punch biopsy
The excised punch biopsy cylinder consists of oral mucosa (**1**) and the subjacent minor salivary glands (**2**) of the lower lip. The orientation of the plane of section is important to permit proper evaluation of all segments of the biopsy.

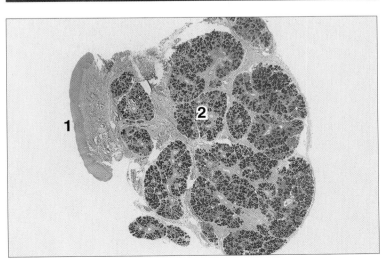

25 Histologic view of the punch biopsy in Fig. 24
In this case, histologic characteristics of Sjögren's syndrome could not be detected (PAS, x 10).

1 Mucosal epithelium
2 Lobules of the labial salivary gland

Excisional Biopsy—Small Lesions

It has already been emphasized, for both incisional as well as excisional biopsies, that it is important to always include a rim of the adjacent, normal mucosa. The reason for this is that the pathologist may find important diagnostic clues in the transitional zone between normal and pathologic oral mucosa.

Excisional biopsies of small lesions are harvested in the form of an elliptical incision, creating a wedge-shaped tissue block. This procedure also guarantees a sufficient quan-

tity of normal tissue. This type of excision also enhances adaptation of the wound margins. The suture material should be 3.0 monofilament or polyfilament thread used with an atraumatic, curved, cutting needle. The distance between the individual sutures is 4–5 mm. These sutures remain *in situ* for one week and are then removed. Disturbances of wound healing following the excisions of small lesions of the mucosa rarely occur.

Excisional biopsy—small lesion

26 Small connective tissue hyperplasia ("fibroma") on the tip of the tongue
The biopsy of lesions of this type is usually also the definitive treatment.

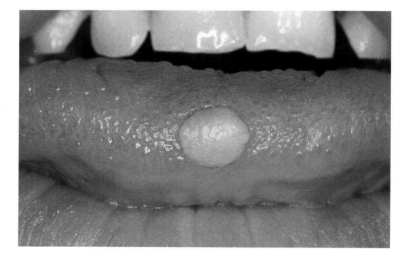

27 Incision
The incision is carried around the designated area. A certain amount of hemostasis is achieved with finger pressure.

Right: Histologic view. Typical exophytic connective tissue hyperplasia with hyperplastic epithelium (Mallory, x 6).

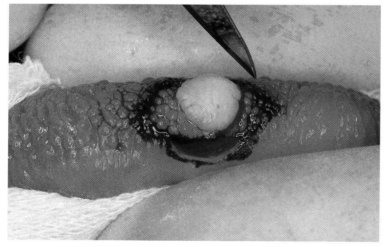
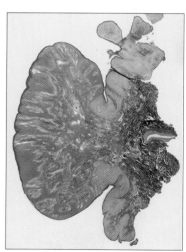

28 Site of the biopsy after removal of the fibromatous hyperplasia
Hemorrhage is minor, thanks to the vasoconstrictor contained in the anesthetic solution. It is not necessary to electrocoagulate any vessels. Three to four individual sutures will be adequate to close the wound.

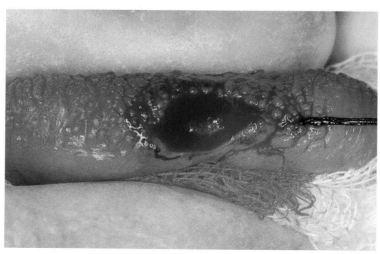

Excisional Biopsy—Large Lesions

As noted earlier, in the case of lesions that exceed a diameter of 1.5–2 cm, it may be necessary to perform two incisional biopsies in order to obtain representative tissue sections. If a mucosal lesion is rectangular in shape, with a length of more than 2 cm, it is prudent to excise it *in toto*. Although the wound may at first appear to be extensive, the course of healing will be satisfactory if the wound margins are well adapted. It may be necessary to undermine the wound margins to achieve tension-free wound closure. The sutures should be placed relatively close together and must be well-knotted, but must not strangulate the wound margins because dehiscences may otherwise occur.

Biopsy wounds on the hard palate cannot be sutured; they must be left to secondary granulation healing. A surgical stent can be fabricated to cover the wound area. Such wounds should be treated with a surgical dressing (iodoform gauze strips). The healing of such palatal soft tissue defects can last up to three weeks.

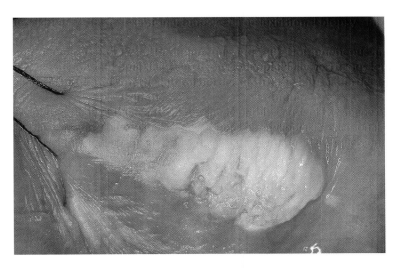

Excisional biopsy—large lesion

29 Homogeneous and partially verrucous leukoplakia of the lateral border of the tongue
Because of the shape of this leukoplakia, excisional biopsy is preferred over incisional biopsy.

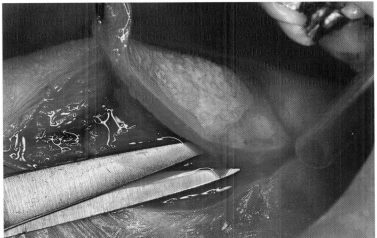

30 Excision of the lesion
After outlining the biopsy with a scalpel incision, the biopsy is freed up from mesial toward distal using a scissors. Note that a rim of normal tissue is included in the biopsy.

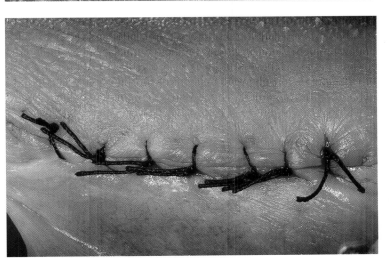

31 Surgical field after suturing
The large size of this excisional biopsy required wound closure with closely spaced sutures that did not strangulate the wound margins. The wound margins should be adapted free of any tension; otherwise dehiscences can occur.

Contraindications

Harvesting a biopsy is a minor surgical intervention. If the patient's medical history reveals any blood dyscrasias or if the patient is undergoing anticoagulant therapy, biopsy is contraindicated.

The general practitioner should *never* take a biopsy of a pigmented lesion. There is a reasonable chance that a dark pigmented oral lesion is a malignant melanoma. As with other oral malignant processes, immediate referral to an appropriate specialist for definitive diagnosis and therapy is necessary. The biopsy of malignant tumors, especially oral carcinoma, is absolutely necessary to secure the diagnosis, but it should be performed in such a way that the danger of metastasis formation is reduced as far as possible.

Preoperatively, a biopsy may be obtained for frozen section diagnosis. The frozen tissue is processed immediately by the pathologist and the diagnosis is secured. For some tumors, especially malignant lymphoma, this type of rapid diagnosis is not sufficient. The technique can also be used intraoperatively to examine tissue margins for the presence of malignant tissue.

Contraindications

32   Suspicion of a malignant melanoma on the gingiva
Biopsy of darkly pigmented lesions should *never* be performed in the general dental practice. Immediate referral with a suspected diagnosis is indicated.

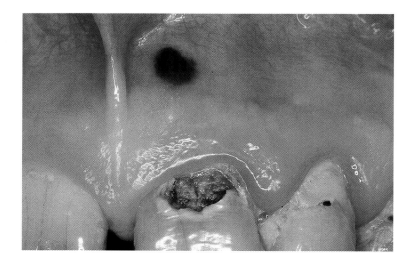

33   Leukoplakia of the floor of the mouth
Even though there is a clear indication for a biopsy in this case, the pigmentation presents a warning sign. The biopsy revealed a hyperpigmentation of the leukoplakia lesion, which had developed into a malignant melanoma over the course of several years.

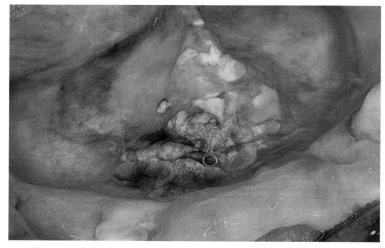

34   Ulcerated, exophytic squamous cell carcinoma of the floor of the mouth
A biopsy should be performed in all cases of malignant changes or lesions about which there is a suspicion of malignancy, but *never* in the general dental practice. Immediate referral to an appropriate oral maxillofacial surgeon or clinic is mandatory.

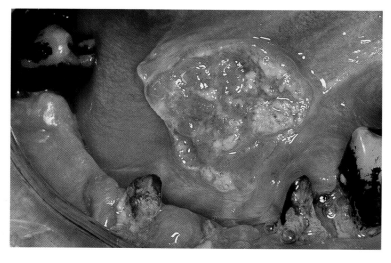

Cytologic Smear Techniques

With many white and erythematous lesions of the oral mucosa, it is possible to collect smears of the surface of the lesion and to submit such material for histopathologic examination. A classic example for the use of this technique are lesions that are suspected of being Candida infections. Material is scraped off the mucosal surface using a metal spatula. The collected material is spread evenly onto a glass slide and fixed immediately with 70% alcohol. Spray fixation is also possible. The fixed smear is packaged in an appropriate container for transfer to the pathology laboratory, accompanied by the appropriate clinical information.

Oral exfoliative cytology for determining epithelial atypia has lost some of its significance during the last decade, especially for the diagnosis of carcinoma, because often only few abnormal cells can be found in such a smear. The number of false negative reports was therefore quite large. The development of quantitative analysis of cytomorphology, DNA analysis, and the demonstration of other tumor markers has recently led to a resurgence of the smear technique (Ogden et al. 1997).

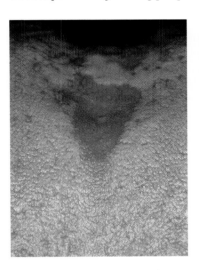
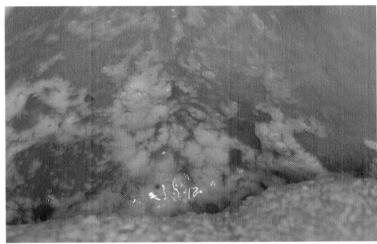

35　Candida infection
The whitish pseudomembranes consist of desquamated epithelial cells, inflammatory cells and Candida organisms, which are easy to diagnose in smear preparations.

Left: Chronic erythematous candidiasis is recognized as the so-called median rhomboid glossitis. Candida organisms can be recognized in the erythematous region, but to a lesser extent than in the pseudomembranous form depicted in the illustration on the right.

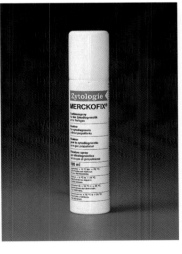
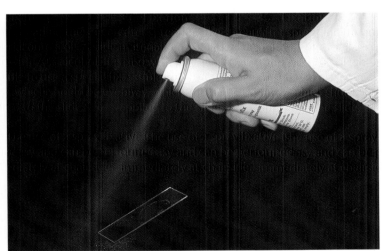

36　Fixation
After spreading the smeared material onto a glass slide, it is fixed with 70% alcohol. It is also possible to use a special fixation spray, which should be evenly applied to the slide.

Left: The use of a spray fixative is quite easy and can be performed immediately at chairside.

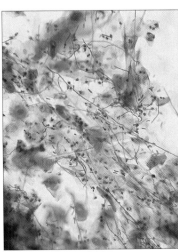
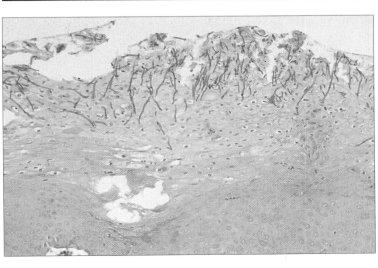

37　Histology and smears
Oral mucosa with superficial infection by Candida albicans hyphae. The Candida organisms penetrate vertically into the parakeratinized epithelium (PAS, x 80).

Left: Smear preparation of a pseudomembraneous candidiasis. This smear reveals desquamated epithelial cells as well as long, red-stained Candida hyphae and several polymorphonuclear granulocytes (PAS, x 80).

Pathology Report

When the pathologist receives biopsy material, it is prepared for microscopic examination. In addition to routine staining, special stains may also be necessary to arrive at a definitive diagnosis. The standard staining method uses hematoxylin and eosin (H & E). Following histologic examination of the stained sections, the pathology report, including the definitive diagnosis, is prepared. This report will often include a section dealing with suggestions for possible treatments, additional examinations, or further biopsies.

The pathology report on soft tissue changes is usually available three to four days after receipt of the biopsy.

Hard tissue biopsies of bone or teeth or soft tissue lesions that include hard tissues must first be decalcified. This can be accomplished very quickly using strong acids, although this is associated with the loss of some cytologic detail. A more gentle decalcification using EDTA requires several weeks.

38 Pathology report
Here is an example of a report that would be received by the dentist a few days after sending in a biopsy.

Dr. W. Jones
Department of Pathology
University of Anystate
Anystate, USA

November 11, 1999

To: Dr. T. Smith

| **Patient:** | Wurzelspitz, Ruth | **Received:** | March 10, 1999 |
| **Date of Birth:** | 12. 09. 1929 | **Returned:** | March 12, 1999 |

Clinical Diagnosis: Nodular leukoplakia of the floor of the mouth

Specimens:
1 15 x 5 x 5 mm biopsy with a papillary surface
2 12 x 2 x 2 mm biopsy with a smooth surface

Observations:

1. The surface of this specimen is lined by a stratified squamous epithelium with hyperparakeratosis and hyperorthokeratosis that varies over various epithelial areas. The epithelium displays a papillary histoarchitecture. Aside from several hyperchromatic nuclei, there are no signs of epithelial atypia. The basement membrane is completely intact. A severe inflammatory infiltrate exists in the adjacent connective tissue.

2. Oral mucosa with hyperparakeratotic, stratified squamous epithelium. With PAS staining, Candida hyphae are seen in the superficial keratinized epithelial layers. The epithelium is hyperplastic, with long, narrow rete pegs. In some areas of pronounced epithelial atrophy, the rete pegs are teardrop-shaped. In addition, mild atypia of the basal cells with hyperchromatic nuclei can be seen. The basement membrane appears to be intact. A more precise examination is rendered difficult because of a dense inflammatory cell infiltrate.

Conclusion:

This partially verrucous, partially papillary lesion of the oral mucosa, with a superficial Candida infection, shows signs of mild epithelial atypia.
Because this mucosal change is derived from a region of the oral cavity that has a high risk of malignant transformation, removal of the lesion in toto is suggested. Whether this should be performed through excision or laser therapy cannot be assessed at this time because the size of the lesion was not known.

Dr. W. Jones

Encl.: Two slides

Cooperation with the Oral Pathologist

It is important for the clinician to correlate the histologic findings with the clinical appearance of the lesion. The responsibility for determining whether the histologic diagnosis fits the clinical situation resides with the clinician. An incompatible histologic diagnosis must never be accepted. It can also happen that the histologic findings do not lead to a definitive answer. If there are discrepancies between the clinical and the histologic diagnosis, the dentist should never hesitate to call the pathologist in order to clarify the situation. The biopsy may not have derived from a charac-teristic or a representative area of the lesion, thus necessitating an additional biopsy.

Even when the pathologist's histologic report states that the tissue alterations are "benign," during the post-biopsy period the clinician should carefully observe the clinical development and course. If healing of the site of the biopsy is delayed or if there is a recurrence of the lesion, a new biopsy is indicated. If the clinician receives a histologic report of malignancy, the patient must be referred *immediately* to a specialist.

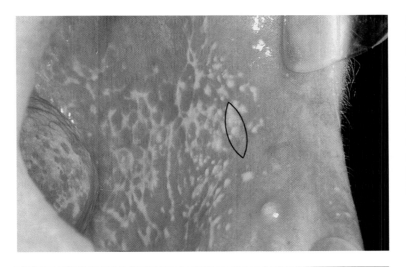

39 Lichen planus with possible biopsy site
If there is insufficient information concerning the clinical picture of the disease process, it may be impossible to differentiate between lichen planus and leuko-plakia, even histomorphologi-cally. If the biopsy findings do not correspond with the clinical picture, a discussion with the pathologist must ensue.

40 The do's and don'ts of tissue biopsies

Do:

● Carefully select the site for an incisional biopsy

● Inject the anesthetic solution away from the biopsy site, never into the biopsy site

● Include adjacent normal tissue in the biopsy

● Immerse the biopsy in fixative immediately upon removal

● Inscribe the transport container and the biopsy report form with the patient's name and that of the clinician

● Provide medical history and clinical findings as well as a clear description of the biopsy site

● Always correlate the clinical and histopathologic di-agnoses

Don't:
● Use electrosurgery or laser, only the scalpel (or punch instrument)

● Create artifacts caused by forceps or other instruments

HIV Infection

In 1981, several unusual opportunistic infections and tumors, such as *Pneumocystis carinii* pneumonia, oral candidiasis, Kaposi's sarcoma, B-cell lymphoma and cytomegalovirus infections were diagnosed in young men in California who led promiscuous lifestyles. These findings were an indication of reduced host immune resistance. In the same year, and on the basis of clinical observations, massive T-cell defects as well as epidemiologic observations, the *acquired immunodeficiency syndrome* (AIDS) was defined. The number of individuals infected with HIV and affected by AIDS grew exponentially. In addition to homosexual men, other groups also became infected, for example, intravenous drug users, recipients of blood or blood products, partners of these risk groups, as well as the newborn of mothers at risk.

An infectious agent was suspected, and it was isolated in 1983 at the Pasteur Institute (Paris, France) as a lymphadenopathy syndrome–associated virus, a lentivirus. Since 1986, various viral isolates have been characterized as human immunodeficiency virus (HIV). Today, HIV infection is a world pandemic. In several areas of the world, however, especially in North America and portions of Western Europe, there have been tendencies for the rate of infection to decrease. In stark contrast, the problems of HIV infection and of AIDS in Black Africa as well as Southeast Asia have shown dramatic increases. The World Health Organization (WHO) recently estimated that 33.6 million persons are infected with HIV (*Wkly. Epidemiol. Rec.* 44, 1999). The rapid discovery of the causative agent in AIDS and the development of test systems and procedures for mass screening of blood and blood products early on led to hope for a rapid stemming of the infection. While remarkable advances have been made in the chemotherapy of HIV infection over the past two years, the early optimism emanating from HIV research that a protective vaccine would be found has proved to be deceptive until this day (end of 1999). Reichart and Gelderblom (1998) published a compendium for dentists that includes clear and concise presentations of all important aspects of the AIDS situation for the dental practice.

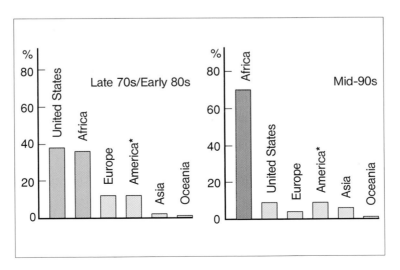

41 Regional dissemination of AIDS
Geographic distribution of reported AIDS cases in adults and children in the late 70s/early 80s (left) and during the mid-90s (right). (*Wkly. Epidemiol. Rec.* 48, 1997)
(* excluding the United States).

Epidemiology

Twice each year, the WHO publishes the cumulative AIDS cases from all countries that report these data. The WHO discriminates between the types of distribution, the so-called *patterns*: Pattern I countries are characterized primarily by disease transmission among homosexuals and bisexuals; Pattern II countries by heterosexual transmission; Pattern I–II is characterized by a mixture of homosexual and heterosexual transfer; Pattern III countries exhibit only a low incidence of infection. In Western Europe and North America, one observes primarily Pattern I, while Pattern II predominates in Black Africa as well as in South and Southeast Asia.

The number of reported AIDS cases is of less importance for the worldwide situation than the estimated number of HIV infected individuals. At the end of 1999, the WHO estimated that 33.6 million adults and children were living with HIV/AIDS. By the end of 1999, it is estimated that a total of 16.3 million adults and children (2.6 million in 1999) will have died because of HIV/AIDS since the epidemic began in the early 1980s. As of November 15, 1999, a total of 2,201,461 AIDS cases had been reported to the WHO.

42   Estimated distribution of HIV/AIDS in adults at the end of 1999
From this graphic it is clear that Black Africa as well as Southern and Southeast Asia have the highest levels of HIV infections, followed by Latin America. On the other hand, East Asia and the Pacific Rim nations exhibit a lower rate of infection.

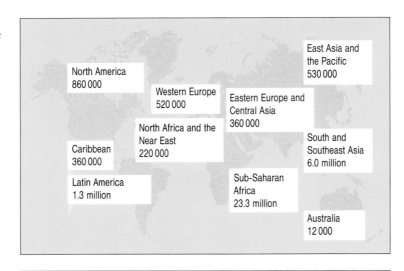

43   Estimated deaths due to AIDS in adults up until the year 2000
The evident increase in Africa is clearly visible as well as in Asia and Latin America.

Right: Various information and estimated figures from the UNAIDS-US, Centers for Disease Control and Prevention.

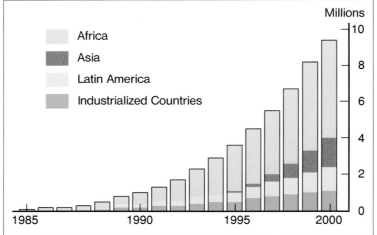

- HIV infections worldwide: 34 million
- HIV infections in the United States: 900 000
- New HIV infections worldwide in 1999: 5.6 million
- New HIV infections per year in the United States: at least 40 000
- Daily new HIV infections worldwide: 8 500
- Daily new HIV infections in the United States: at least 110
- Annual cost for anti-HIV therapy: up to $16 000 per patient
- Available vaccine: not yet known

44   Cumulative incidences in Europe
This graph shows cumulative incidences in European countries according to infection risk. In Spain (E) and Italy (I), the number of HIV-infected individuals who are intravenous drug users (IVDA) is high. To date there has been no satisfactory explanation for this phenomenon. (D* pertains only to the previous West German areas).
(Source: RKI-AIDS/HIV Bi-annual Report I/99. Date: June 30, 1999)

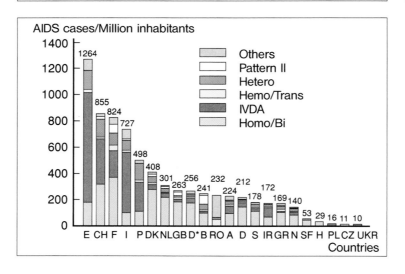

Epidemiology in Europe and Germany

In Western Europe, referring to the incidence per million inhabitants, the countries of Spain, France, Italy, Denmark, but also Switzerland, England and Germany are severely affected. However, during the last few years a decline in reported AIDS cases has been observed in some industrialized countries, such as the United States, Spain, Italy and others. The dramatic change of progression rates of HIV to AIDS are due to the introduction of HAART (Highly Active Anti-Retroviral Therapy) in 1995–1996, which has contributed to decreases of up to 70% in the number of reported AIDS cases and AIDS-related deaths.

Up until the end of June 1999, a total of 18,239 AIDS cases were reported in Germany. Of these, 8,870 were men and 12% were women (*RKI AIDS/HIV Bi-annual Report* I/99, 1999). As in most other countries, the major population centers are the most heavily affected.

In 1999, the AIDS Center in Germany predicted that a total of 2000–2500 infections per year would occur (*RKI AIDS/HIV Bi-annual Report,* 1999). Since the beginning of this epidemic, a total of 50–60,000 individuals in Germany have been infected.

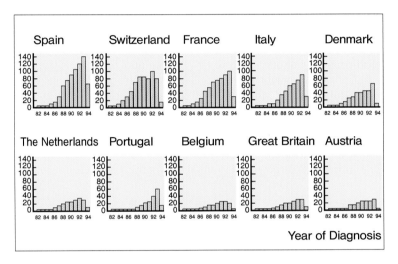

45 Decline in reported AIDS cases in selected industrialized countries
During the past three to four years, a decline in the incidence of AIDS has been noted in some industrialized countries. Antiretroviral combination therapies are marked by reduced morbidity and mortality of patients who receive this type of treatment.

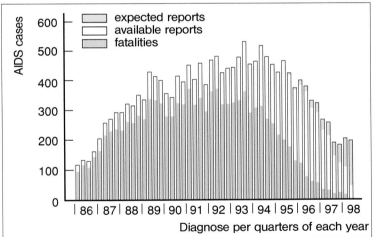

46 AIDS in Germany
This graph reveals statistics about AIDS in Germany between 1986 and 1999. The dates reveal the number of reported AIDS cases with the number of deaths in the reported groups as well as the delay in reporting, quarter by quarter. The continuous reduction of registered AIDS cases since 1994–95 can be attributed to the new combination therapies.

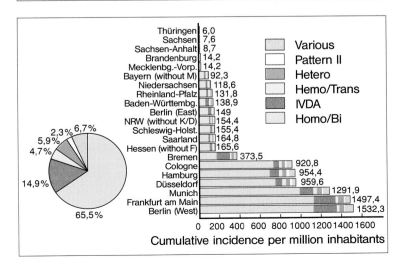

47 Epidemiologic data from Germany
The AIDS/HIV Bi-annual Report I/99, published by the Robert Koch Institute, depicts the cumulative AIDS incidence per million inhabitants as a function of infection risk in geographic areas of Germany as well as selected large population areas.

Left: Distribution of the reported AIDS cases according to infection risk groups (N = 18,239). A total of 118 children with AIDS was reported (0.5%).

HIV Virology

The human immunodeficiency virus belongs to the category of retroviruses, which are characterized by their RNA genome and the reverse transcriptase as well as a virus-coded RNA- and DNA-dependent polymerase. The morphology as viewed in the electron microscope is characteristic (Reichart and Gelderblom 1998). The HIV-1 and HIV-2 strains are related to the lentiviruses of the chimpanzee and the mandrill or Syke's monkey, respectively. Both trace their origins to Africa. They are, however, variously distributed throughout the African continent: while HIV-1 is predominant in central Africa, HIV-2 predominates in West Africa.

The distribution of HIV in its new host species, namely man, was enhanced by certain sociocultural influences, such as mobility and promiscuity. In addition to its high replication rate, the variability of HIV is of importance. A number of subtypes have been identified, primarily in tropical Africa. HIV exhibits a determined cellular tropism, and targets the immune system and the central nervous system. CD4$^+$ T helper cells, as well as antigen-presenting cells such as macrophages, provide the necessary receptors for an infection. The CD4$^+$ surface protein is the sole identifier of a cell that can be infected with HIV-1.

48 HIV ultrastructure
This transmission electron photomicrograph reveals the structure of the virus. Working from the outside inward, it is possible to differentiate the virus capsule (large arrow), the wedge-shaped virus core that is typical for lentiviruses as well as the so-called lateral body (arrowhead). On the surface one can observe the so-called virus knobs (small arrows) (TEM, x 150 000).

Courtesy H. G. Gelderblom

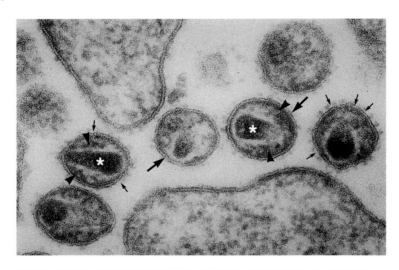

49 HIV structure—molecular components
This graph depicts the structure of an HI-virus with the virus envelope (coded from the ENV gene), the knobs as well as the inner body of the virus, which is surrounded by matrix proteins. The matrix and the core consist of gag-gene and gag-pol-gene coded structural proteins.

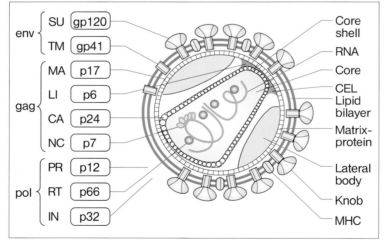

50 HIV interaction with host cells
This graph depicts the docking of the HI-virus to the CD4$^+$ receptor. The HIV enters into the host cell; the reverse transcription by means of the reverse transcriptase (RT) occurs with subsequent virus replication and the assembly of virions and the process of budding, followed finally by maturation.

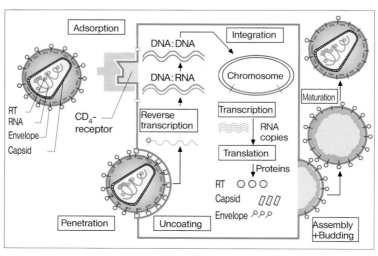

Various subtypes of HIV-1 and HIV-2 have been detected, primarily in sub-Saharan Africa. On the other hand, only one or two HIV-1 subtypes dominate worldwide. In Europe and North America, subtype B is responsible for more than 80% of all new HIV infections.

Clinical Course and Classification

AIDS is defined through various typical diseases. In acquired immunodeficiency, three stages can be differentiated: 1. Primary infection, 2. Phase of clinical latency, and 3. The "acquired immunodeficiency syndrome" (AIDS). The classification system proposed in 1993 by the Centers for Disease Control and Prevention has achieved widespread acceptance. This classification applies whenever an HIV infection is established through laboratory findings, and takes into consideration the clinical symptoms (categories A, B, C) and also the number of CD4$^+$ T helper cells (categories 1, 2, 3). Category A corresponds to an asymptomatic HIV infection without AIDS-defined diseases or weaknesses of cell-mediated immunity. Category B applies to an HIV infection with a serious defect of cell-mediated immunity. Category C consists of the typical AIDS-defined diseases.

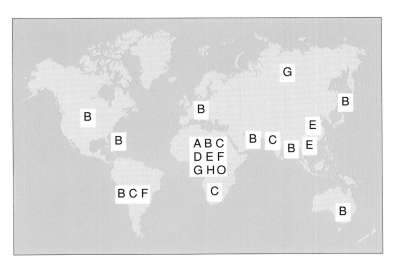

51 Distribution of the HIV-1 subtypes
The subtypes are categorized in groups A–J (primary groups), M and 0 ("outlier groups"). The latter are encountered most frequently in tropical Africa. HIV subtype E was ascertained in the heterosexual population of Thailand. Presently, there is no worldwide threat to the heterosexual population by subtype E.

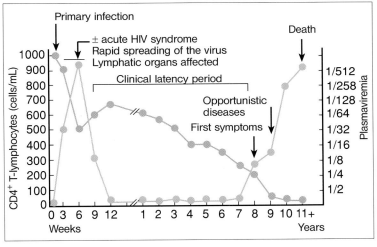

52 HIV infection—clinical course
The graph depicts the decrease of CD4$^+$ T-cell lymphocytes. This correlates with viremia over the course of clinical latency and on to symptoms of opportunistic diseases, and finally to death.

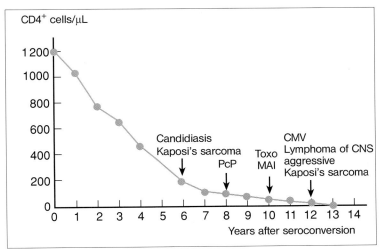

53 Opportunistic infections
This graph shows how the progressive loss of CD4$^+$ cells as well as opportunistic infections and also opportunistic neoplasms occur. Oral candidiasis often occurs early on and can be viewed as a marker disease.

CMV Cytomegalovirus
MAI Mycobacterium avium intracellulare
Toxo Toxoplasma
PcP Pneumocystis carinii

Classification of Oral Manifestations

The first classification of oral manifestations (Pindborg 1989) was grouped according to causative factors into: 1. Bacterial, 2. Mycotic, 3. Viral Infections, 4. Neoplasias, and 5. Lesions of unknown origin. In 1993, this classification was modified (EC 1993). The current classification is as follows:

- Lesions strongly associated with an HIV infection (Group I)
- Lesions less commonly associated with HIV infection (Group II), and
- Lesions seen in HIV infection (Group III).

The occurrence of oral manifestations depends upon a number of factors. In addition to geographic, ethnic, gender-related and age-related aspects, the stage of the disease process plays a significant role. Certain oral diseases have achieved the status of *marker diseases* for HIV infection, particularly oral candidiasis and hairy leukoplakia.

Greenspan et al. (1992) formulated preliminary and definitive diagnostic criteria for the various oral manifestations. For some of them, such as erythematous candidiasis, definitive diagnostic criteria are difficult to establish.

54   Classification of the oral manifestations of HIV infection
The current classification describes the diseases of the oral cavity that have been documented to date. New entities were frequently observed at the beginning of the HIV epidemic, but in more recent years the list of oral manifestations has remained relatively constant. This is partially due to the fact that a reduction in the rate of HIV infection has been observed in Western Europe and in North America. Also, effective antiretroviral therapies have reduced morbidity of HIV-infected patients.

Group I
Lesions strongly associated with HIV infection

- Candidiasis
     Erythematous
     Pseudomembranous
- Hairy leukoplakia
- Kaposi's sarcoma
- Linear gingival erythema
- Necrotizing (ulcerative) gingivitis
- Necrotizing (ulcerative) periodontitis
- Non-Hodgkin's lymphoma

Group II
Lesions less commonly associated with HIV infection

- Bacterial infections
     Mycobacterium avium intracellulare
     Mycobacterium tuberculosis
- Melanotic hyperpigmentation
- Necrotizing (ulcerative) stomatitis
- Salivary gland disorders
     Dry mouth due to reduced salivary flow
     Unilateral or bilateral swelling of the major salivary glands
- Thrombocytopenic purpura
- Ulcerations not otherwise specified (NOS)
- Viral infections
     Herpes simplex virus
     Human papilloma virus (wart-like lesions)
       – Condyloma acuminatum
       – Focal epithelial hyperplasia
       – Verruca vulgaris
     Varicella zoster virus
       – Herpes zoster
       – Varicella

Group III
Lesions seen in HIV infection

- Bacterial infections
     Actinomyces israelii
     Escherichia coli
     Klebsiella pneumoniae
- Bacillary epithelioid angiomatosis (BEA)
- Drug reactions (ulcerations, erythema multiforme, lichenoid, toxic epidermolysis)
- Fungal infections (excluding candidiasis):
     Cryptococcus neoformans, Geotrichum candidum
     Histoplasma capsulatum, Mucoraceae (mucormycosis),
     Penicillium marneffei, Aspergillus flavus
- Neurological disturbances
     Facial paresthesia
     Trigeminal neuralgia
- Recurrent aphthous stomatitis
- Viral infections
     Cytomegalovirus (CMV)
     Molluscum contagiosum

Diagnostic and Therapeutic Aspects of Oral Manifestations of AIDS

The occurrence of HIV infections and of AIDS has significantly altered and expanded the diagnostic spectrum of oral manifestations. The basic immunodeficiency permits the occurrence of opportunistic infections and neoplasias to an extent that has not been witnessed up until now in the dental practice with such frequency or severity.

It is of extreme importance to note also that diseases occur in individuals who, were they immunocompetent, would never be observed. It is also noteworthy that most individuals infected with HIV are between the ages of 18 and 45, an age in which oral candidiasis, Herpes zoster or Kaposi's sarcoma would normally not be expected. In the daily practice of oral diagnosis, therefore, it is prudent to consider that the occurrence of uncommon diseases with regard to age and gender should always be considered as a possible consequence of immunodeficiency in the sense of an HIV infection.

It is also very important to note that many manifestations of immunodeficiency occur *primarily* in the *oral cavity*, especially oral candidiasis. Because the oral cavity is easily accessible for both clinical inspection and palpation, particular care should be exercised during clinical examination.

An additional important aspect of the care of patients with HIV infection or AIDS is the fact that the immunodeficiency is persistent. Therapeutic measures, especially the prescription of antimycotics or antibiotics must be considered differently than for patients who are immunocompetent. Thus, practitioners often do not bear in mind that when the therapeutic measures are ceased because of an inadequate immune response, the disease process will quickly recur. This is especially true for viral and mycotic infections (Reichart 1999).

As the immunodeficiency increases, the number and also the severity of opportunistic infections also increase, so that in many cases long-term medication or so-called "on-and-off" therapy will be instituted.

Prevention, for example with use of antimycotics against oral candidiasis, is for the most part not performed today because experience has shown that over the course of years, therapy-resistance can occur, which is no longer treatable. A most basic principle is that the treatment of an oral manifestation must not disregard other, more important aspects, because it is possible that the prescription of an antibiotic for treatment of necrotizing gingivitis or periodontitis could compromise a significantly more important infectious disease, and its consequent therapy (Reichart 1999a; Reichart 1999b).

Also of importance is the fact that the newly-implemented triple or multiple therapy for HIV infection—using inhibitors of the reverse transcriptase of the virus, and using non-nucleoside reverse transcriptase inhibitors as well as HIV protease inhibitors—apparently drastically reduces the number of oral manifestations (Schmidt-Westhausen et al. 2000).

The absolute number of HIV-infected individuals will continue to decrease in the West. Furthermore, the time span between infection and the manifestation of AIDS-defined diseases will increase. The practitioner of dentistry, especially in large population centers, will continue to be confronted with HIV-infected and AIDS patients. While the purely dental treatment of such patients is unproblematic, diagnostic and therapeutic difficulties related to the oral manifestations in terms of opportunistic infections or opportunistic neoplasias will continue to be confounding elements of diagnosis.

In this atlas, we will make reference to various oral manifestations of HIV infection. The various phenomena will be demonstrated using typical clinical examples. A recently published AIDS compendium for dentists provides further diagnostic and therapeutic details (Reichart and Gelderblom 1998).

Facial Region

The external facial skin and its multiplicity of diseases does not rank as a major focus of diagnosis for the practitioner of dentistry. However, because of excellent dental operatory illumination, each time the dentist sees a patient, there is an opportunity to recognize possible alterations of the facial skin. Arriving at a definitive diagnosis is not the primary goal, but rather recognizing suspicious changes of the skin and making the patient aware of them. Even a short medical history can often provide clues about the type of pathologic alteration. It is important to keep in mind that the skin is subject to a great number of alterations during the course of life. This chapter will present only a few examples of such diseases. The reader is also referred to the dermatologic (Hornstein 1996) and the maxillofacial-surgical literature (Härle 1993).

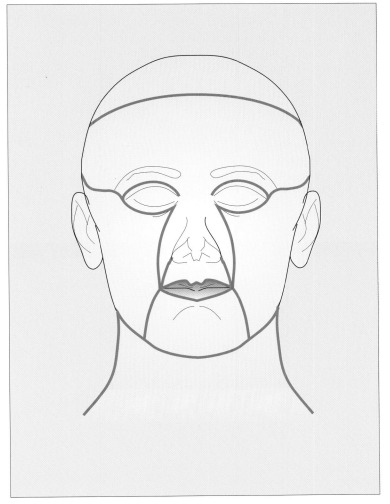

55 Facial skin areas
This schematic diagram shows the various facial skin areas: perioral, perinasal, periorbital, the areas of the temporal bones and the forehead as well as the cheeks. Many diseases tend to affect certain areas of the facial skin and are detected more frequently in these areas. A particular example is the basal cell carcinoma, which appears particularly in the perinasal area.

Infections—Bacterial

Odontogenic Abscess and Extraoral Fistula

Inflammation of odontogenic origin leads most frequently to submucous infiltrates and abscesses, but may also penetrate into the soft tissues of the face. Odontogenic infections may be acute or chronic and in addition to soft tissues infections may also involve bone. The spectrum of causative agents include Gram-positive streptococci, staphylococci and Gram-positive and Gram-negative bacteria, both aerobic and anaerobic, as well as fungi and viruses (Machtens and Bremerich 1995).

Knowledge of the spread of such infections along anatomic borders is of extreme importance for the therapy. Surgical opening and drainage of an abscess remains the therapy of choice. Antibiotics, especially penicillin, represent supportive therapy. The very severe abscesses that were observed in previous eras, sometimes with deadly consequences, have become much more rare today.

56 Acute odontogenic abscess
Note the erythematous, shiny skin covering the right side of the chin. This represents an initial abscess formation, which emanated from the mandibular right canine.

Right: Massive swelling of the left cheek, the upper and lower eyelids as well as portions of the nose. The odontogenic abscess originated from the maxillary left canine. The danger of thrombophlebitis formation is acute.

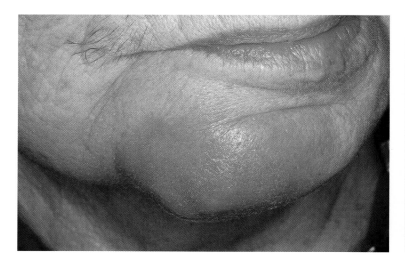
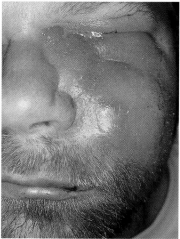

57 Extraoral fistula
A circumscribed swelling with spontaneous opening is evident on the ventral surface of the right mandible. All of the molar teeth exhibited a high degree of mobility due to osteomyelitis. During the removal of these teeth, several large osseous sequestra were extirpated.

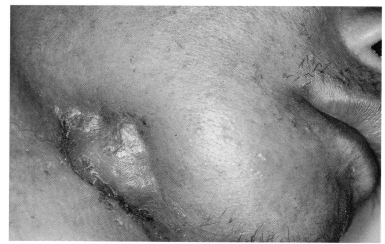

58 Extraoral fistula of a chronic, granulating inflammatory process of odontogenic origin
This type of fistula is often detected in the area of the mandibular border, emanating from non-vital molars, which are affected by chronic, periapical, granulating inflammatory processes. Simply excising the fistula is inadequate treatment; the tooth of origin must also be either removed or treated (endodontically).

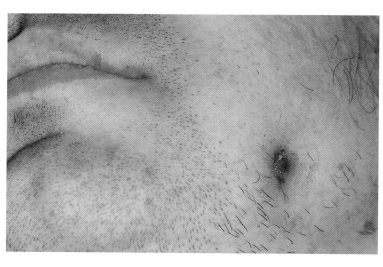

Acne Vulgaris

Up to 90% of all cases of acne vulgaris of the papulopustulous type are observed in young patients. The forehead, nose and the cheek regions are most often affected.

Contagious Impetigo

Contagious impetigo is an acute skin infection caused by staphylococci or by beta-hemolytic Streptococcus A. This disease process affects mainly children; the lips and perioral region are the most frequent sites.

Noma

Noma (Cancrum oris) is seen primarily in children in Africa and Southeast Asia. Predisposing factors include malnutrition, gastrointestinal parasite infestation, and other underlying diseases that reduce host defense mechanisms. There exist etiopathogenic similarities between noma and Plaut–Vincent fusospirochaetosis. Enormous soft tissue destruction is often observed. In many cases, noma is a lethal condition (Prabhu and Praetorius 1992).

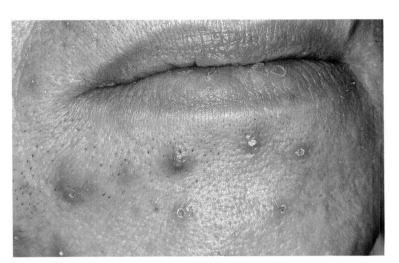

59 Acne vulgaris
Multiple pustules at various stages of development are apparent in the region of the lower lip and the adjacent facial skin. The infected pustules derive from the typical sebum retention. Acne is hormone-dependent and generally subsides after puberty.

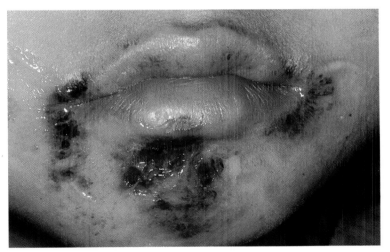

60 Contagious impetigo
Note the extensive, confluent, and partially scabbed erosions in the perioral region and on the chin. This six-year-old hill-tribe girl from the mountains of Thailand suffered from vitamin deficiency as well as nutritional deficiency. Impetigo is highly contagious, but can be successfully treated using topical antibiotics.

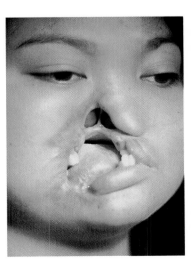
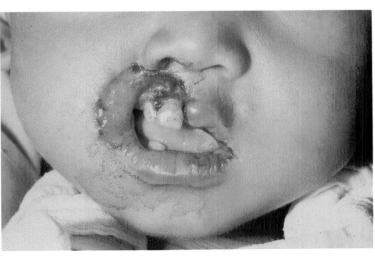

61 Noma
This subacute case of noma in a hill-tribe child from northern Thailand had already been treated antibiotically. The right upper lip and a portion of a corner of the mouth had already been lost.

Left: Late consequences of noma, with extensive soft tissue loss of the lips, the cheek as well as the right portion of the nose. An extended period of plastic surgical reconstruction is required in such cases (Reichart 1974).

Leprosy

Leprosy (Hansen's disease), which is caused by *Mycobacterium leprae*, affects over 12 million people, mostly in tropical countries. Leprosy has also had a resurgence in Europe as a result of immigration and worldwide travel by Europeans. The clinical manifestations of leprosy take several forms, depending upon the individual's immune status:

- Tuberculoid leprosy
- Lepromatous leprosy
- Borderline leprosy

In addition, there exist undetermined transition types and leprosy reactions. The face is most often affected, but the oral mucosa is only affected in cases of lepromatous leprosy (20–60% of cases) (Reichart 1974, 1976; Reichart et al. 1992).

A very basic problem for leprosy patients is the *loss of sensitivity*, which leads to extensive mutilations, especially of the fingers. Because the peripheral nervous system is almost always affected, facial paralysis often occurs, with subsequent infection and damage to the conjunctiva, often leading to blindness.

62   Lepromatous type of leprosy
Left: Patient during a leprosy reaction. Multiple extensive leprosy lesions lead to the clinical picture of "facies leonina."
The eyebrows and eyelashes have been completely lost. This type of leprosy is highly contagious.

Right: Multiple small leprotic lesions in the region of the lower lip and chin.

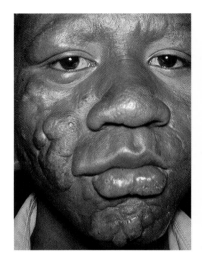 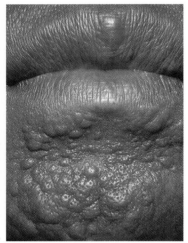

63   Leprosy
Note the almost complete loss of the fingers, which resulted from lost sensitivity and specific leprosy-associated granulomatous processes.

Right: "Burned-out leprosy" with bilateral facial paralysis, blindness, "saddle nose," loss of sensitivity in the trigeminal region, and loss of the maxillary anterior teeth (Reichart et al. 1976, 1982).

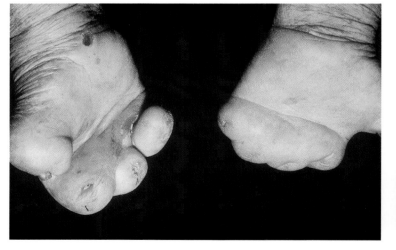 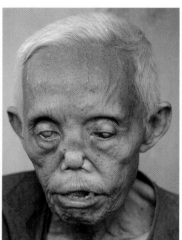

64   Tip of the tongue in a patient with lepromatous leprosy
On the tip of the tongue as well as on the lower lip one observes a whitish lesion which looks silvery; this is leprosy-specific. Leprosy affecting the uvula is often associated with massive tissue loss.

Right: This skull of a person with leprosy exhibits shortened roots of the anterior teeth caused by specific granulomatous processes in the area of the anterior segment of the maxilla ("facies leprosa").

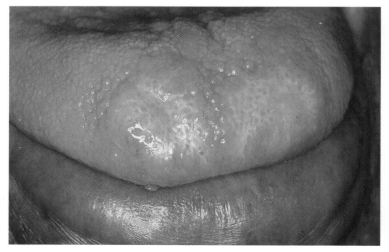 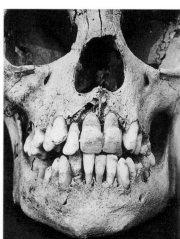

Infections—Protozoal, Viral

Leishmaniasis

Leishmaniasis is caused by a protozoa (Prabhu 1992). About 12 million people are infected worldwide. Various infectious species and clinical disease manifestations can be differentiated. Disease transmission occurs by means of sand fly bites; both humans and animals may serve as sources of infection. The South American form of leishmaniasis is most often characterized by involvement of the mucosa (nasal, oral and pharyngeal). The clinical course of mucocutaneous leishmaniasis is associated with infiltrative, ulcerous, perfo-

rating, vegetative polyposis and multilocal foci (Hornstein 1996).

Nasal Herpes and German Measles

Herpes nasalis is less common than Herpes labialis (see p. 46); the course of the disease is similar.
German measles (Rubella) leads to a classic exanthema with occipitocervical lymphadenitis. An intraoral erythema may rarely be observed.

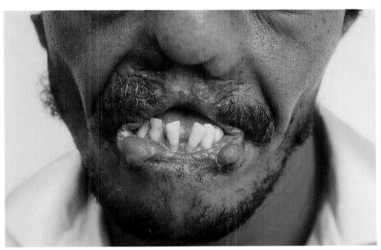

65 Leishmaniasis
This Brazilian patient suffered extensive loss of both upper and lower lips as well as portions of the nose. It is no longer possible for him to completely close his mouth. Plastic surgical measures are indicated for functional and esthetic reasons.

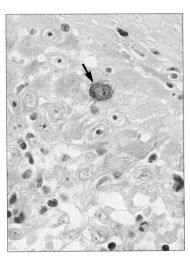

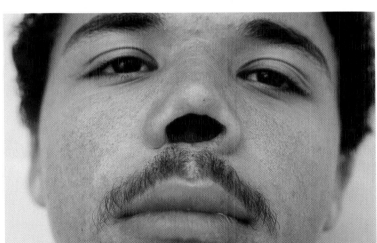

66 Mucocutaneous Leishmaniasis
In this young Brazilian, there has been complete loss of the nasal septum as well as portions of the internal nasal anatomy.

Left: Granulation tissue from mucocutaneous leishmaniasis, demonstrating a histiocyte (arrow) containing Leishman–Donovan bodies and Leishmania braziliensis (Toluidine blue, x 200).

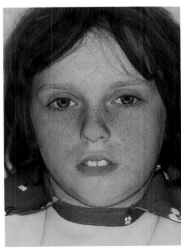

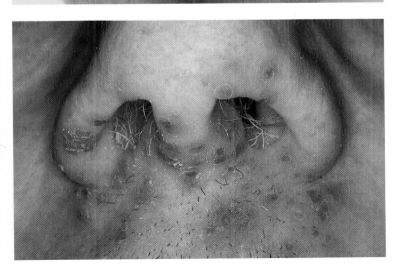

67 Viral infection of the facial skin
In this female, who suffered from nasal herpes, one observes multiple erythematous lesions with crust formation.

Left: The typical macular rash is observed on both cheeks. Embryopathologic effects may occur during pregnancy. Pre-pubertal immunization is necessary.

Infections—Mycotic

Dermatophytosis (or trichophytosis), especially in the facial region, is relatively common and also referred to as tinea. The causative agents are either anthropophilic or zoophilic, with the latter becoming more common:

- *Trichophyton rubrum* is common the world over and is characterized by inflammatory changes in the region of the beard, the hair and the skin of the chin. The lips are less often affected.
- *Trichophyton mentagrophytes* is zoophilic and is commonly found in house pets.

- Dermatophytosis (or trichophytosis) caused by infection with *Microsporum canis* most frequently affects children, especially in the hair of the head (Tinea capitis; Prabhu et al. 1992).

Typical signs and symptoms of fungal diseases of the facial skin include itching, erythema and exfoliating areas. Intraoral manifestations have not been described to date. Appropriate antimycotic treatment must also be applied to the infected house pet.

68 Trichophyton Rubrum
Here, *Trichophyton rubrum* has elicited a case of Tinea barbae, which commonly manifests itself as circular areas of erythema. This condition has also been called "ringworm of the beard."

Right: Trichophyton rubrum culture.

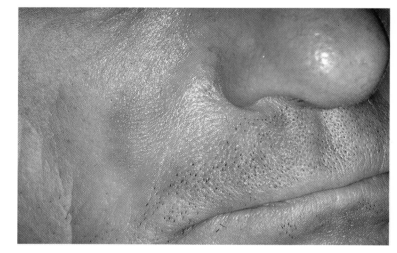
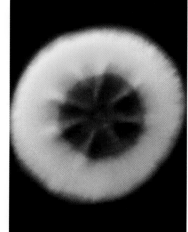

69 Microsporia
This patient experienced multiple, periorbital and facial areas of erythema that itched severely. The causative agent was *Microsporum canis*.

Right: Microsporum canis culture; typical configuration and color.

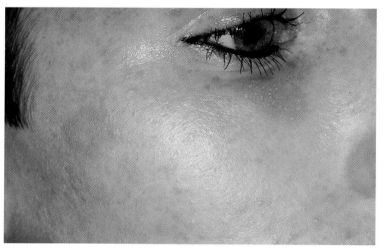
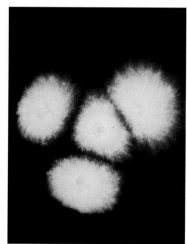

70 Trichophytosis of the cheek
This erythematous lesion in a young person was caused by *Trichophyton mentagrophytes*. Such lesions are typically erythematous, exfoliative and itchy.

Right: Trichophyton mentagrophytes culture, of the granulosum variant.

Courtesy H.-J. Tietz

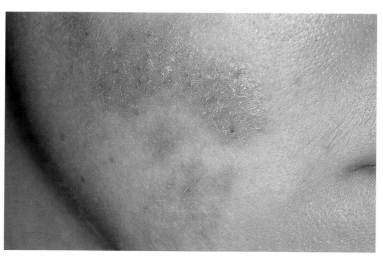
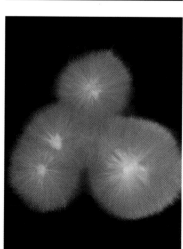

Mechanical, Physical, Chemical and Other Causes

Post-traumatic hematoma of the jaws and facial area is a common consequence of all severe trauma. If a patient suffers from a clotting disorder, even minor surgical procedures can be accompanied by massive hematoma (Baer and Boese-Landgraf 1997). The condition is characterized by hemorrhage into the tissue spaces, and is usually resorbed within a relatively short period of time if there is no infection of the hematoma.

The term *automutilation* refers to self-inflicted damage or injury to portions of the body, which may be located intraorally or extraorally (Reichart and Köster 1978). As a result of neurotic disturbances, such patients inflict themselves with various types and severities of injuries to attract the attention of their surroundings or of their physician. The treatment for such disturbances falls within the realm of psychotherapy.

Following the application of local anesthesia, *areas of ischemia of the skin* may be observed near the injection site or at some distance from the site.

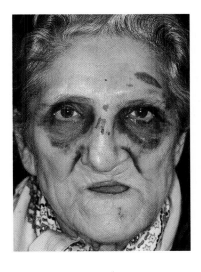
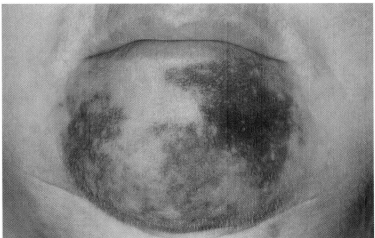
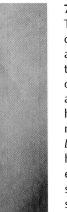

71 Hematoma
This case of hematoma in the chin region occurred following apicoectomy on the left side of the mandible. If there is a danger of infection, systemic antibiotics are indicated. Local application of heat can lead to more rapid resorption of the hematoma. *Left:* This severe, periorbital hematoma occurred after the elderly patient fell. Note also that she had previously undergone surgery to correct a cleft lip.

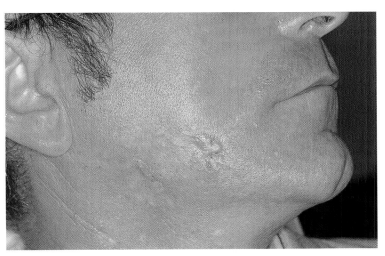

72 Automutilation
This neurotic patient injured himself on both cheeks by constantly scratching the skin with his fingernails and causing injuries; note the scar tissue that has resulted from the healing process. The diagnosis of such situations can be quite difficult. Self-induced lesions are also known as "Münchhausen syndrome" (see p. 71; Tyler et al. 1995).

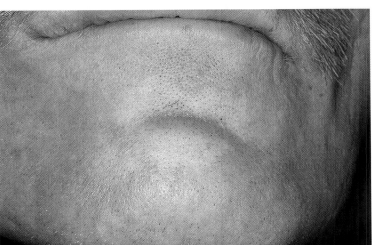

73 Ischemia
Depicted here is an area of local ischemia in the region of the lower lip and the middle of the chin. This occurred following administration of local anesthesia. In many cases, such ischemia may involve large tissue areas, especially the cheeks. Such reactions usually occur immediately following injections. The ischemia usually persists for only a few minutes.

Benign Tumors

Lymphangiomas are congenital hamartomas of the lymphatic vessels. It is possible to differentiate between deep, cavernous and superficial, cystic lymphangioma. In addition, the cystic hygroma is well-known. Oral lymphangiomas are usually observed on the tongue, floor of the mouth, and in the vestibulum. The clinical appearance is of a translucent vesicle with either a clear or a hemorrhagic content.

The so-called nevus flammeus ("port-wine mark") may be one component of the *Sturge–Weber syndrome*. It is charac-

terized by a unilateral *hemangioma* following the distribution of the trigeminal nerve; in 30% of such cases the oral mucosa is involved (Cohen 1995).

Several cysts or odontogenic tumors can produce facial asymmetry (Schmidt-Westhausen et al. 1991).

74   Lymphangioma
In the region of the gingiva and the vestibulum of the patient illustrated on the right, one can observe multiple, blister-like changes of the mucosal surface, as a typical clinical picture of lymphangioma.

Right: In this patient, one can observe a pronounced asymmetry, in which the left cheek is primarily affected. If injury occurs in an area of lymphangioma, there is a danger of secondary infection.

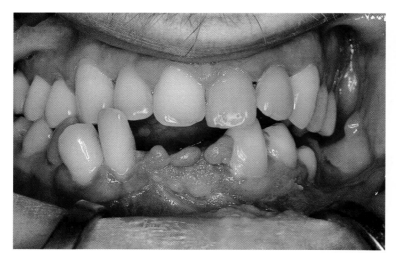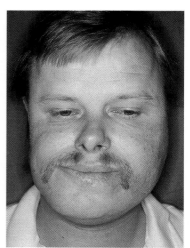

75   Nevus flammeus (port-wine nevus)
Left: This young male exhibited a hemangioma extending along the course of the first and second branches of the trigeminal nerve. In such cases, laser therapy can provide cosmetic improvement.

Right: Nevus flammeus on the right side of the face, primarily in the region of the second trigeminal branch. The oral mucosa of the right side of the maxilla, including the gingiva, was also affected.

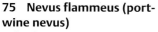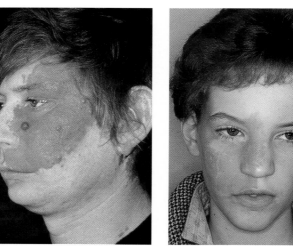

76   Ameloblastic fibroma
This panoramic radiograph reveals a multicystic, radiolucent lesion extending from the first premolar into the ascending ramus of the right side of the mandible. Two molars had already been removed.

Right: Pronounced facial asymmetry resulting from expansion of the horizontal and ascending rami of the mandible, which is afflicted by a large ameloblastic fibroma, an odontogenic tumor of the jaw.

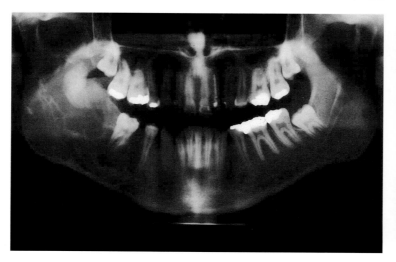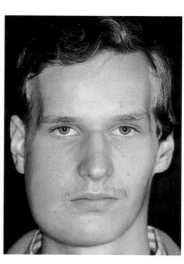

Nevus; Malignant Tumors

The so-called "*Mongolian macula*" of the facial skin is rarely observed and must be distinguished from other skin nevi when making a differential diagnosis. Recurrence of such lesions usually does not occur.

Basal cell carcinomas (Ulcus rodens) are locally destructive, but do not disseminate metastases. Ninety percent of such lesions occur in the upper two thirds of the face. These tumors generally occur after the age of 40 and are found only in areas of the skin with hair follicles.

The most common is the nodular form, which exhibits many types of growth (Härle 1993).

The *malignant melanoma* is found in 7–8% of all cases in the face or neck. Over the last 25 years, the malignant melanoma has increased four-fold in central Europe. In the facial region, the lentigo maligna melanoma is the most frequently encountered (Hornstein 1996). The lentigo maligna with intraoral localization has occasionally been described.

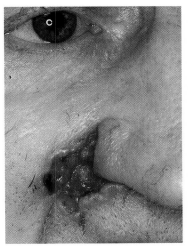
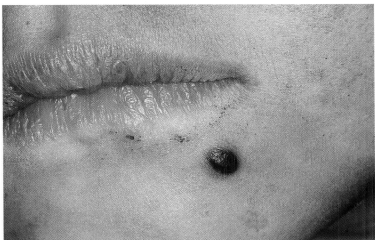

77 "Mongolian macula"/basal cell carcinoma
A pigmented nevus is obvious near the lower lip in a young boy from Thailand. This lesion is harmless, even though it presents clinical similarities to a melanoma.

Left: Basal cell carcinoma. The nasolabial junction is a typical location for the basal cell carcinoma. This patient exhibits a type referred to as a terebrating ulcer.

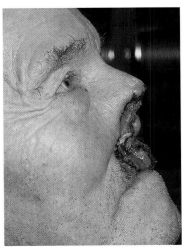
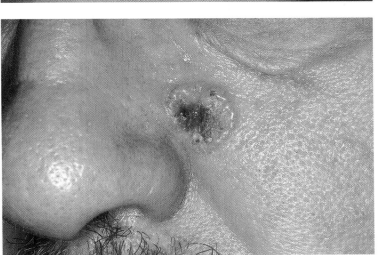

78 Basal cell carcinoma
Note the ulcer in the area of the nasolabial groove exhibiting a central area of ulceration with a crust.

Left: Loss of the upper lip and part of the nose due to an extensive terebrating ulcer. This type of basal cell carcinoma has a tendency to form local recurrences and is also occasionally associated with extensive tissue destruction of the midface.

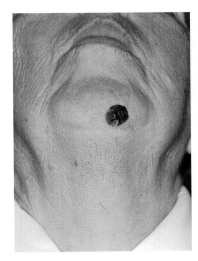
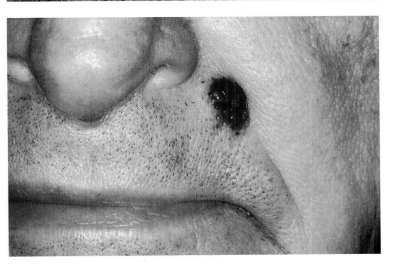

79 Malignant melanoma
In the area of the left upper lip there is a black-bluish, nodular neoplasia which, in this case, was not preceded by a lentigo maligna.

Left: In the chin region of this elderly woman one can observe a lentigo malignant melanoma. The early recognition of pigmented lesions of the facial skin is one of the dentist's important roles.

Syndromes

The *nevus sebaceus syndrome* is rare, and manifests itself as a linear lesion on the skin of the face or scalp. The oral mucosa and gingiva can also be affected (Reichart et al. 1983). The nevus is harmless, but can be esthetically objectionable.

Bourneville–Pringle disease (tuberous sclerosis) is a neurocutaneous syndrome of neuroectodermal origin, which is classified with the phakomatoses. As a result of glial hyperplasia within the central nervous system, consequent symptoms such as mental retardation can ensue. In the mid-face and lower face, one often observes small, multiple angiofibromas, which sometimes also appear on the gingiva. Hyperplastic changes of the enamel have also been reported. Other manifestations may also be present, even including dysontogenetic neoplasias of the internal organs (Gorlin et al. 1976).

80 Nevus sebaceous syndrome
The nevi originate at the corner of the mouth and run a linear course, exhibiting slightly raised plaques. The lesion exhibits surface characteristics resembling warts. This condition exists from birth and enlarges in pace with normal growth.

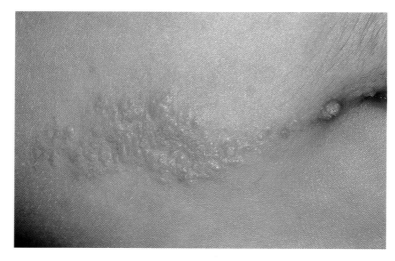

81 Nevus sebaceous syndrome
In addition to the linear sebaceous nevus on the right cheek, note also an additional field of nevi in the midline of the forehead to the tip of the nose of this 15-year-old female.

Right: Biopsy of a gingival lesion reveals multiple epithelial papillary projections exhibiting orthokeratotic epithelium (H & E, x 80).

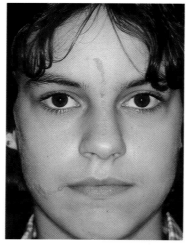
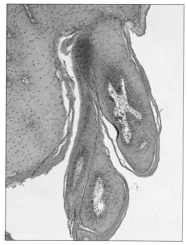

82 Bourneville–Pringle syndrome
In this female patient, note the multiple small nodules in the area of the midface, especially in the nasolabial groove. This woman did not exhibit any neurological symptoms or characteristic oral manifestations, but did exhibit the typical subungual angiofibroma on many of her fingers.

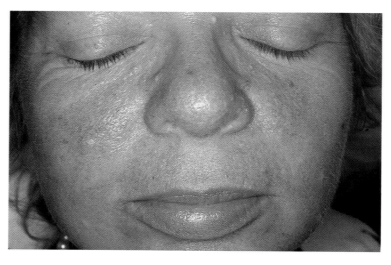

Epidermolysis bullosa includes inherited diseases in which defects of cellular structural proteins of the basement membrane of the skin lead to the appearance of blisters. Various forms of epidermolysis bullosa have been differentiated:

- Epidermolytic epidermolysis bullosa (simplex type with five subtypes)
- Junctional epidermolysis bullosa
- Dermolytic epidermolysis bullosa
- Acquired epidermolysis bullosa

The primary symptoms of *ectodermal dysplasia* include anhidrosis or hypohidrosis as well as dysplasia of hair, nails and teeth. Numerous forms of inherited ectodermal dysplasia are known (Hornstein 1996).

Crouzon's syndrome (craniofacial dysostosis) is characterized by typical malformations of the skull.

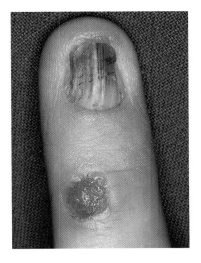
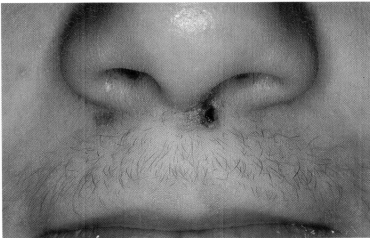

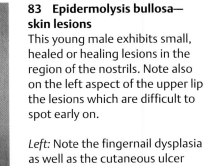

83 Epidermolysis bullosa—skin lesions
This young male exhibits small, healed or healing lesions in the region of the nostrils. Note also on the left aspect of the upper lip the lesions which are difficult to spot early on.

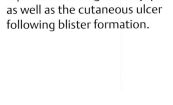

Left: Note the fingernail dysplasia as well as the cutaneous ulcer following blister formation.

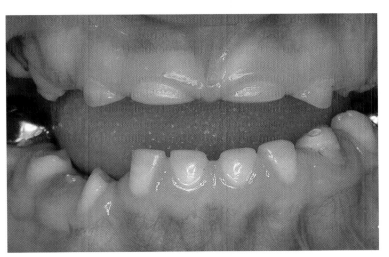

84 Epidermolysis bullosa—dentition
This photograph shows the teeth of the patient in Fig. 83. Especially the maxillary anterior teeth exhibit dysmorphology. Enamel defects have been described in various forms of epidermolysis bullosa, most often in the more severe forms.

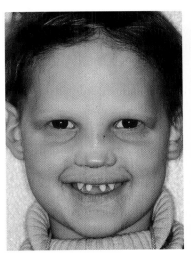
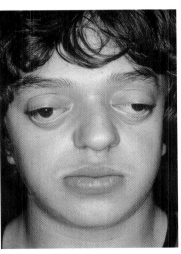

85 Ectodermal dysplasia—Crouzon's syndrome
Left: Ectodermal dysplasia. The eyebrows are poorly developed. There is hypoplasia of the midface, with depressed nasal bridge and oligodontia.

Right: This young male exhibits the typical features of Crouzon's syndrome, including hypertelorism, hypoplasia of the midface, exophthalmia, and prognathism. Abnormalities of tooth position are frequently observed.

Other Lesions

Pemphigus vulgaris can also occur as a primary lesion on the facial skin. In this autoimmune disease, autoantibodies against desmosomal glycoprotein (130 kDa) and plako-globin (85 kDa) circulate as antigenic structural proteins of the desmosomes. Following the formation of immune complexes, the proteases release intercellular substances, primarily to the suprabasal keratinocytes. This leads to acantholysis with consequent blister formation.

The *dermoid cyst* is usually localized in the floor of the mouth. The cyst is lined by keratinizing squamous epithe-lium, and commonly contains hair follicles and sebaceous glands.

Partial facial paralysis can result from various factors. It is necessary to differentiate a central from a peripheral facial paralysis. The so-called "idiopathic" peripheral facial para-lysis is most common. This is assumed to represent a mononeuritis of viral origin (Herpes virus).

86 Pemphigus vulgaris—dermoid cyst
Left: Pemphigus vulgaris; note a fresh lesion following rupture of a bulla.

Middle: Dermoid cyst of the floor of the mouth. The swelling was soft.

Right: Dermoid cyst. Histology reveals the cystic lining exhibiting foreign body giant cells. The lumen contains desquamated epithelial cells (H & E, x 80).

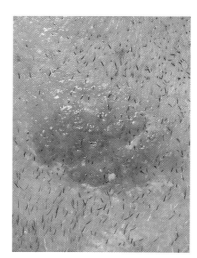 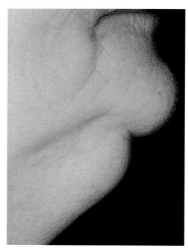 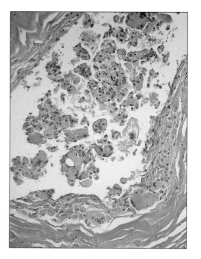

87 Peripheral facial paralysis—ocular involvement
This patient cannot close her right eye. The so-called Bell's phenomenon can also be observed. When attempting to close the eyelid, the eyeball rotates upward. If facial paralysis of the middle branch persists, inflammation and injury to the conjunctiva can result.

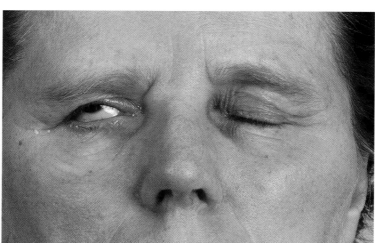

88 Peripheral facial paralysis—oral region
In this female (the same as shown in Fig. 87), the mouth is also affected. The patient is unable to whistle or purse the lips. In most cases, complete or at least partial restitution of nerve function can be expected.

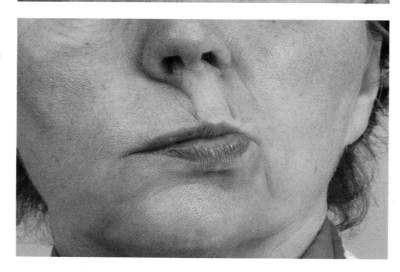

Piercing

Piercing of various parts of the human anatomy is a practice that has increased dramatically in recent years. While piercing of the ears and also the nose have been commonly observed, in more recent times piercing and subsequent insertion of jewelry within the oral cavity and in perioral regions, especially the tongue, have become more common. This type of "body jewelry" appears not to be detrimental to the intake of foodstuffs or speaking. Host reactions following the piercing procedure, such as allergy or inflammation, have been only infrequently observed. Only future studies will reveal whether or not this type of body ornamentation in the oral cavity, especially when base metals are used, will lead to long-term complications.

Several cases of body piercing in Malaysia have been described recently in which sarcoid-like foreign body reactions in the areas of the cheek and the oral mucosa were observed (Ng et al. 1997).

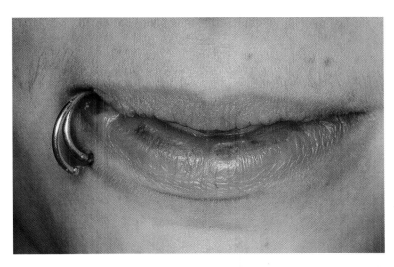

89 Piercing of the right corner of the mouth
In this young female, one can observe two piercing rings at the corner of the mouth, which appear to have caused no clinical evidence of cutaneous or mucosal reactions.

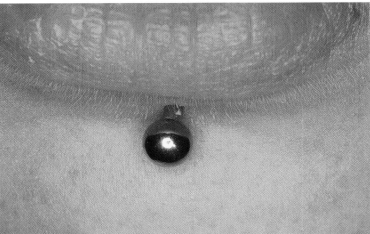

90 Piercing of the lower lip
In this case, the lower lip was pierced through to the intraoral vestibulum two years previously (see Fig. 91). Up until this time, no untoward reactions to this piercing jewelry had been noted.

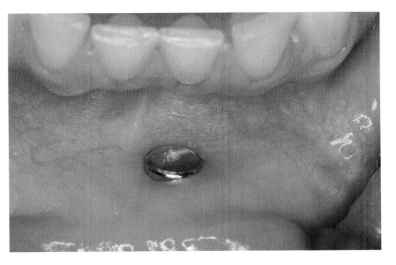

91 Piercing of the lower lip
This photograph shows the perforation in the labial vestibulum. A flat cap secures the jewelry. Note that the oral mucosa of the vestibulum surrounding the cap is unremarkable.

Lips

Definition—Anatomy

The lip is divided into vermilion border, labial commissures, labial mucosa, and the labial sulci. The *vermilion border* (the "lipstick region") represents the area between the labial mucosa and the skin. The *labial commissures* consist of an approximately 1.5 cm square of mucous membrane immediately behind the corners of the mouth. The *labial mucosa* covers a rectangular area extending from the vermilion border to 1 cm from the deepest part of the labial sulcus, bordered laterally by the corners of the mouth. The *labial sulci* comprise a rectangular area mesial to the distal surfaces of the upper/lower canines and extending from the mucogingival reflexion to the deepest part of the sulcus and then approximately 1 cm toward the labial mucosa (Kramer et al. 1980).

The lips represent a transition zone between intra- and extraoral surfaces. Pathologic alterations in this region may originate from structures in both the skin and the mucosa.

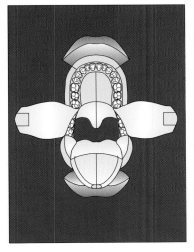
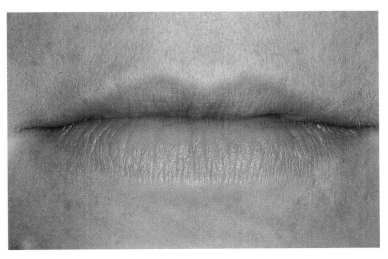

92 External anatomy of the lip
The upper lip displays the typical Cupid's bow. The difference in color between the vermilion border and the immediately adjacent skin results from the thin epithelial layer that covers the vermilion border.

Left: Schematic depiction of the lip region showing the vermilion border, the labial mucosa as well as the upper and lower sulci.

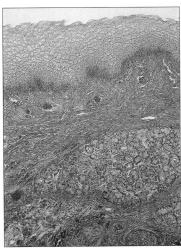
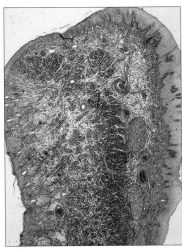
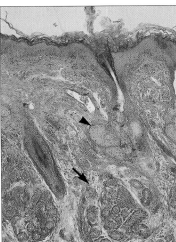

93 Histology of the lip
Left: Labial mucosa exhibiting salivary glands in the submucosa (Mallory, x 30).

Middle: Sagittal section through the upper lip. The mucosa can be seen on the right (Mallory, x 6).

Right: The skin-covered portion of the lip exhibits accessory structures, such as hair follicles, sebaceous glands (arrowhead), and sweat glands (arrow) (Mallory, x 30).

Courtesy K. Kalz

Anomalies

Congenital lip pits are rare anomalies of the lower lip and are occasionally seen at the corners of the mouth. They usually appear as symmetrical fistulae, varying in depth from 0.5–2.5 cm. Such lip pits are generally asymptomatic, although secretions may exude from the depths of the pits, and this may bother the patient. In such cases, it is necessary to perform an excision that includes the glandular tissue.

The so-called *double lip* occurs on the inner mucosal surface of the upper lip. When the mouth is slightly opened, the redundant soft tissue comes into view. A double lip can also appear as one manifestation of the Ascher's syndrome, which itself may be associated with blepharochalasis and goiter.

Labial fissures are cracks predominantly of the lower lip midline area caused by trauma or dehydration. These cracks may persist for long periods of time. They are most often observed in young individuals.

94 Lip pits
Lip pits in a young female who complained of the watery secretion that accumulated in the pits. The surgical specimen revealed the existence of fistulous tracts connecting the surface of the lip with subjacent salivary glandular tissue.

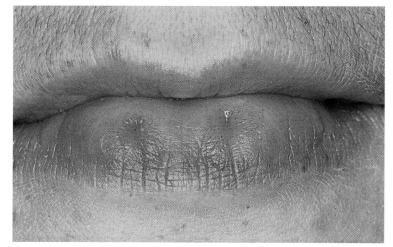

95 Double lip
Double lip in a 12-year-old boy. The curtain-like soft tissue emanates from the inner surface of the upper lip. This condition is usually treated surgically for purely cosmetic reasons.

Right: The section through the excised tissue reveals that the bulk of the redundant mass consists of hyperplastic salivary gland tissue. Note a large vessel (arrow) at the left edge of the section (H & E, x 40).

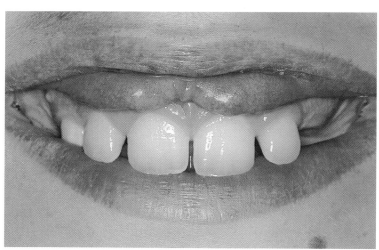
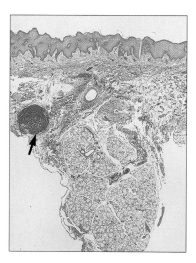

96 Labial fissure
Median lower lip fissure or crack in a young man who was continously exposed to cold and dry weather. The fissure bled easily and, because of constant lip movement, the healing process was often protracted. Frequent use of protective lip balms can assist in preventing the formation of labial fissures and cleft formation.

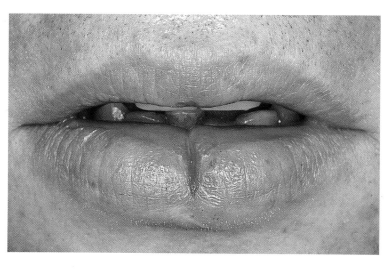

Infections—Mycotic

Angular cheilitis is characterized by fissures that emanate from the corners of the mouth and are often associated with white plaques. Superficial ulceration and bleeding are common. Patients sometimes complain of pain and a gagging reflex.

In the past, angular cheilitis was observed almost exclusively in elderly patients who wore full dentures and who experienced a reduced vertical dimension. Today, however, one also observes this disorder in younger individuals who are infected with HIV. Constant moisture at the corners of the mouth present excellent conditions for the growth of Candida albicans, which is the primary etiologic agent.

Chronic *mucocutaneous candidiasis* is known to be associated with heterogeneous endocrine disturbances and immunological defects. Afflicted patients suffer from infections of the skin, the nails, and the mucous membranes by various species of Candida.

- Candida albicans
- Staphylococcus aureus
- Constant moisture
- Loss of vertical dimension
- Avitaminosis
- Immunosuppression

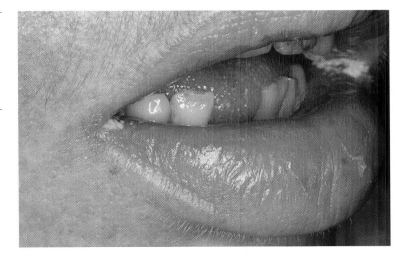

97 Angular cheilitis
This HIV-infected, drug-dependent female presented with white plaques in the area of the corner of the mouth bilaterally. This patient also exhibited a pseudomembranous candidiasis of the oral cavity. The lower lip exhibited exfoliative cheilitis (Reichart et al. 1997).

Left: Etiologic factors in angular cheilitis.

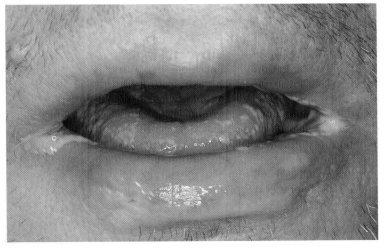

98 Angular cheilitis
AIDS patient with pronounced plaque formation and diffuse erythema at the corners of the mouth. Candida infections usually involve all of the oral mucosa. In the early stages of HIV infection, topical antimycotic agents are usually sufficient, but with increasing immunodeficiency, systemic antimycotic agents, such as fluconazole, must be prescribed (Greenspan 1994).

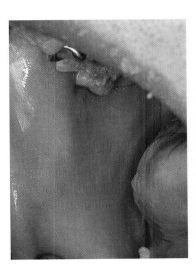

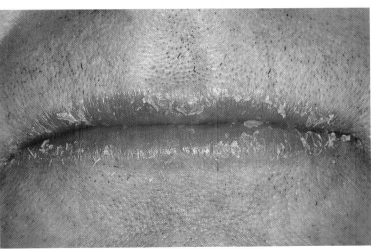

99 Chronic mucocutaneous candidiasis
Both lips of this elderly patient exhibit pronounced exfoliation, and the vermilion borders are highly erythematous, which is typical for exfoliative cheilitis.

Left: The right buccal mucosa exhibits an erythematous candidiasis. Treatment is rendered more complicated by the underlying immunodeficiency.

Infections—Viral

Labial Herpes

Labial herpes is characterized by vesicle formation on the skin and the vermilion border. This disorder begins with the formation of blisters, which often coalesce and lead to ulcerations and scab formation. Labial herpes was observed in 3% of an unselected Swedish cohort (Axéll 1976). The prevalence rate increases to 17% if a 2-year history of labial herpes is included. The causative organism is *herpes virus hominis*, type 1 (HSV-1).

Seldom, but especially in HIV-infected patients, HSV-2 may also infect the perioral regions; HSV-2 is usually associated with genital herpes infection.

In its "dormant" phase, the herpes simplex virus resides in neural ganglia such as the Gasserian ganglion; it is reactivated by factors such as UV-light, fever, or hormonal dysfunctions. In immunocompromised patients, all oral ulcerations should be examined for herpes simplex virus (Woo and Lee 1997). (See also pp. 96, 132, 152)

100 Labial herpes
Vesicles developing on the skin near the left corner of the mouth. An itching sensation 12 hours prior to blister formation is a characteristic initial symptom.

Right: Cycle of infection. Following reactivation, the HSV-1 in the neural ganglia regroup and migrate into the area served by the nerve.

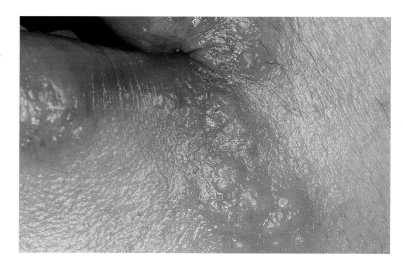

101 Labial herpes in an HIV-infected patient
As a result of the immunodeficiency, labial herpes and other HSV infections can be quite extensive and persistent. Even areas of the skin and mucosa that are usually not involved in immunocompetent patients may exhibit quite severe lesions.

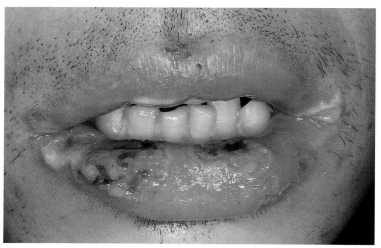

Herpes simplex virus
↓
Infection of epithelial cells
↓
Primary infection
Acute infection · Subclinical infection
Clinical manifestation
↓
Latent Infection.
The virus persists in the ganglia of 70–90% of the population.
↓
Reactivation
Provoked by:
Fever
Allergy
Trauma
Sunlight
Immunosuppression
Psychological stress
Chemical substances
Hormonal changes
↓
Recurring manifestations
↓
Release of the infectious virus

102 Labial herpes in late stage, with crust formation
This is an immunocompetent, elderly female patient. Without any treatment whatsoever, the lesions healed spontaneously and without scarring within 14–21 days.

Right: Immunohistochemical depiction of HSV-1 (stained red) in the epithelium of the vermilion border and the labial skin (APAAP, x 40).

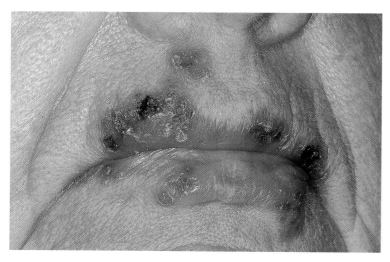

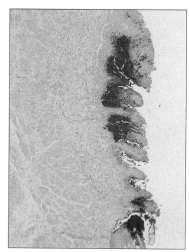

The treatment for labial herpes must be initiated at the earliest possible time. The most often employed antiviral medication is Aciclovir; it can effectively inhibit blister formation when applied topically during the prodromal stage. The use of systemic anti-viral medications is only indicated in patients who are immunocompromised (Scully 1996).

Herpetiform Aphthae

Herpetiform ulcerations can affect any area of the oral mucosa. Lesions 1–2 mm in size may number 10 to 100. Such multiple lesions can coalesce and enlarge. The sur- rounding mucosa appears intensely erythematous. Despite the terminology that is currently employed, the relationship between HSV-1 and the herpetiform ulcerations remains unclear.

Actinic Cheilitis

Actinic cheilitis is caused by intensive exposure to UV rays. It is characterized by ulceration, edema and scab formation.

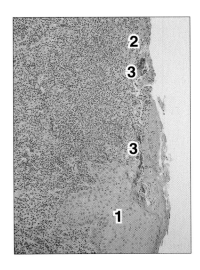
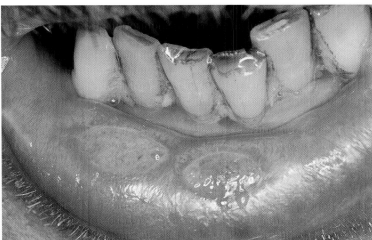
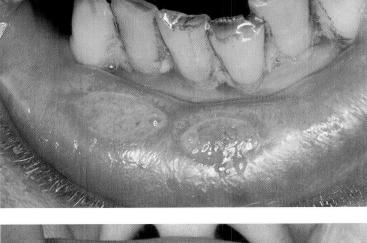

103   Labial herpes on the vermilion surface of the lower lip
Fibrin-coated ulceration following confluence and bursting of the blisters. Vesicles in this region of the lip usually burst early on.

Left: Histologic picture of a herpetic mucosal lesion with ulceration (**2**) and several (red-stained) HSV-1-positive epithelial cells (**3**) in the upper layers (**1** = epithelium). A pronounced inflammatory reaction can be noted in the subepithelial region (APAAP, x 40).

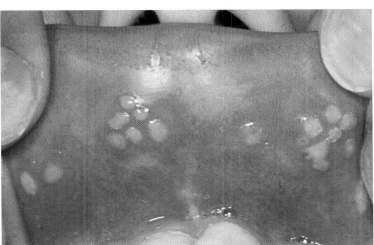

104   Herpetiform ulceration
Herpetiform ulcerations on the mucosa of the upper lip. The appearance of small aphthoid ulcerations in clusters upon an erythematous background is typical. In the absence of a defined cause, purely symptomatic therapy is the treatment of choice.

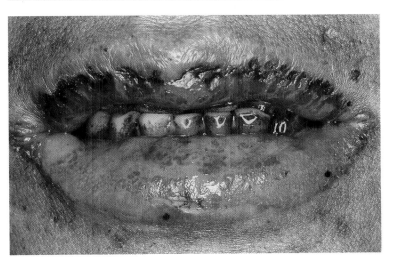

105   Actinic cheilitis
Actinic cheilitis in a Himalayan mountain dweller. Due to lack of sun protection, a severe cheilitis with pronounced edema developed. The blurred transition zone between the vermilion border and the skin provides visual evidence of earlier similar occurrences. There have been rare reports of actinic glossitis: Mountain climbers at high altitude had exposed the tongue to sunlight because of their labored breathing.

Contagious Molluscum

Contagious molluscum is sometimes observed on the facial skin of children. The oral mucosa is exceedingly rarely affected. In HIV-infected patients, however, perioral and intraoral lesions have been observed (Sugihara et al. 1990, Ficarra and Gaglioti 1989). The lesions are characterized by soft and flesh-colored, white, translucent or yellowish papules which are 3–10 mm in size. These lesions are painless and often occur in clusters.

The condition is caused by a pox virus or one of the Nakano group II pox viruses. Such viruses are encountered worldwide. The condition is contagious, and transfer normally occurs through direct contact, which can be sexual or nonsexual. Autoinnoculation is also suspected.

The lesions are harmless, but may indicate a certain degree of immunodeficiency. Treatment consists of surgical excision. Recurrence is frequent.

Contagious Molluscum

106 Clinical picture
In this HIV-infected young male, multiple papules of various sizes are obvious on the vermilion border and adjacent labial skin of both upper and lower lips. Additional lesions were also detected on the facial skin, especially in the periorbital region. Identical lesions were detected in this man's partner.

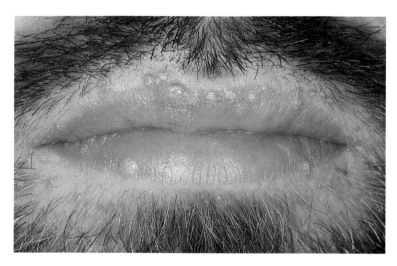

107 Histology
Histologic view of a representative contagious molluscum papule from the lip. Note the masses of basophilic intracytoplasmic inclusion bodies in the epithelium (H & E, x 80).

Right: Contagious molluscum of the lip. Intracytoplasmic inclusion bodies can also be seen on the surface of the lesion (H & E, x 60).

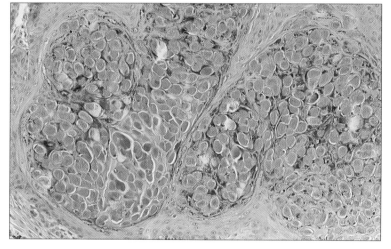
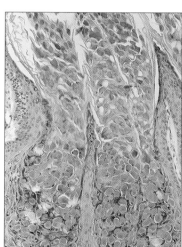

108 Virus particles
Electron microscopy confirms the diagnosis. In the region of the keratinocytes, one can observe tightly packed, completely developed, and mature pox virus particles (TEM, x 40 000).

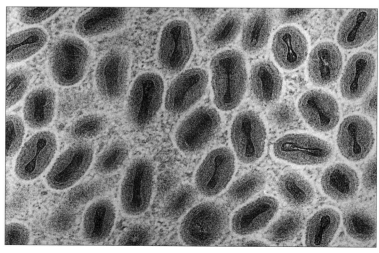

Focal Epithelial Hyperplasia

Focal epithelial hyperplasia (FEH, Heck's disease) is characterized by the appearance of multiple, flat, white nodules on the oral mucosa. This condition was first observed and described among American Indians of New Mexico and Brazil. The condition was also found later in Canadian and Greenland Eskimos. Several cases have also been observed in Europeans (Reichart et al. 1982).

The surface of the lesions is finely stippled and mildly keratinized. The color of the nodules corresponds to that of the adjacent mucosa. If the mucosa is stretched, the lesions seem to disappear. Most commonly the lesions are found on the mucosa of the lips, the buccal mucosa as well as the labial commissures. The human papilloma virus types 13 and 32 are always associated with focal epithelial hyperplasia (Scully 1996). The "therapy" consists simply of repeated observation because, especially in children, these lesions are self-limiting (see also pp. 69 and 99).

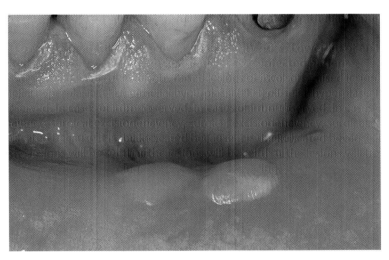

Focal epithelial hyperplasia

109 Lower lip of an HIV-infected patient
Two soft, raised lesions of focal epithelial hyperplasia (FEH) can be observed. In cases of immunodeficiency, surgical excision may be indicated because it is unlikely that the lesions will be self-limiting.

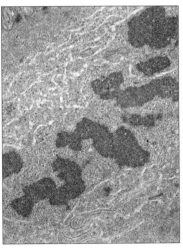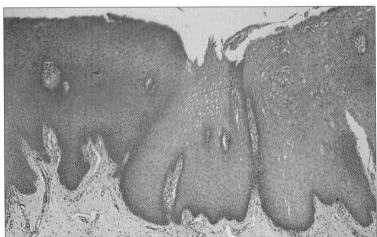

110 Histology
Histologic picture of the FEH from the patient in Fig. 109. The epithelium is hyperplastic, with broad, acanthotic rete pegs ("elephant foot" morphology) (H & E, x 60).

Left: Electron microscopic view of the labial epithelium from Fig. 109. Note the clumping of the nuclear chromatin in the so-called mitosoid cells of the spinous layer (TEM, x 6000).

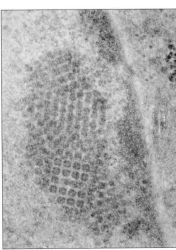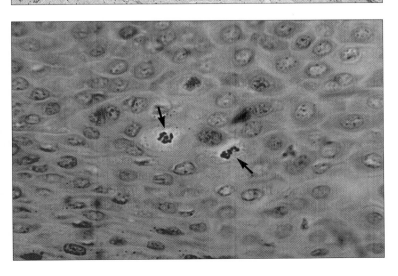

111 Histology
Histologic picture exhibiting the stratum spinosum, with two mitosoid cells (arrows) which exhibit the typical cellular changes caused by the HPV infection (H & E, x 300).

Left: Electron microscopic picture of a virus particle. Particularly evident is the crystalline structure and configuration of the virus particle (TEM, x 20 000).

Other Infections

Recurrent Aphthous Ulcers (RAU)

This common type of oral ulceration is characterized by recurrent ulcers upon nonkeratinized oral and oropharyngeal mucosa. The prevalence of RAU varies between 10 and 65%, with females more commonly affected than males and nonsmokers more commonly than smokers. In most cases, the medical history will reveal a familial pattern. The individual ulcer is covered superficially by fibrin and is surrounded by a red halo. It is possible to differentiate between minor and major variants.

The precise etiology remains unclear (Pedersen 1993), but the ulcerations may be caused by mechanical trauma and certain food products. The prodromal stage begins with a burning sensation; the established ulceration can be quite painful. Following the first occurrence of aphthous ulcers, usually at about age 20, patients can expect to experience RAU in intervals of years, months or weeks, or the lesions may persist almost constantly. RAU is a common manifestation in HIV-infected individuals (MacPhail et al. 1991, Phelan et al. 1991).

Recurrent aphthous ulcers

112   Labial aphthae of the minor type
The lesion is coated with fibrin and exhibits the characteristic hyperemic periphery. This localization, as well as that depicted in Fig. 113, is most commonly observed, followed by lesions of the cheek, the tongue, and the floor of the mouth.

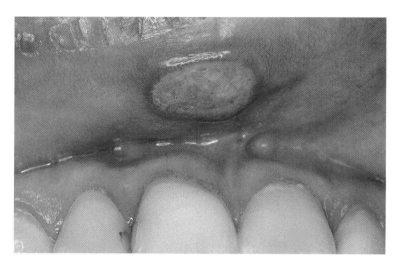

113   Minor aphthae of the mucosa of the lower lip
With the lesion in this location, near the vestibulum and the labial frenum, every movement of the lip elicits pain.

Right: Histologic picture of the initial ulcer formation. The epithelium is split, and ulcer formation occurs after complete epithelial disruption. The resulting cavity is filled with serous fluid and some polymorphonuclear leukocytes (H & E, x 80).

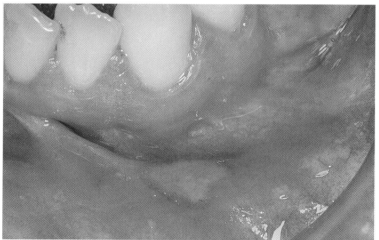
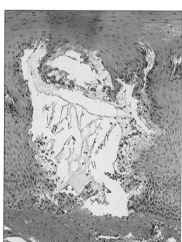

114   Major aphthae
Major aphthous ulceration, with a crater-like, fibrin-covered defect. The healing period of an ulceration of this size can extend over three weeks. Numerous treatments for RAU have been suggested, including topical corticosteroids, disinfectants and antibiotics, all of which provide only symptomatic relief (Saxon et al. 1997).

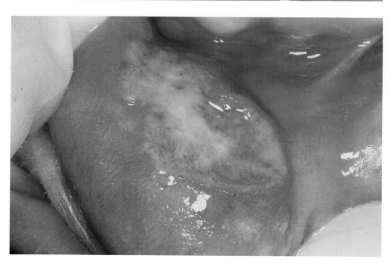

Mechanical and Physical Causes

Lip Biting

Lip biting, often associated with cheek biting, is a mild form of self mutilation. These patients bite or chew upon their own oral mucosa, or suck on it. When formulating a differential diagnosis, it is important to remember that only mucosal areas that approximate the plane of occlusion will exhibit pathologic alterations. Injured tissues exhibit irregular, white tags of desquamating epithelium. Such mucosal lesions are not precancerous (Pindborg et al. 1997).

Mucocele

The mucocele, or mucosa cyst, results from trauma, giving rise to retention or extravasation phenomena, during which local accumulation of salivary secretion within the submucosa occurs. The lower lip is more often affected than the upper lip, followed by the floor of the mouth and the ventral aspect of the tongue. Mucoceles are soft, painless, fluctuant, and often exhibit a bluish color (see also p. 263).

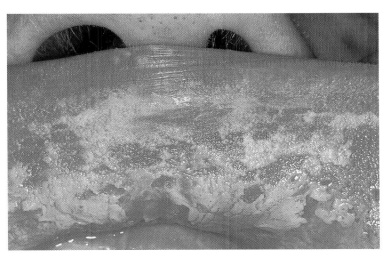

115   Lip biting
The upper lip of this young patient exhibits irregular, white areas with small mucosal erosions. The patient admitted that she had developed the lip-biting habit and chewed almost constantly on both upper and lower lips. The treatment involved the fabrication of an "oral screen" to assist in breaking the habit. Two months later, the labial lesions had completely subsided.

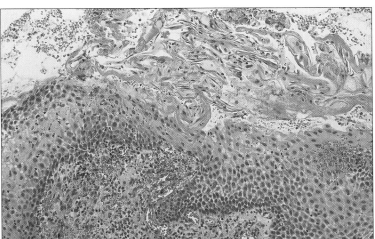

116   Lip Biting—histology
Histologic picture of a typical epithelial alteration. The superficial layers are in the process of desquamation, so that the epithelial layer appears to be reduced in thickness. A moderate inflammatory infiltrate can be seen in the subepithelial area. Several vessels exhibit hyperemia and diapedesis (H & E, x 100).

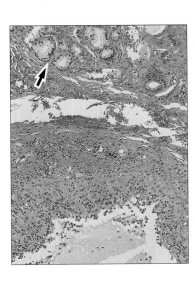
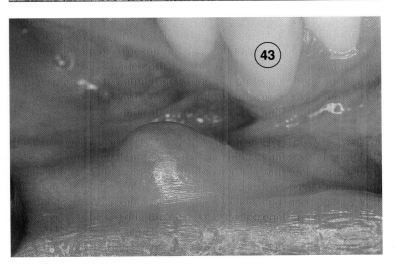

117   Mucocele
Mucocele of the lower lip in its most frequent location, adjacent to tooth 43. Mucoceles sometimes burst spontaneously, but in most cases surgical removal is indicated.

Left: The cystic wall consists of compressed granulation tissue with proliferating fibroblasts. The lumen contains mucous secretion and macrophages. Within the wall, one can observe acini and ductal structures of the mucous salivary glands (arrow) (H & E, x 80).

Disturbances of Keratinization

"Snuff Dipper's Lesion"

In some areas of the world, especially in Scandinavia and North America, individuals use "smokeless tobacco" by placing it in the labial or buccal vestibulum. This causes leukoplakia-like manifestations of those areas of the mucosa that come into contact with the tobacco quid. Pronounced alterations of the epithelium can ensue. In contrast to bona fide leukoplakia, the "snuff dipper's lesion" seldom transforms malignantly (Andersson 1991). If tobacco use is stopped, the oral mucosal lesions are completely reversible.

Leukoplakia

Leukoplakia of the lip is rare and is usually limited to the labial mucosa, without infringing upon the vermilion border. Labial carcinoma, on the other hand, normally originates from the vermilion border. The topic of oral leukoplakia is treated in detail in the chapters "Cheek/Sulcus" (p. 73), "Tongue" (p. 100), "Floor of the Mouth" (p. 117), and "Gingiva" (p. 154).

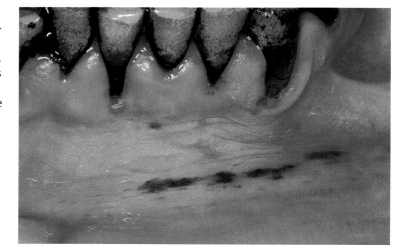

118   "Snuff Dipper's Lesion"
For over thirty years, this 48-year-old male placed snuff daily into the mandibular labial vestibulum. One can observe a homogeneous leukoplakia with brownish discoloration from the tobacco. Intense dark staining of the lower incisor teeth is also characteristic of this habit.

Courtesy T. Axéll

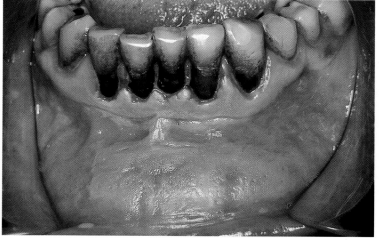
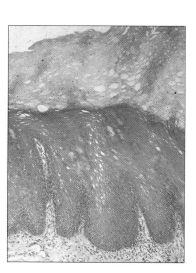

119   "Snuff Dipper's Lesion"
Note the lesions on the attached gingiva, the labial sulcus and the labial mucosa. The labial mucosa is characterized by a yellowish, stippled surface, the "fingerprint" of smokeless tobacco use.

Right: "Snuff dipper's lesion" with pronounced hyperplasia of the epithelium and massive hyperorthokeratosis. The subepithelial inflammatory infiltrate is moderate (H & E, x 40).

Courtesy T. Axéll

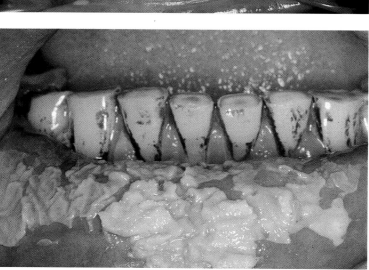

120   Labial leukoplakia
Homogeneous leukoplakia with a verrucous surface. The hyperkeratotic layer is almost leather-like and exhibits cracks that are caused by lip movements. This case of labial leukoplakia was observed in a person from India, and could be traced to intensive smoking by way of the indigenous Hookah pipe.

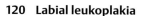

Benign Tumors

Adenoma, Hemangioma and Lymphangioma

Benign tumors of the lips, such as adenoma, are rare. The most common benign tumor of the labial salivary glands is the *pleomorphic adenoma* (see also p. 140). Fifteen percent of all intraoral salivary gland tumors occur on the lips. The upper lip is more commonly afflicted than the lower lip.

Hemangioma and lymphangioma are both hamartomatous in nature, and are frequently congenital. The *hemangioma* is bluish-red in color. It may be capillary or cavernous in nature, depending upon the diameter of the affected vessels. If pressure is applied to the lesion, it blanches.

Lymphangioma is less common than hemangioma. It appears as irregular nodules, sometimes appearing as gray, red or yellow-brown papillary lesions that are similar in color to serum.

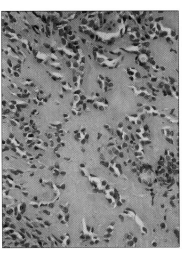
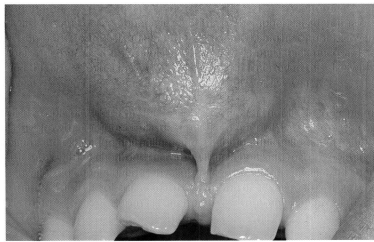
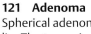

121 Adenoma
Spherical adenoma of the upper lip. The tumor is covered by normal labial mucosa. The tumor achieved this size within a period of five years.

Left: Microscopic picture of the neoplastic growth, composed of epithelium and exhibiting duct-like structures within a homogeneous, hyalinized connective tissue matrix. This type of adenoma is referred to as "tubular" (H & E, x 100).

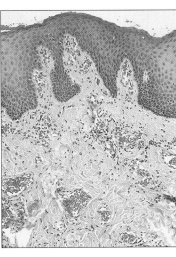
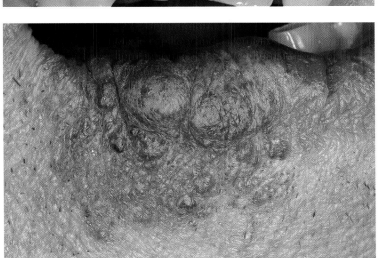

122 Hemangioma
Mixed capillary and cavernous hemangioma of the lower lip. The cavernous form determines the pebbly clinical appearance. This hemangioma involved only the lip. Labial hemangioma can be quite extensive, for example in the Sturge–Weber syndrome.

Left: Histologic picture of the hemangioma. The vascular spaces reveal that this section derives from the more capillary region of the tumor (H & E, x 80).

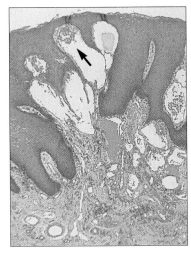
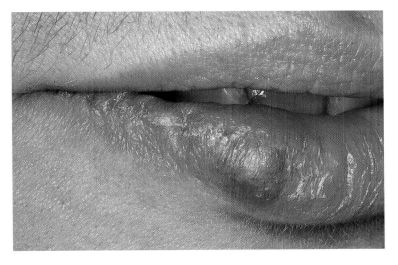

123 Lymphangioma
Depicted is a small, circumscribed, light bluish lymphangioma of the lower lip. The bluish color indicates that the lymphatic channels contain a certain level of erythrocytes.

Left: Histologic picture of the lymphangioma with large, thin-walled lymph vessels (arrow) immediately below the epithelium. Some of the lymph vessels contain erythrocytes. This confirms the clinical impression (H & E, x 60).

Malignant Tumors

Carcinoma

By definition, labial carcinoma is limited to the vermilion border, and occurs in 95% of cases on the lower lip (Pindborg 1982). It is more common in fair-skinned individuals; the ratio of affected males to females varies between 10:1 and 20:1. There are large geographic differences in the incidence rate—from 0.7% (Germany) to 27% (Newfoundland). The tumor exhibits varying clinical characteristics: from harmless-appearing ulcerations to large exophytic lesions. Induration of the peritumor area is an important diagnostic criterium.

Labial carcinoma is a tumor of the elderly. Tumors that are smaller than 2 cm in diameter are only seldom associated with metastases, while larger tumors metastasize about as often as carcinoma of the floor of the mouth or of the tongue. Well-differentiated labial carcinomas metastasize in 6% of cases, while poorly differentiated tumors metastasize in 52% of cases. A comprehensive review of labial and oral cavity carcinomas was presented by Jovanovic (1994). (See also pp. 79, 108, 120, 170, 198)

124 Incidence rates of labial carcinoma
This bar graph depicts selected regions or countries exhibiting varying incidence rates of labial carcinoma, some high, some low.

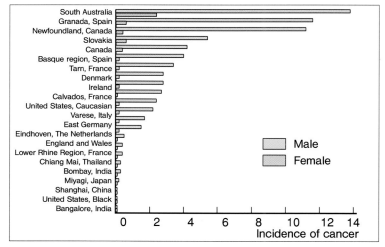

125 Topography of labial carcinoma
The dark pink-colored segments of the lower lip indicate the most frequent localization of labial carcinoma. Any changes of the lips that give the practitioner a suspicion of carcinoma should be immediately referred to a maxillofacial surgeon. The surgeon will be responsible for definitive diagnosis as well as treatment; the treatment usually involves primary surgical excision.

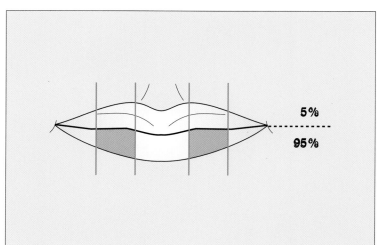

126 Etiology of labial carcinoma
The graphic illustration depicts the significance of the various factors.

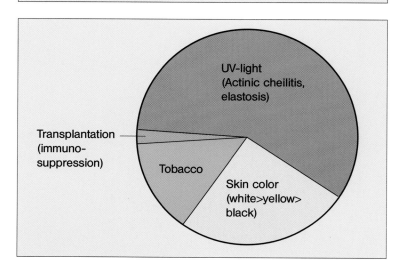

Important *etiologic factors* are ultraviolet light and skin color (race). Individuals with a darker skin color exhibit a low incidence rate of labial carcinoma, probably because of the melanin pigment, which provides a certain protective influence. In contrast to this, individuals with a lighter skin color who work in the open and are therefore exposed to sunlight, such as farmers or seafarers, are especially frequently affected.

Because the upper lip is less exposed to direct sunlight than the lower lip, the frequency of carcinoma is significantly lower on the upper lip.

Tobacco is an additional etiologic factor, especially pipe smoking. Other factors such as viral infection (HSV-1/2; HPV) and immunologic disturbances must also be considered (Jovanovic 1994). Labial carcinoma has also been described in patients who receive organ transplants, particularly kidney transplants (de Visscher et al. 1997).

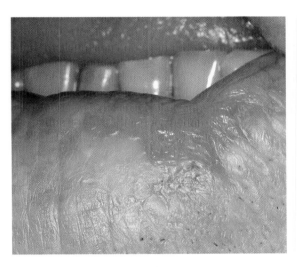
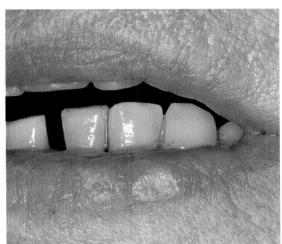

127 Labial carcinoma

Left: The demarcation between the vermilion border and the skin has disappeared. One can observe a whitish change and a small scab-covered area, which appears to be an initial ulceration. These rather non-spectacular clinical changes should, however, be watched carefully.

Right: Small, whitish, harmless-appearing alteration on the lower lip. In this case, it was an early carcinoma. Palpation revealed definite induration.

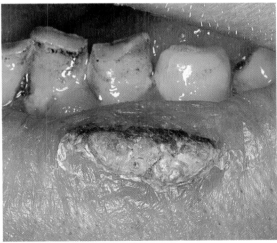
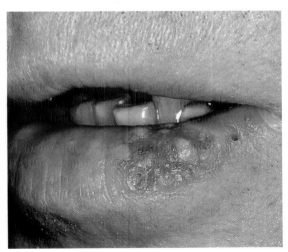

128 Labial carcinoma

Left: Clearly demarcated ulceration with thick scab formation exhibits scaling and a tendency towards desquamation on the indurated borders. The ulceration is surrounded by an erythematous halo.

Right: Note the reddened area of the vermilion border with some scab formation and small nodules. Such erosions and non-healing ulceration represent an important symptom of malignancy.

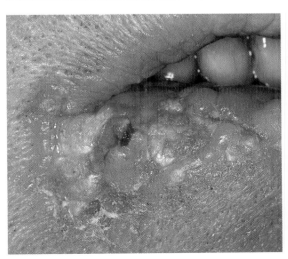
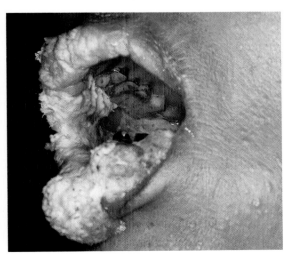

129 Labial carcinoma—verrucous carcinoma

Left: Large carcinoma of the lower lip. The border between the vermilion border and the skin has been completely lost. The histologic examination revealed a squamous cell carcinoma.

Right: Pronounced and extensive verrucous carcinoma of the upper and lower lips and the buccal mucosa in a female from Thailand who had chewed betel quid for over 40 years (from Pindborg et al. 1997).

Verrucous Carcinoma

The verrucous carcinoma, or the so-called Ackerman tumor, comprises 2–20% of all oral cavity carcinomas, but is rare on the lips. Verrucous carcinomas are characterized by exophytic, papillomatous, slow growth. In most cases, verrucous carcinomas are strongly related to tobacco habits, such as pipe smoking or the chewing of betel quid. Especially with betel quid chewing, the lesions may be pronounced and extensive.

The treatment for verrucous carcinoma is total excision. Metastases are relatively seldom.

Basal Cell Carcinoma

While the basal cell carcinoma of the facial skin is a frequent neoplasm in the elderly, basal cell carcinoma of the oral cavity is extremely rare. As with the squamous cell carcinoma of the lip, frequent exposure to sunlight appears to be an important etiologic factor.

Treatment for basal cell carcinoma is excision, and metastasis is relatively rare. However, if removal of the tumor is incomplete, recurrence is likely.

130 Verrucous carcinoma
Histologic picture revealing excessive hyperplasia of the epithelium as well as massive hyperorthokeratosis. The rete pegs are broad; epithelial atypia, including elevated mitotic activity is seldom observed. The tumor growth occurs expansively but not by infiltration ("pushing as an advancing front") (H & E, x 10).

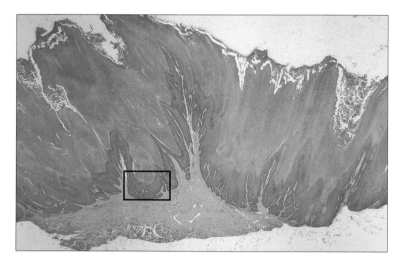

131 Verrucous carcinoma
Higher magnification of the squared area outlined in Fig. 130. The rete pegs are broad. The well-differentiated epithelium shows no signs of atypia. The basal membrane is intact. The epithelial islands represent cross-section cuts through the irregular rete network and are not signs of infiltrative growth. The inflammatory reaction is minimal (H & E, x 120).

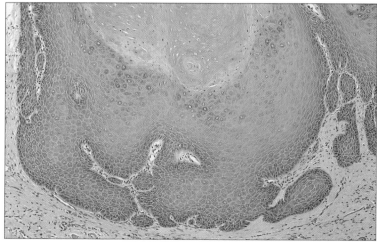

132 Basal cell carcinoma
This quite unusual case of basal cell carcinoma exhibits severe destruction of the upper lip with exposure of the maxillary alveolar process. The lesion had been present for six years and had slowly increased in size. The patient, a 76-year-old male, exhibited another basal cell carcinoma in the region of the right temple.
Right: Histologic section with infiltrating islands and strands of epithelial basal cells. A moderate to severe inflammatory infiltrate is also observed (H & E, x 80).

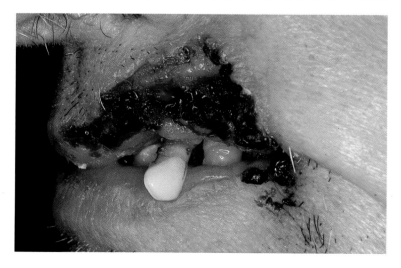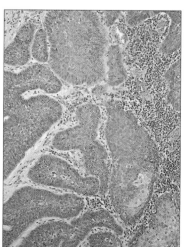

Syndromes

Melkersson–Rosenthal Syndrome

The clinical picture of unilateral (partial) facial paralysis, labial swelling and fissured tongue is known as the Melkersson–Rosenthal syndrome (MRS). It affects males and females equally and there is no racial predilection. All aspects of the syndrome do not always occur simultaneously. The swelling, which is the dominant symptom of this syndrome, is not painful, is firm to palpation and may become very large (Winnie and de Luke 1992, Zimmer et al. 1992).

The term *orofacial granulomatosis* describes a comprehensive diagnosis including the Melkersson–Rosenthal syndrome, Crohn's disease and sarcoidosis with an identical histologic appearance. Noncaseating epithelioid cell granulomas are observed histologically.

The etiology is unknown, but factors such as nutrition, flavoring and local immune response may be involved.

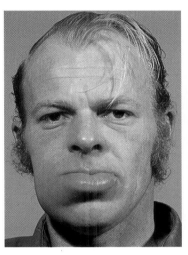
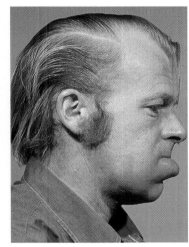

Melkersson–Rosenthal syndrome

133 Pronounced edema of the lower lip
This patient had already experienced several episodes of facial swelling. He had a fissured tongue (Fig. 134), but no facial paralysis.

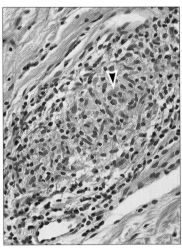
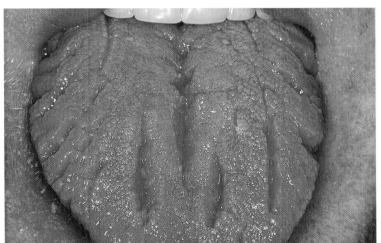

134 Fissured tongue with mild edema—histology of the labial edema
Patient from Fig. 133.

Left: Higher magnification of the epithelioid cell granuloma of the edematous labial lesion. The periphery of the granuloma consists of lymphocytes and proliferating fibroblasts, while the center harbors mainly macrophages. Some of the macrophages appear to be in the process of forming giant cells (arrowhead) (H & E, x 120).

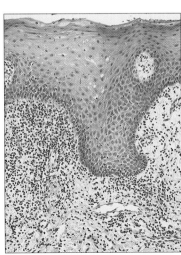
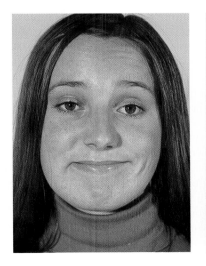
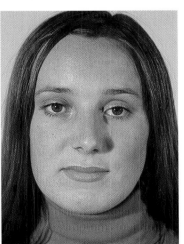

135 Young female with facial paralysis
Left: Histologic picture of the buccal mucosa from MRS, exhibiting pronounced infiltration by lymphocytes and macrophages (H & E, x 80).

Middle and Right: Young woman with MRS showing signs of facial partial paralysis. The edema presents in the form of a pillow-like thickening of the buccal mucosa. She had experienced identical symptoms four times.

Exudative Erythema Multiforme

Exudative erythema multiforme, or Stevens–Johnson syndrome, is a chronic inflammatory, mucocutaneous disease that can occur in both males and females at any age. The etiologic factors remain unclear, but various antigens and other factors such as herpes virus, other infections as well as medicaments have been suspected. The most conspicuous characteristics of this disease are stomatitis, conjunctivitis, balanitis, and skin lesions (Farthing et al. 1995). In most cases, the disease is self-limiting within one to several weeks. The clinical picture is often preceded by an infection of the upper respiratory tract, with fever. The skin lesions vary from small papules to extensive lesions that have been described as iris-like. The oral manifestations consist of macular, bullous and pseudomembranous manifestations that are less well circumscribed than the corresponding skin lesions.

Lyell Syndrome

Lyell syndrome, or *toxic epidermal necrolysis* (TEN), is a rare disease of the skin and oral mucosa.

Exudative Erythema multiforme

136   Characteristic lesions of the upper and lower lips
Note the appearance of erosions, scab formation and hemorrhage on the vermilion border. Treatment is nonspecific, whereby the systemic administration of corticosteroids can significantly shorten the course of the disease.

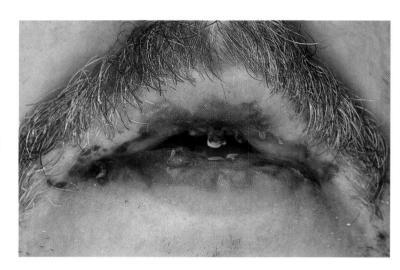

137   Buccal mucosa
Pseudomembranous (arrowhead) and bullous lesions (arrow) of the buccal mucosa in the patient depicted in Fig. 136. In addition, one observes a diffuse stomatitis and edema of the entire oral cavity.

Right: Cutaneous lesions on the palmar surface of the left hand. Notice the "target" configuration of the individual elements.

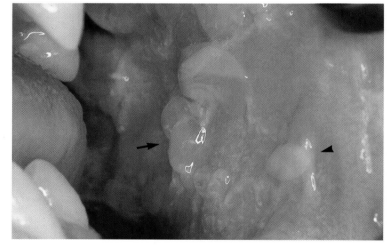
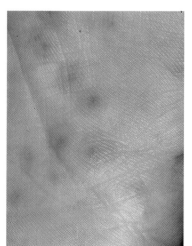

138   Ocular manifestations
This is the same patient depicted in the two figures above. The conjunctiva are heavily inflamed; this patient suffers from photophobia.

Right: Schematic diagram showing the areas of initial manifestations in the face. It is the conjunctiva and the lips that are affected above all.

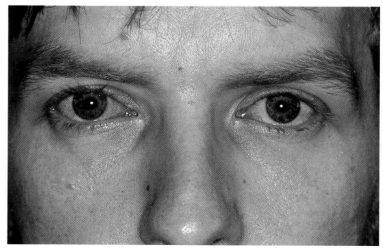
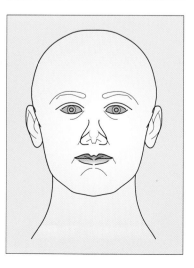

It is comparable to the Stevens–Johnson syndrome, but the clinical course is considerably more severe, and often fatal. Lyell syndrome is characterized by pronounced lysis of surfaces that are covered by stratified squamous epithelium.

Cases of toxic epidermal necrolysis are observed for the most part in patients with AIDS (Schmidt-Westhausen et al. 1998). In these patients, the cause is usually poly-chemotherapy, especially when sulfonamides are taken. The mortality rate for patients with TEN is 30–50%.

Graft Versus Host Reaction

The graft versus host reaction (GVHR) is a complex, multi-systemic, immunologic phenomenon that occasionally manifests following transplantations (Nakamura et al. 1996). The acute form of GVHR is characterized by a skin rash and mucosal erythema with pronounced ulceration and lysis of the epithelium.

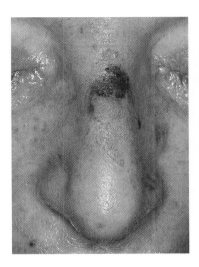
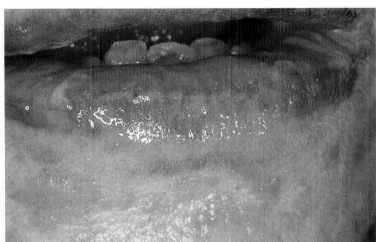
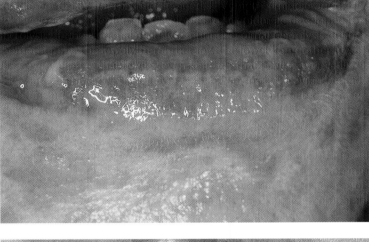
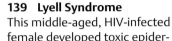

139 Lyell Syndrome
This middle-aged, HIV-infected female developed toxic epidermal necrolysis during a course of polychemotherapy. The lower lip exhibits several blisters that have burst, leaving behind an eroded, fibrin-coated surface. The adjacent skin also exhibits several small blisters.

Left: On the bridge of the nose, one notes erosion immediately adjacent to an area of epidermal lysis; this is comparable to Nikolsky's sign.

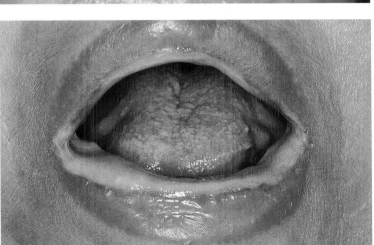
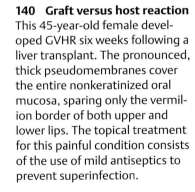

140 Graft versus host reaction
This 45-year-old female developed GVHR six weeks following a liver transplant. The pronounced, thick pseudomembranes cover the entire nonkeratinized oral mucosa, sparing only the vermilion border of both upper and lower lips. The topical treatment for this painful condition consists of the use of mild antiseptics to prevent superinfection.

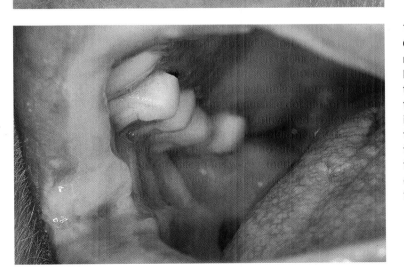

141 Graft versus host reaction
Corner of the mouth and buccal mucosa of the patient depicted in Fig. 140. Notice that the keratinized mucosa of the palate and the dorsum of the tongue are not involved. Following systemic treatment with corticosteroids, the lesions subsided and no further complications were experienced following retransplantation.

Dermatologic Manifestations

Hereditary Epidermolysis Bullosa

Epidermolysis bullosa is a rare disease that is characterized by vesicular and bullous eruptions on the skin and mucous membranes. Various subtypes are recognized, such as dystrophic or mild forms. This disease is inheritable in an autosomal dominant or recessive pattern. The primary symptom of the dystrophic form is blister formation. These occur in areas of pressure or trauma, but may also occur spontaneously. After healing, keloids may form. The oral mucosa often exhibits combinations of bullae, infiltrated areas,

ecchymosis, and white, thickened plaques (Hornstein 1996).

Pemphigus Vulgaris

Pemphigus vulgaris may affect the labial mucosa (see also p. 40). A comprehensive review of the literature was published in 1997 (Robinson et al. 1997). (See also p. 157)

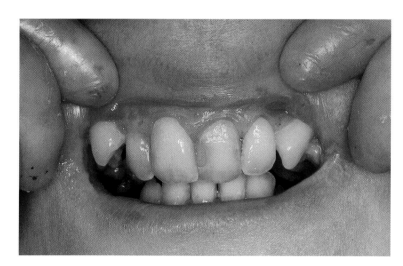

142 Hereditary epidermolysis bullosa
Due to scar formation in the region of the labial vestibule following numerous episodes of bulla formation, this female patient was no longer able to open her mouth properly. Her fingers exhibit the typical glove-like "epithelial covering" that results from healing of earlier phases of epidermolysis.

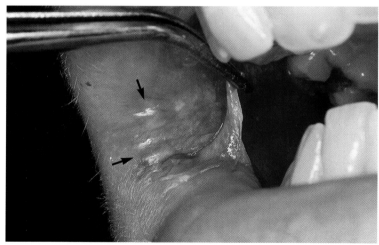

143 Hereditary epidermolysis bullosa
During the extraction of a mandibular molar, the soft tissue at the corner of the mouth was traumatized; a subepithelial cleft formed that led subsequently to sloughing. A portion of the traumatized epithelium remains in situ (arrows), while a smaller portion has been lifted using forceps to demonstrate the sloughing.

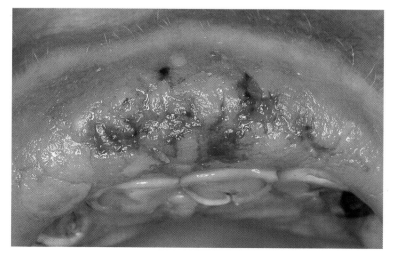 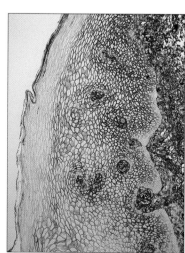

144 Pemphigus vulgaris
Note the obvious ulcerations and bulla formation on the labial mucosa of the upper lip.

Right: Immunohistochemical depiction of IgM in a biopsy from an early pemphigus lesion. The epithelium exhibits characteristic intercellular staining for this marker (PAP, x 60).

Pigmentation

Peutz–Jeghers Syndrome, Osler's Disease, Tattooing

Peutz–Jeghers syndrome is characterized by mucocutaneous melanotic pigmentation and intestinal polyposis; the latter is significant because of the possibility of malignant transformation of the polyps. About one-half of all individuals with this condition exhibit brown to black spots on the perioral tissue and the vermilion border. Intraoral pigmentation is usually observed on the buccal mucosa (Loff et al. 1995).

Osler's disease, also known as hereditary hemorrhagic telangiectasia, results from a disturbance of capillary formation and is characterized by telangiectatic lesions and hemorrhagic diathesis. Lesions of the skin and mucosa appear red or violet in color.

Tattooing deposits exogenous pigmentations into the skin and mucosa. Together with so-called piercing (see also p. 41), tattooing has become a trend in modern society.

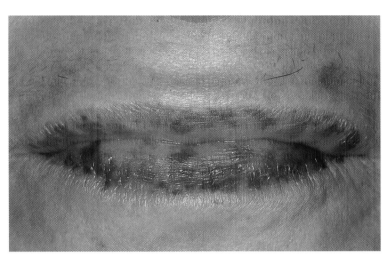

145 Peutz–Jeghers syndrome
Endogenic pigmentation of the vermilion border in a case of Peutz–Jeghers syndrome. The brown, melanin pigmentations are irregularly distributed. Dentists should watch closely for this type of pigmentation in order to establish a diagnosis of the syndrome and to permit appropriate referral of the patient to a gastrointestinal specialist.

Courtesy G. Bethke

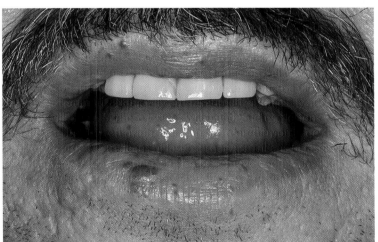

146 Osler's disease
Telangiactatic, slightly raised lesions are noted on the upper and lower lips. Several similar small lesions were found on the mucosa of the tongue. Often, especially after traumatization, these lesions will bleed. Such hemorrhage can be treated by means of laser surgery; small lesions can also be removed using this technique.

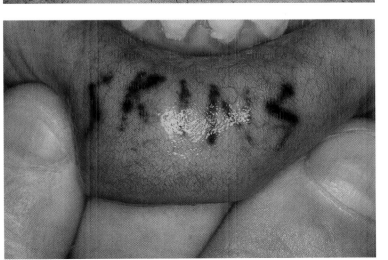

147 Tattooing
This "semi-ritualistic" pigmentation was observed on the lip of a young male, who belonged to a skinhead group. Tattoos of this type are difficult to remove and usually have to be excised. As an alternative, laser therapy can be considered.

Buccal Mucosa/Sulcus

Definition—Anatomy

The *buccal mucosa* is located between the maxillary and mandibular buccal sulci, and extends forward to the corners of the mouth. The areas defined as labial commissures are excluded. The left and right, upper and lower *buccal sulci* comprise a rectangular area posterior to the distal surfaces of the canines, back to the anterior tonsillar pillar and extending from the mucogingival reflexion to the deepest part of the sulcus, and then approximately 1 cm toward the mucosa of the buccal mucosa (Kramer et al. 1980).

The buccal mucosa may exhibit characteristic variations in clinical appearance, such as leukoedema or heterotopic sebaceous glands, the latter being particularly prominent in this location. A common pathologic alteration is the so-called fibroma, a hyperplasia of connective tissue usually induced by trauma.

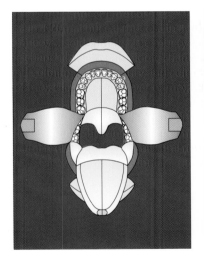
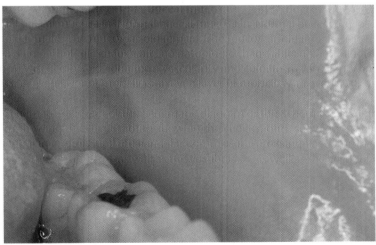

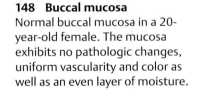
148 Buccal mucosa
Normal buccal mucosa in a 20-year-old female. The mucosa exhibits no pathologic changes, uniform vascularity and color as well as an even layer of moisture.

Left: Schematic diagram of the mouth showing the cheeks, the retroangular commissural areas as well as the vestibula.

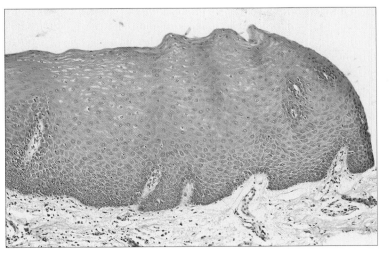
149 Buccal mucosa—histology
Histologic preparation of normal buccal mucosa with a regular epithelial layer and the formation of small rete pegs. The surface layer is parakeratotic, or may be altogether absent. A few scattered inflammatory cells can be noted in the subepithelial area. Textbooks of anatomy often describe the oral mucosa as nonkeratinizing. This is not true, however, for the palate, the gingiva, and also partially the buccal mucosa (H & E, x 80).

Anomalies

Fordyce's Granules, Physiologic Pigmentation

Heterotopic sebaceous glands, also known as *Fordyce's granules*, are sebaceous glands that occur in the oral mucosa, especially in the buccal mucosa. Fordyce's granules are small, slightly raised, yellow or white nodules found either individually or in clusters. They are not observed in children, rather they appear only in the second or third decade of life. Between 80 and 90% of the adult population may be affected. The extent of the glands is greater, the density higher, and the size of the granules larger in males than in

females. These glands are harmless, and their secretion may have a protective function (Sewerin 1975).

Physiologic pigmentation of the oral mucosa occurs more frequently in dark-skinned individuals and in Blacks. All areas of the oral cavity may be affected. This pigmentation is harmless. A histologic evaluation is not indicated for cases of physiologic pigmentation.

150   Fordyce's granules
The buccal mucosa in this female patient exhibits extensive expansion of the heterotopic sebaceous glands, which appear in small clusters that tend to coalesce. The differential diagnosis should include white lesions.

Right: Pronounced Fordyce's granules near the maxillary buccal vestibulum, a typical localization of mucosal sebaceous glands.

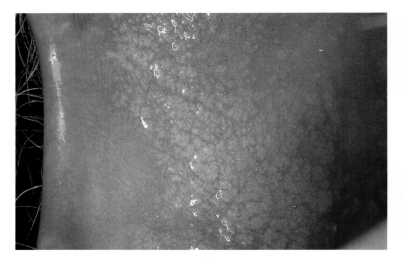 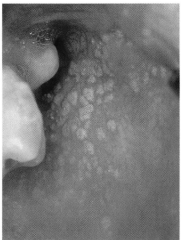

151   Physiologic pigmentation
The buccal mucosa in this elderly, hill-tribe female from the mountains of Thailand exhibits retroangular, circumscribed, brown pigmentation. Very apparent is the pale appearance of the entire oral mucosa, which is an indication of severe anemia.

Right: The histologic picture reveals a characteristic heterotopic sebaceous gland in the oral mucosa. This one lies deeper than those which are clinically apparent (H & E, x 80).

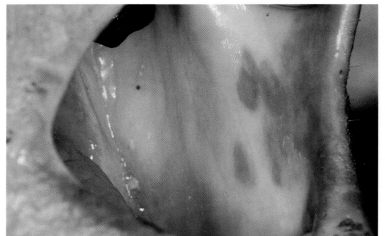 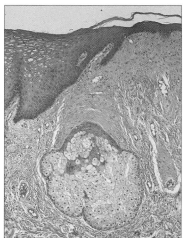

152   Physiologic pigmentation
This photograph depicts the buccal mucosa of a farmer from Thailand, exhibiting heavy pigmentation. The pigmentation is diffuse and is masked by a superficial leukoedema.

Right: Histologic picture of physiologic pigmentation. Note the melanin granules of the basal cells (H & E, x 150).

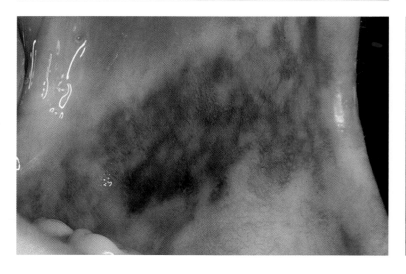 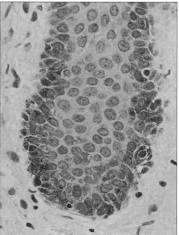

Phlebectasia, White Sponge Nevus, Peutz–Jeghers Syndrome

Phlebectasia of the buccal mucosa is less common than that of the ventral aspect of the tongue. The lesions appear as hemispherical, small, round, bluish-red elevated areas, which are often multiple and which may appear like "beads on a string." They are more common in people over 60 years of age and there is a relationship between oral phlebectasia and cardiopulmonary diseases.

White sponge nevus is an inherited autosomal dominant alteration of the mucosa. It usually occurs bilaterally, is whitish-gray, thickened, and often exhibits deep fissures. Other mucosal regions of the body may be affected (Bánóczy et al. 1973, Jorgensen and Levin 1981).

Peutz–Jeghers syndrome consists of mucocutaneous pigmentation and intestinal polyposis. This disease is transmitted as an autosomal dominant trait.

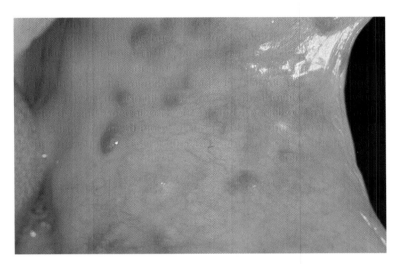

153 Phlebectasia
The buccal mucosa exhibits multiple, bluish-red nodules that correspond to venous dilatations. With increasing age, dilatation of small vessels may occur, also in the oral mucosa and especially on the ventral surface of the tongue. Therapeutic measures are not required.

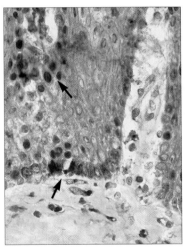
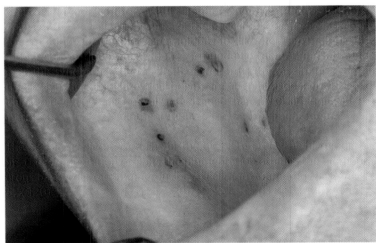

154 Peutz–Jeghers Syndrome
In the area of the buccal mucosa, there are multiple dot-like pigmentations surrounded by erythema. In this syndrome, the intestinal polyps are of greater medical significance than the oral pigmentation.

Left: The histologic picture exhibits the pigmentation of numerous basal cells (arrows) (H & E, x 120).

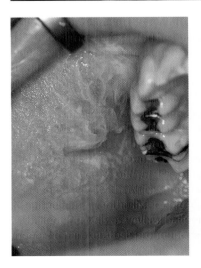
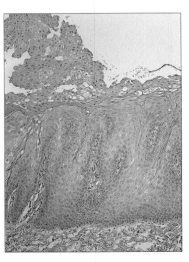

155 White sponge nevus
Left: The buccal mucosa appears thickened, white and fissured. For the differential diagnosis, it is important to remember that this lesion may extend deeply into the vestibulum. Such extensive lesions do not occur with cheek biting. In this young patient, the contralateral side was similarly affected.
Right: Histologic picture of the white sponge nevus, with hyperplastic epithelium, acanthosis, several ballooning cells as well as a pronounced parakeratosis (H & E, x 80).

Infections—Mycotic

Candidiasis

The classification of oral candidiasis has been revised numerous times in recent years. The most often cited classification is that of Lehner (1967). This classification differentiates between acute pseudomembranous, acute atrophic, and chronic hyperplastic as well as chronic atrophic candidiasis. The chronic hyperplastic form is further subdivided into four subcategories. Today the term "erythematous candidiasis" is used more frequently than "atrophic candidiasis."

It is difficult to differentiate between acute and chronic forms, especially in patients with HIV. To date, there is no clear definition of the term "chronic." It is important to remember that species of Candida occur in the oral cavity of 3–48% of all healthy adults and from 45–65% of all healthy children (El-Kabir and Samaranayake 1993). In 17% of cases only *Candida albicans* is detected. This is the most important organism for oral candidiasis, although other species, such as *Candida glabrata* and *Candida krusei*, often appear in connection with HIV infection.

156 Primary oral candidiasis— classification
The classification differentiates between primary and secondary (not shown) forms of oral candidiasis (Axéll et al. 1997). *Secondary* oral candidiasis includes systemic mucocutaneous forms of candidiasis, for example resulting from absence of the thymus or candidiasis as a part of an endocrinopathy syndrome.

Acute Forms	Candida-associated alterations
● Pseudomembranous ● Erythematous	● Denture stomatitis ● Angular cheilitis ● Median rhomboid glossitis
Chronic Forms	**Primary keratinized alterations**
● Hyperplastic ● Nodular ● Plaque-like ● Pseudomembranous	● Leukoplakia ● Lichen planus ● Lupus erythematosus

157 Candida albicans
Candida albicans forms typical white colonies. Candida can be quantified following smears and culture, using the so-called colony forming unit (CFU) technique. The clinical picture does not necessarily correspond to the quantitative analysis.

Right: Important Candida species and other fungi that occur frequently in the oral cavity.

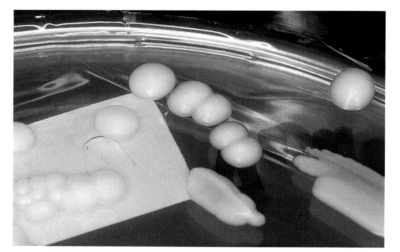

● Candida albicans
● Candida tropicalis
● Candida glabrata
● Candida parapsilosis
● Candida krusei
● Candida dubliniensis

● Rhodotorula
● Saccharomyces

158 Candidiasis—smear
Taking a cytologic smear is advantageous for the diagnosis of candidiasis. Using a spatula, the affected mucosa is lightly scraped and the harvested material is smeared onto a glass slide. Following drying and fixation in 70% alcohol, staining is carried out using PAS to identify hyphae and pseudohyphae.

Right: Carrier tube for the microbiological diagnosis, which should be performed to support the cytologic smear test.

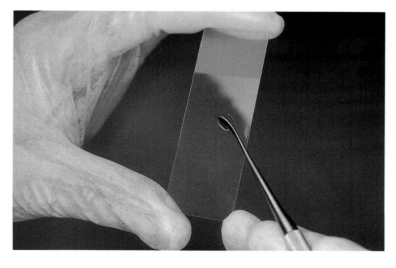

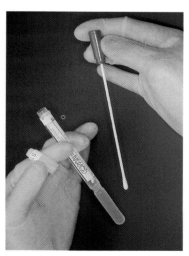

Although it is not yet known why various clinical forms of oral candidiasis occur, there exists a body of knowledge concerning pathogenicity, adhesions, and defense mechanisms (Challacombe 1994, Soll et al. 1994):

- Candida organisms produce enzymes, which permit penetration into the oral mucosa. Phospholipases, which are localized primarily on the tips of the hyphae, as well as extracellular proteases play the most important role in *Candida albicans*.
- The adhesion of Candida species onto mucosal surfaces is of special importance for the establishment of the disease. Hyphae appear to adhere better than conidia.

- The host's attempt to combat Candida species involves immune and nonimmune factors. Nonimmune factors include iron, lysozyme, histidine, lactoferrin and salivary glycoproteins (McCullough et al. 1996). Phagocytosis represents the most important cellular mechanism for the control of *Candida albicans*.

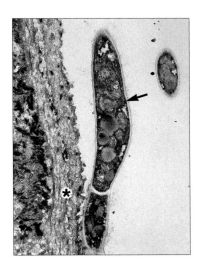 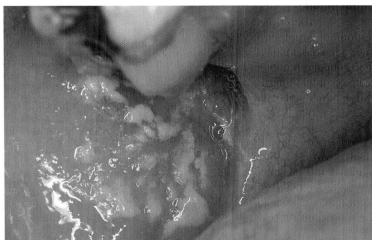

159 Pseudomembranous candidiasis
Pseudomembranous candidiasis is characterized by white, loosely adherent plaques that are situated upon an otherwise unchanged mucosal surface (see pp. 96, 129).

Left: Electron microscopy of hyphae (arrow). The hyphae penetrate into the epithelium (*) by means of enzymes and a complicated mechanism known as thigmotropism.

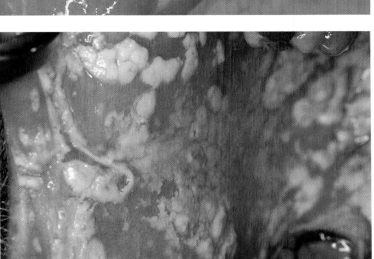

160 Pseudomembranous candidiasis—chronic type
This HIV-infected patient presented with a pseudomembranous candidiasis of the chronic type. The problem had persisted for several weeks, and the lesions could be scraped off only with difficulty. This form of candidiasis often proves to be therapy-resistant in the later stages of AIDS. In some of these cases, *Candida krusei* and *Candida glabrata* are involved, in addition to *Candida albicans*.

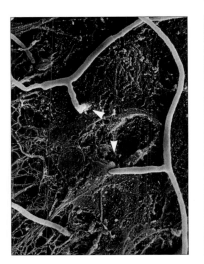 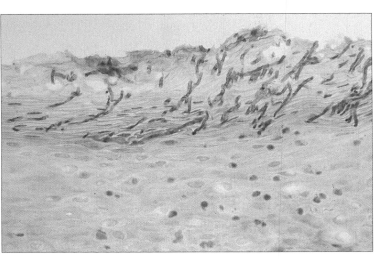

161 Candidiasis—histology
The histologic picture reveals that hyphae infiltrate the parakeratotic epithelium perpendicular to the surface.
Left: Scanning electron micrograph of the epithelial surface in a case of pseudomembranous candidiasis. Several hyphae penetrate into the epithelium (arrowheads). Enzymes secreted at the tips of the hyphae break down the keratin protein, thus permitting the penetration of the hyphae deeper into the tissue (SEM, x 7000).

Predisposition

A large number of factors may serve to predispose toward oral candidiasis. Included here, of course, are nutritional, mechanistic, and iatrogenic factors. In addition to local irritation and poorly fitting dentures, immunologic and endocrinologic diseases may play a role (Romagnoli et al. 1997). Chronic and malignant diseases, severe blood dyscrasias, irradiation, as well as age and smoking can act as predisposing factors.

Prevention and Therapy

Prevention and treatment of oral candidiasis is an important task for the dentist. Good oral hygiene as well as denture cleansing for elderly patients are absolutely necessary for the prevention of, for example, denture stomatitis. The use of a 0.12% chlorhexidine digluconate solution leads to a reduction of inflammatory factors. The therapy may include polyenes and azoles; both topical and systemic therapy may be indicated (Greenspan 1994).

162 Erythematous candidiasis
Buccal mucosa exhibits diffuse erythema with no white spots.
Right: Diagram of the histologic picture of erythematous candidiasis in an immunodeficient patient. Note pronounced local epithelial atrophy (*) and moderate infiltration by macrophages and lymphocytes.

1 Blastospores
2 Langerhans cells
3 Macrophages
4 Lymphocytes
5 Vessels

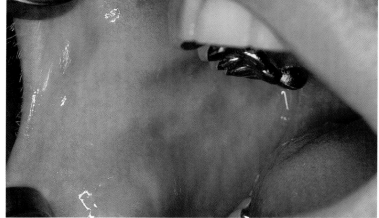
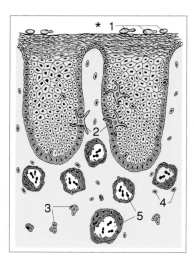

163 Hyperplastic candidiasis
AIDS patient exhibiting hyperplastic, therapy-resistant candidiasis.

Right: The epithelium is hyperplastic and acanthotic. There is infiltration by hyphae on the surface. There is an inflammatory infiltrate in the subepithelial area.

1 Hyphae and pseudohyphae
2 Langerhans cells
3 Macrophages
4 Lymphocytes
5 Vessels

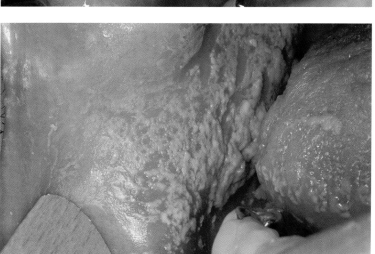
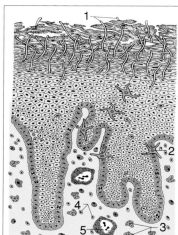

164 Candida in the electron microscope
Transmission electron microscopic picture of a penetrating hypha (arrow), which has dissolved the interepithelial contact and squeezed itself between two epithelial cells (*) into the tissue (TEM, x 25 000). (from Reichart et al. 1995)

Right: Scanning electron microscopic picture of an infiltrating hypha in the middle of a primarily orthokeratinized epithelial cell (SEM, x 6000).

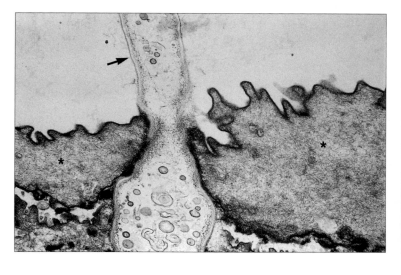
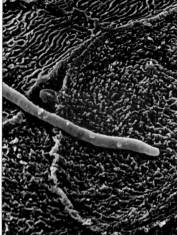

Infections—Viral

Focal Epithelial Hyperplasia

Focal epithelial hyperplasia (FEH; Heck's disease) is caused by the human papilloma virus subtypes 13 and 32; it appears also to have a genetic component. In 1972, Praetorius-Clausen reported that 20% of Greenland Eskimos and almost 34% of Venezuelan Indians were affected with FEH. The disease is asymptomatic and is often detected only fortuitously. The mucosa of the cheeks, lips, and tongue are most often affected. No treatment is indicated (see also pp. 49 and 99).

Herpetic Gingivostomatitis

Primary herpetic gingivostomatitis is caused by HSV-1. Recurrences caused by reactivation of the infection usually appear as labial herpes (see p. 46). In Western countries, herpetic gingivostomatitis usually appears in adolescents or young adults, and is associated primarily with HIV-infected patients. Blisters of 2–3 mm in diameter appear early on, then quickly burst and ulcerate.

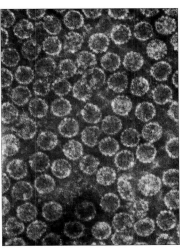
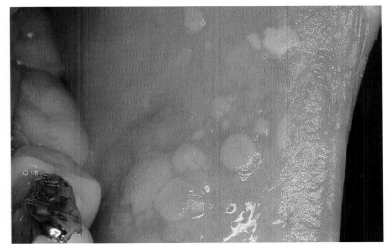

165 Focal epithelial hyperplasia
Note on the cheek mucosa the multiple, flat, pale and well-circumscribed areas of hyperplasia. If the mucosa is stretched using two mouth mirrors, the hyperplastic areas disappear into the level of the mucosal surface.

Left: Human papilloma virus as seen in the electron microscope after negative contrasting (TEM, x 100 000).

Courtesy H.-G. Gelderblom

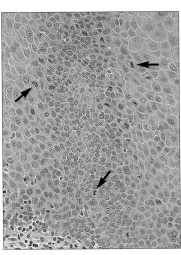
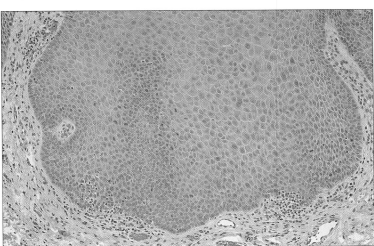

166 Focal epithelial hyperplasia—histology
The histologic picture of FEH demonstrates epithelial hyperplasia with mild parakeratosis and cells with pyknotic nuclei. The rete pegs are broad, providing the term "elephant foot–like" (H & E, x 100).

Left: Within the epithelium, note the mitosoid epithelial cells (arrows) that cannot be interpreted as atypical mitoses (H & E, x 200).

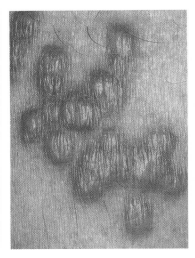
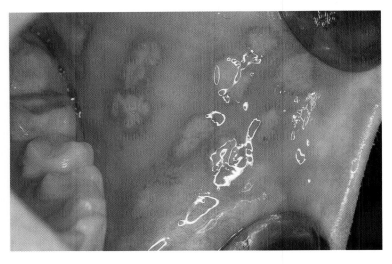

167 Herpetic gingivostomatitis
There are multiple aphthoid ulcerations on the surface of the cheek; the patient had a primary HSV-1 infection. Because the blisters quickly burst, they are seldom actually observed in the mouth. Superinfections can be inhibited by the use of disinfectant mouth rinses.

Left: Skin vesicles of HSV-1 infection in an HIV-infected patient. Aciclovir and similar, newer preparations can be instituted therapeutically.

Mechanical, Physical, Chemical and Other Causes

Cheek Biting

Cheek biting is usually observed in younger individuals and involves traumatization of the buccal mucosa; it is a chronic habit with psychogenic components. Patients repeatedly bite upon the cheek or labial mucosa, and pull the tissue between the teeth. The result is epithelial hyperkeratosis, which can give the appearance of leukoplakia or candidiasis. In the differential diagnosis, it is important to note that the extent of the white lesions in cheek and lip biters is always limited to those areas that can be reached by the teeth.

Betel quid Chewing

At least 20 million South- and Southeast Asians chew a peculiar betel "quid" composed of areca nuts, betel leaves, slaked lime (calcium hydroxide) and tobacco. Intensive chewing leads to lesions that appear red on the oral mucosa and which become black in color on the teeth with time (Reichart and Philipsen 1996, 1998).

168   Cheek biting
The buccal mucosa exhibits leukoedema and small, whitish creases and ridges, which are caused by sucking and chewing on the cheek.

Right: Histologic picture of a cheek bite lesion. Noteworthy is the extreme epithelial hyperplasia with detached portions of epithelium. The incorporation of darkly-staining bacteria (arrowheads) is also characteristic (H & E, x 80).

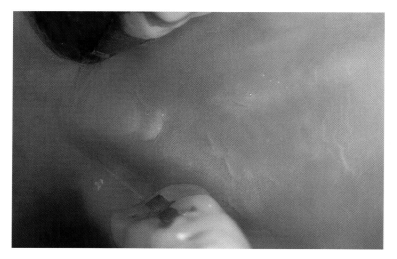
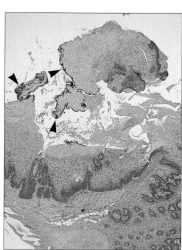

169   Cheek biting/betel quid chewing
The left cheek exhibits the typical picture of a cheek biting patient. The epithelial surface is irregularly coated and "shredded." If such patients are asked about the habit, they usually admit to it.

Right: The buccal mucosa is covered by a red layer that results from betel quid chewing; this layer quickly separates. Polyphenols from the areca nut provide the basic material for this discoloration.

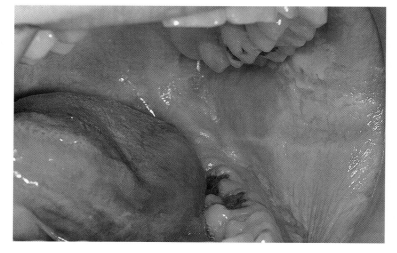
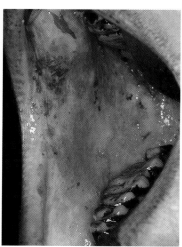

170   Cheek biting/betel quid chewing
The clinical picture of cheek biting can vary. A biopsy is not absolutely indicated. The tissue change is harmless. After insertion of a protection shield, the white lesions usually disappear within 10–14 days.

Right: Histologic picture of the oral mucosa of a betel quid chewer, revealing incorporation of calcium particles (arrows) derived from the betel quid (von Kossa, x 200).

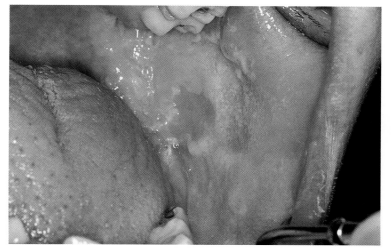
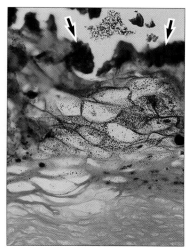

Submucous Fibrosis

Submucous fibrosis (Reichart et al. 1994) is associated with betel quid chewing. It leads to fibrosis of the subepithelial connective tissue, resulting in limitations of mouth opening and tongue mobility. The incidence of carcinoma of the oral cavity is elevated in these patients.

Self mutilation (Münchhausen Syndrome)

Self-inflicted oral injuries are rare (automutilation, Münchhausen syndrome). Self-inflicted injury is attributable to psychiatric disturbances. In extreme cases, patients inject their own urine and feces to attract the attention of the physician. The diagnosis is difficult because such patients adapt a deliberately misleading persona (Lamey et al. 1994).

Chemical Burns

Chemical burns in the oral cavity result from topical application of irritating substances, especially analgesic tablets. Such topical application in the oral cavity leads to desquamation of the epithelium and possible ulcer formation.

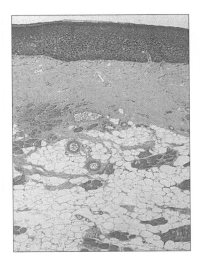
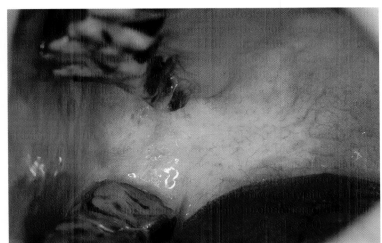
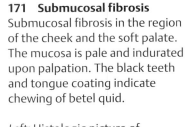

171   Submucosal fibrosis
Submucosal fibrosis in the region of the cheek and the soft palate. The mucosa is pale and indurated upon palpation. The black teeth and tongue coating indicate chewing of betel quid.

Left: Histologic picture of submucous fibrosis. Beneath the atrophic epithelium there is a homogeneous, eosinophilic band which typifies a fibroelastic alteration of the lamina propria (H & E, x 60).

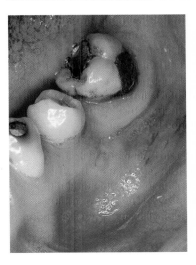
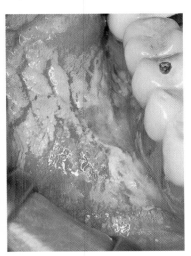

172   Self mutilation/chemical burn
Left: A small ulcer with a white border can be seen near the transition zone between the attached gingiva and the mobile mucosa. This patient constantly poked a pointed pencil into this area.

Right: This chemical burn appeared shortly after application of an aspirin tablet in the buccal vestibulum. Treatment is usually not necessary.

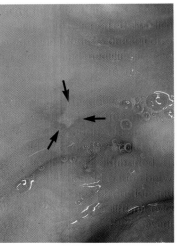
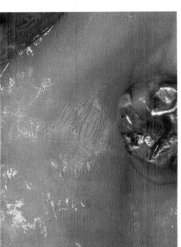

173   Lichenoid reaction
Left: The lichenoid reaction arises due to corrosion products or local allergic reactions and medicaments.

Right: Following extraction of the molar, which had a large, old amalgam restoration, this lichenoid reaction (arrows) subsided. The histologic differentiation between lichenoid reaction and true lichen planus is difficult (McCartan and McCreary 1997, Savage 1997).

Lichenoid Reaction/Gold Allergy

In recent years, the oral lichenoid reaction has re-emerged as a topic of discussion. A wide spectrum of causes is known. The clinical picture is similar to that of true oral lichen (Savage 1997, McCartan and McCreary 1997).

Oral reactions such as allergic stomatitis are rare. Reactions similar to cutaneous allergic eczema do not occur. Patients who, for example, are allergic to nickel seem to tolerate this metal in the oral cavity. The patient may experience a rash, but no oral lesion will occur. (So-called acrylic allergy is usually not a hypersensitivity to acrylic materials, but rather

a Candida infection.)

Particularly gold and antimalarial substances such as methyl dopa can elicit lichenoid reactions. Local reaction of the oral mucosa to gold is extremely rare (Holland-Moritz et al. 1980).

174 Gold allergy—lichenoid reaction
On the gingival papilla mesial to the gold crown on the first molar, whitish lesions are observed (arrows). A true allergy to gold was detected in this patient.

Right: A lichenoid reaction is obvious on the cheek mucosa adjacent to the gold crown. A suspicion of hypersensitivity to gold should only be addressed in exceptional cases.

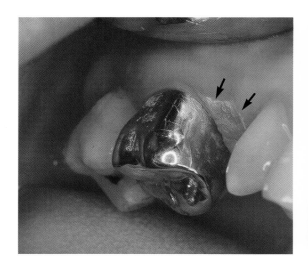
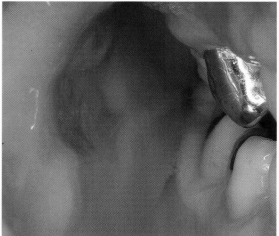

175 Gold allergy/Münchhausen syndrome
After removal of the gold crown (see Fig. 174, right), a reduction of the lichenoid reaction was evident six weeks later (arrows).

Right: These whitish lesions, similar to the white sponge nevus, are actually manifestions of the Münchhausen syndrome in this case of unknown etiology. Corrosive liquids are often involved.

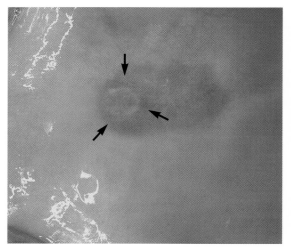
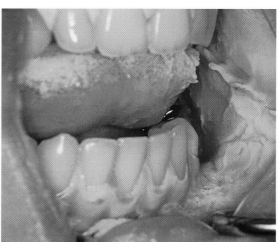

176 Münchhausen syndrome
This young female patient (shown in Fig. 175, right) exhibited not only white, swollen lesions of the buccal mucosa, but also similar lesions on the gingiva, especially on the interdental papillae.

Right: It is often extremely difficult to prove that intraoral lesions have been self-inflicted. Psychotherapeutic support during treatment of the patient is absolutely necessary (Reichart and Köster 1978).

Courtesy B. Hoffmeister

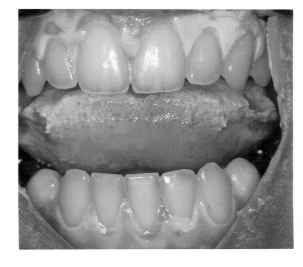
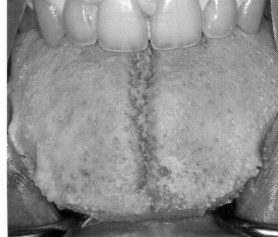

Disturbances of Keratinization

Leukoplakia

The classification of oral leukoplakia was revised in 1994 (Schepman and van der Waal 1995, Axéll et al. 1996, Pindborg et al. 1997). In the book published by the World Health Organization entitled *Histological Typing of Cancer and Precancer of the Oral Mucosa,* leukoplakia is classified as well as defined as *mainly white lesions of the oral mucosa which cannot be characterized as any other lesion.* Some leukoplakias are precancerous (Pindborg et al. 1997).

In diagnosing oral leukoplakia, it is necessary to differentiate between a preliminary and a definitive diagnosis. If the leukoplakia is of long-standing, a histopathologic examination should be performed. Lesions that subside following elimination of causative factors are appropriately named. These are, for example: frictional keratosis, tobacco-associated lesions, or candidiasis. In addition, leukoplakias are differentiated into homogeneous and non-homogeneous forms. (See also pp. 52, 100, 117, 137, 154).

Homogeneous leukoplakia

- Flat, corrugated
- Fissured
- Pumice-like

Non-homogenous leukoplakia

- Verrucous
- Nodular
- Ulcerated
- Erythroleukoplakia

- Frictional keratosis
- Glass blower lesion
- Cheek biting
- Leukoedema
- Chemical burn
- White sponge nevus
- Lichen planus
- Hairy leukoplakia
- Pseudomembranous candidiasis

177 Leukoplakia

Clinical classification/differential diagnosis
Left: Ninety percent of all oral leukoplakias are of the homogeneous type. They may occur in all regions of the oral cavity (Pindborg et al. 1997).

Right: Important differential diagnoses of oral leukoplakia.

Country	N	Prevalence (%)	Author(s)
India	7 286	4.2	Wahi et al. (1970)
India	101 761	0.7	Mehta et al. (1972)
India	57 518	11.7	Smith et al. (1975)
India	5 449	1.6	Bhonsle et al. (1976)
Sweden	20 333	3.6	Axéll (1976)
Germany	4 000	2.2	Wilsch et al. (1978)
Burma	6 000	1.7	Lay et al. (1982)
United States	23 616	2.9	Bouqout and Gorlin (1986)
USSR (former)	1 569	8.0	Zaridze et al. (1986)
Thailand	1 866	1.1	Reichart et al. (1987)
Netherlands	1 000	1.4	Hogewind and van der Waal (1988)
Hungary	7 820	1.3	Bánóczy and Rigo (1991)
Germany	1 000	0.9	Reichart and Kohn (1996)

178 Epidemiology
But for a few exceptions, most clinical studies from numerous countries provide prevalence rates but not incidence rates for oral leukoplakia.

Country	n	Commissure	Cheek	Lip	Tongue	Hard Palate	Floor of the Mouth	Gingiva/ Alveolar Process	Author(s)
Denmark	560	24.4	32.3	8.9	7.3	3.8	6.5	15.1	Roed-Petersen and Renstrup (1969)
India	161*	52.2	81.1	0.3	0.3**	3.2***	****	15.1	Mehta et al. (1972)
United States	3256	****	21.9	10.3**	6.8	10.7***	8.6	41.8	Waldron and Shafer (1975)
Hungary	670	37.5	25.3	6.8**	8.2	8.5	5.7	6.7	Bánóczy (1977)
Germany	200	****	23	16**	19	17	6	19	Maerker and Burkhardt (1978)
United States	682	****	23.6	1.5	9.1	4.3	6.2	23.7	Bouquot and Gorlin (1986)
Sweden	1607*	89.3	38.6	1.7	1.1	0.5	0.8	2.7	Axéll (1987)
Germany	1362	****	60.6	*****	15.3	7.6	2.4	14.1	Schell and Schönberger (1987)

179 Localization
This table presents a selected list of publications dealing with the localization of leukoplakia (Hogewind 1990). The values are presented as percentages.

    * Several possible localizations

    ** No differentiation between the vermilion border and the labial mucosa

    *** No differentiation between hard and soft palate

    **** Not classified separately

    ***** Not included in this survey

Diagnosis of Leukoplakia

The diagnosis of oral leukoplakia is based upon inspection, palpation, the medical history (especially the history of tobacco and alcohol use) as well as the biopsy. If there is a suspicion that the leukoplakia has become infected with *Candida albicans*, a cytologic smear should be taken to demonstrate Candida hyphae.

In recent years, there has been increasing discussion of the use of mouth rinsing with toluidine blue for the detection of oral cancer and precancerous lesions (Warnakulasuriya and Johnson 1996). While the specificity and sensitivity of this

method for detecting oral carcinoma are high, the results for oral leukoplakias with epithelial dysplasia are less favorable. The false-negative rate of 20.5% would appear to be excessively high. Nevertheless, the toluidine blue technique can be applied for screening in high risk patients.

A representative biopsy with inclusion of healthy tissue is a *conditio sine qua non*. It must be emphasized that harmless-appearing homogeneous leukoplakias can transform into cancer. About 3–6% of all oral leukoplakias transform.

180 Leukoplakia
Left: The buccal mucosa and the edentulous alveolar ridge exhibit white, folded and patchy lesions that are not easily wiped away and which are relatively well demarcated. This patient did not wear a partial denture, so friction keratosis was not included in the differential diagnosis.

Right: Similar lesion with clear demarcation and a "cobble-stone" appearance. This is characteristic of tobacco use.

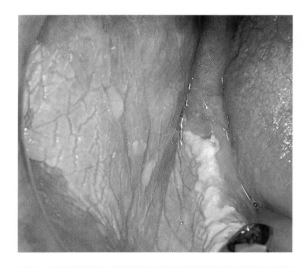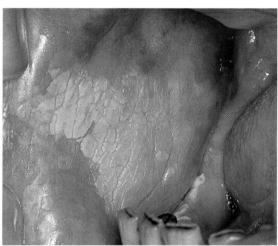

181 Leukoplakia
Left: This retroangularly located leukoplakia occurred bilaterally. This form of leukoplakia is frequently superinfected by Candida, a condition referred to as candida-leukoplakia or hyperplastic candidiasis.

Right: Homogeneous, sharply demarcated leukoplakia with a surrounding leukoedema. If tobacco use is discontinued, homogeneous leukoplakia may completely disappear. This takes up to one year.

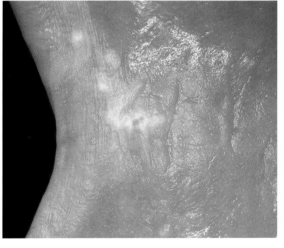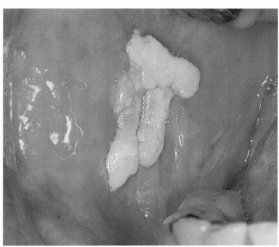

182 Non-homogeneous Leukoplakia
Left: Non-homogeneous leukoplakia is characterized by ulceration (arrow), a nodular type (arrowhead), and the pumice-like form (empty arrowhead).

Right: Non-homogeneous, nodular leukoplakia of the left corner of the mouth. This form of leukoplakia presents the danger of malignant transformation. This patient developed multifocal carcinomas of the oral cavity.

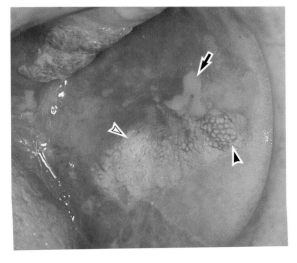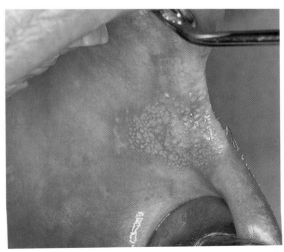

Erythroleukoplakia, Erythroplakia, and Proliferative Verrucous Leukoplakia

Erythroleukoplakia is characterized by red and white areas. Red areas exist due to epithelial atrophy or through secondary infection with *Candida albicans*. Following topical antimycotic treatment, a non-homogeneous erythroleukoplakia may become a homogeneous leukoplakia.

Erythroplakia is defined as a red spot which does not fit with the clinical and histopathological characteristics of any other defined lesion (Pindborg et al. 1997). The differential diagnosis should include erythematous candidiasis, atroph-

ic lichen planus, and other forms of mucositis, such as blister-forming diseases.

Proliferative verrucous leukoplakia was first described by Hansen et al. (1985). More recent studies (Zakrzewska et al. 1996) demonstrated that within a period of 7.7 years, 70.3% of 54 patients developed an oral carcinoma (Silverman and Gorsky 1997).

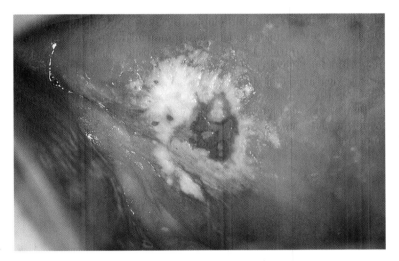

183 Erythroleukoplakia
The non-homogeneous leukoplakia expresses itself in the form of white and red lesions. The red area is partially ulcerated. This type of erythroleukoplakia often exhibits severe epithelial atypia or dysplasia early on, and sometimes even a carcinoma in situ.

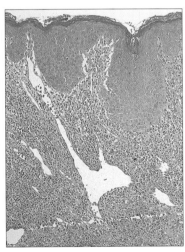

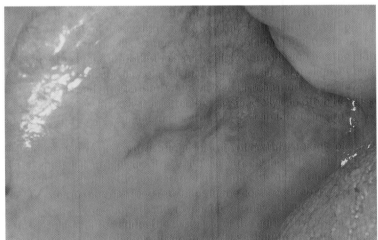

184 Erythroplakia
The diffuse, red spot on the cheek mucosa is erythroplakia. This lesion has the highest probability of malignant transformation, and when viewed histologically can often be classified as a carcinoma in situ.

Left: Histologic picture of erythroplakia. The epithelial atrophy and the appearance of droplet-shaped rete pegs in the connective tissue are characteristic signs. The dysplasia of the epithelium is pronounced (H & E, x 80).

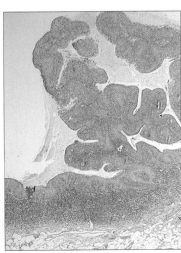

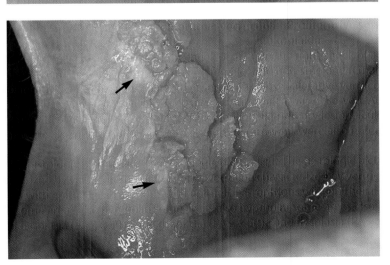

185 Proliferative verrucous leukoplakia
On the right cheek of a 73-year-old non-smoking female, a typical proliferative verrucous leukoplakia was observed. Anterior to the primary lesion, leukoplakic regions were also noted (arrows).

Left: The histologic picture is characterized by verrucous proliferations with epithelial atrophy, and in some areas also hyperplasia and dysplasia (PAS, x 50).

Leukoplakia—Histology

The term leukoplakia is a purely clinical diagnosis and contains no implication with regard to histological findings. A histologic report should always address the question of epithelial dysplasia and its degree of severity.

Most *homogeneous* leukoplakias are hyperorthokeratotic or parakeratotic and exhibit acanthosis without epithelial dysplasia. Signs of inflammation may be present in the lamina propria. The mitotic activity in hyperparakeratosis is higher than that in hyperorthokeratosis. It is characteristic that hyperparakeratotic lesions exhibit a much thicker epithe-

lium than hyperorthokeratotic lesions.

Non-homogeneous leukoplakias are frequently associated with epithelial dysplasia and may already exhibit a *carcinoma in situ* or a squamous cell carcinoma. The same holds true for erythroleukoplakias and erythroplakias.

Leukoplakia—histology

186 Hyperorthokeratosis
This histologic picture is an enlargement of the central box of Fig. 187. The surface exhibits a massive hyperorthokeratosis above the spinous cell layer. In some areas, the epithelium is pushed up into a form that is described as a "chevron type of keratinization" (arrow) (H & E, x150).

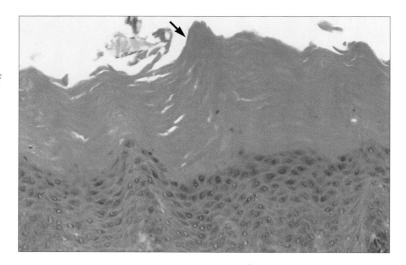

187 Histologic overview
In this low power view, it is easy to recognize the hyperorthokeratosis with acanthosis and hyperplasia of the epithelium. The rete pegs are well-formed and display a nearly normal configuration. An inflammatory cell reaction is evident in the subepithelial region (H & E, x 80).

Right: Higher magnification from Fig. 187 (right box). The basal cells appear normal and there are no signs of dysplasia (H & E, x 150).

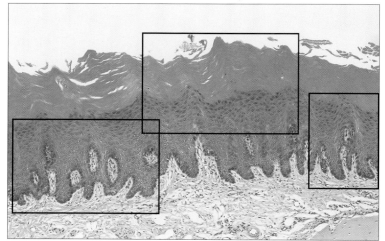
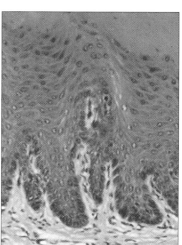

188 Basal cell area of the epithelium
This picture is an enlargement from the left basal area of Fig. 187. In the basal cell region of the epithelium, one notes regular layering and no mitotic activity. There is also no basal cell hyperplasia or any other signs of epithelial atypia (H & E, x 150).

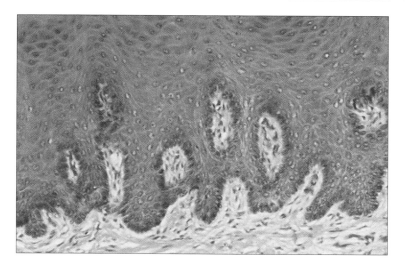

Squamous epithelial dysplasia is characterized as a precancerous lesion by cellular atypia and loss of the normal epithelial maturation and stratification. The epithelial dysplasia encompasses a broad range of changes (Fig. 191). The more pronounced and more frequent these lesions, the greater the severity of the dysplasia.

When considering the severity of dysplasia, there is relative subjectivity with regard to the recognition and interpretation of the significance of minor or more pronounced changes (Abbey et al. 1998). Cellular atypia may also occur during the course of inflammatory reactions. Nevertheless, any degree of epithelial dysplasia, even a mild degree, may indicate an elevated risk of malignant transformation.

Severe epithelial dysplasia can transform into a *carcinoma in situ*. This is characterized by the fact that the entire epithelial layer is involved and the histologic picture corresponds to squamous epithelial carcinoma. Infiltration through the basement membrane has not yet occurred. (Amagasa et al. 1985).

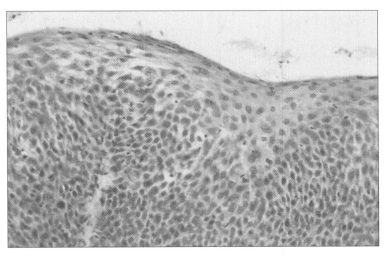

189 Epithelial dysplasia
This picture represents the central framed area from Fig. 190. The surface of the epithelium exhibits parakeratosis and the regular stratification has been lost. The epithelial cells of varying size and varying stain intensity represent signs of a severe epithelial dysplasia
(H & E, x 150).

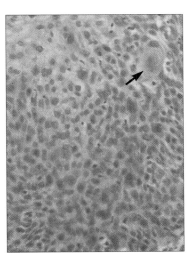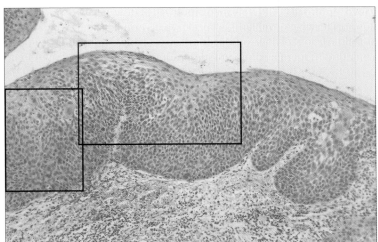

190 Histologic overview
Severely dysplastic epithelium, with loss of stratification. The basement membrane remains intact (H & E, x 80).

Left: Enlargement of the left framed area. The large differences in the sizes of the individual epithelial cells (cellular polymorphism) can be clearly observed. An especially large epithelial cell with nuclear polymorphism is indicated by the arrow (H & E, x 150).

- Loss of polarity of the basal cells
- Basal cell hyperplasia
- Elevated nuclear-cytoplasmic ratio
- Droplet-shaped rete pegs
- Irregular epithelial stratification
- Increased number of mitoses
- Atypical mitotic figures
- Mitoses within the upper epithelial layers
- Cellular and nuclear polymorphism
- Hyperchromatic nuclei
- Enlarged nucleoli
- Loss of intercellular adherence
- Keratinization within the spinous cell layer

191 Criteria for dysplasia
The criteria for dysplasia can occur in varying combinations. The higher the number of individual criteria found in a biopsy, the greater is the severity of the dysplasia.

Transformation of Oral Leukoplakia

The potential for malignant transformation of oral leuko-plakias has been variously reported in numerous publications. There are many reasons for these disparities, such as different definitions and classifications of the clinical and histologic characteristics of leukoplakia. The dentist must carefully document and evaluate all clinical risk factors that might indicate transformation to malignancy.

In recent years, a large number of possible *risk markers* for transformation even to squamous cell carcinoma have been investigated. Many studies focussed especially on the p53-

tumor suppressor gene (Piffkó et al. 1995, Reithdorf et al. 1997, Gopalakrishnan et al. 1997). In addition to integrin receptors (Kosmehl et al. 1995), the proliferating cell nuclear antigen (PCNA) has received particular attention (Schliephake et al. 1992, Tsuji et al. 1995). A comprehensive discussion of the various risk markers, especially at the cellular and molecular level, can be found in the reviews by Johnson et al. (1993, 1996).

Leukoplakia—histology

192   Hyperorthokeratosis
The stratum spinosum and the stratum granulosum are unrecognizable and the architecture of the epithelium is disturbed. The basal cell layer is in some sections doubled or tripled. A moderate inflammatory cell infiltrate is observed in the subepithelial region (H & E, x 80).
Right: Parameters and clinical symptoms of an enhanced risk of malignant transformation of leukoplakia.

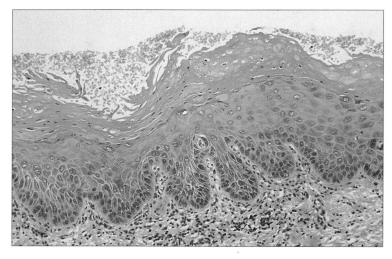

- Symptoms, complaints
- Absence of causative factors
- Long-term persistence of the leukoplakia
- Localization on the floor of the mouth and tongue
- Non-homogeneous leukoplakia
- Presence of epithelial dysplasia
- Medical history of previous oral carcinoma
- Females more frequently affected than males

193   Parakeratosis with pronounced focal epithelial dysplasia
The normal epithelial layering has been lost. The subepithelial infiltrate is pronounced. Lymphocytes can also be observed intraepithelially (H & E, x 80).

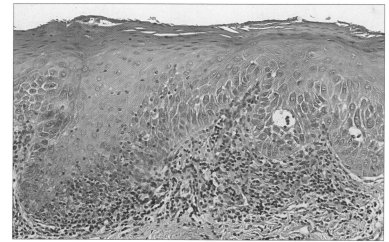

194   Pronounced epithelial atrophy with severe dysplasia
This histologic picture exhibits parakeratosis with loss of normal epithelial stratification. In some regions, enlarged atypical epithelial cells (arrowhead) are observed in the upper epithelial layers. The droplet-shaped epithelial rete ridges exhibit the "dropping-off" phenomena without disruption of the basement membrane (arrows) (H & E, x 80).

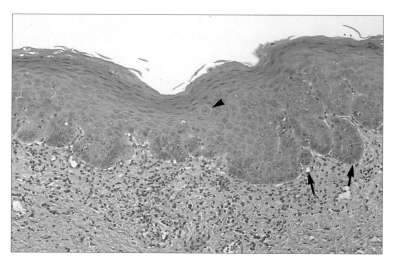

Malignant Tumors

Therapy and Prevention of Oral Leukoplakia

A histologic diagnosis of a *carcinoma in situ* demands immediate surgical treatment, including radical excision. The spectrum of therapy for leukoplakia includes the classical surgical excision (Vedtofte et al. 1987), but recurrence can be expected in 35% of cases. In recent years, CO_2 laser therapy has been increasingly recommended, with a recurrence rate of between 4 and 22% being observed (Hogewind 1990).

Most recently, there have been reports concerning so-called chemoprevention (Sankaranarayanan et al. 1997). For such treatment, retinoids, vitamin A, and above all beta carotene have been used (Kaugars et al. 1996). Most important, however, is that tobacco use must cease (Gupta et al. 1995). Future efforts should be targeted toward primary and secondary prevention of oral leukoplakias and the dentist will play an important role in this effort. (For further information concerning oral leukoplakia, see pp. 54, 79, 108, 120, 170, 198).

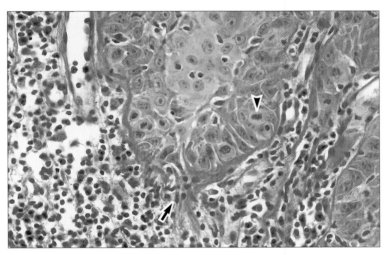

195 Carcinoma in situ
Histologic picture of carcinoma in situ with initial destruction of the basement membrane. The arrow indicates the disruption of the irregular basement membrane, which is partially doubled and in some cases tripled in thickness. The epithelium is dysplastic to a high degree and exhibits multiple mitoses (arrowhead) (PAS, x 80).

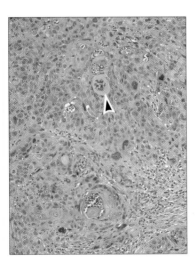
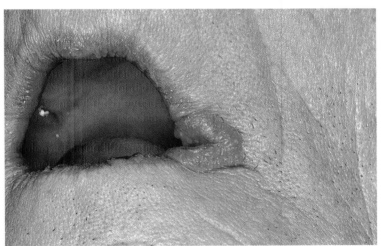

196 Carcinoma of the buccal mucosa
Note the tissue mass at the corner of the mouth. This is not labial carcinoma, but a carcinoma of the cheek which has extended beyond the corner of the mouth (see Fig. 197).

Left: Histology of an undifferentiated squamous epithelial carcinoma with cellular polymorphism. Note the atypical tripolar mitotic figure (arrow head) (H & E, x 80).

197 Carcinoma of the buccal mucosa
This clinical view of the left cheek of the patient in Fig. 196 reveals an extensive squamous cell carcinoma of the buccal mucosa with central ulceration. The typical characteristics of carcinoma are present: central ulceration and an indurated periphery. Due to secondary infection, this squamous cell carcinoma was extraordinarily painful. The size of the tumor required an extensive resection with subsequent plastic surgical reconstruction.

Dermatological Manifestations

Lichen Planus

The term "lichen" derives from botany and refers to one of an order of flowerless plants (moss). It is a dermatological disease with a broad spectrum of clinical manifestations (Jungell 1991). The oral lesions are reticular, papular, bullous, plaque-like, atrophic, erosive and/or ulcerating.

Most patients who experience this disorder are in middle age, and 60% are female. Only 17% experience spontaneous remission. The atrophic and erosive forms are seen most often in elderly patients. The plaque-type of lichen planus is observed primarily in smokers and may be difficult to differentiate from homogenous leukoplakia.

Lichen planus involves not only the oral cavity, but also the skin; 0.5–2.5% of caucasians are affected (Eversole 1995). Between 5 and 45% of patients with oral lesions also exhibit skin involvement.

198 Lichen
A yellow-orange lichen grows upon this cut section of a log in the Swiss Alps. The color spectrum ranges from gray through yellow to varying shades of green. The term "lichen" is also used in the nomenclature of dermatologic disease.

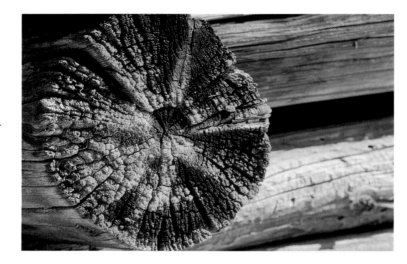

199 Lichen planus—skin
Lichen planus of the skin occurs primarily on the flexor aspects of the extremities. The characteristic red skin lesions appear especially on the lower arm and the wrist. Oral lesions do not necessarily accompany skin involvement.

Right: Schematic diagram of the distribution and main areas of localization of dermal lichen.

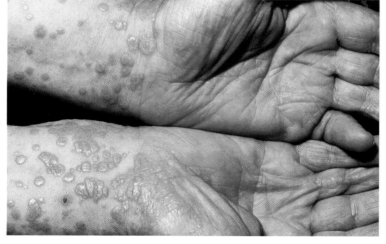
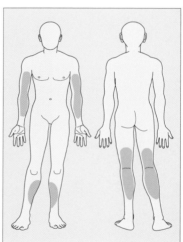

200 Lichen planus of the vermilion border
In the region of the vermilion border, especially of the lower lip, one observes the typical fine, whitish stripes known as Wickham's striae. These are an indication of intraoral involvement. Involvement of the lips is relatively infrequent.

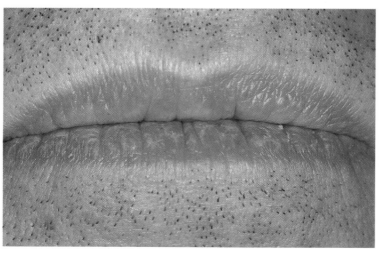

The *reticular type* of lichen planus is the most common; it is characterized by Wickham's striae. In most cases the buccal mucosa is affected, followed by the tongue, lips and palate. The floor of the mouth is virtually never involved. The lesions are often symmetrical (Voûte 1994).

The *etiology* remains unclear even today. The infiltrate that derives primarily from T-lymphocytes indicates a cell-mediated, immunological disturbance of the epithelium. Various types of antigens lead to a cascade of molecular biological processes in the form of cytokine expression, chemotactic factors, and up-regulation of adhesion molecules on the keratinocyte membranes and extracellular matrix protein

on the basement membranes. These adhesive molecules serve as ligands for leukocytic integrins (Eversole 1995).

The traditional belief that lichen planus is in some way associated with emotional stress has not been supported by the scientific data (McCartan 1995).

(Additional information about lichen planus can be found on pp. 19, 101, 137, 156.)

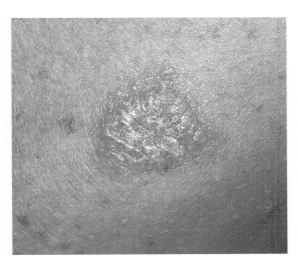 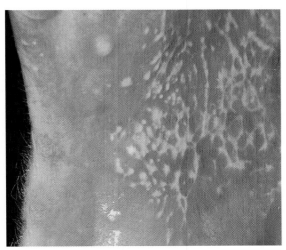

201   Lichen planus
Left: Lichen planus of the skin with a red background and white, scaling epithelium on the surface. The differential diagnosis should include psoriasis.

Right: The buccal mucosa exhibits the classic pattern of papular and reticular lichen. Oral lichen planus may remain unchanged for decades. In many cases, the clinical manifestation changes with the patient's advancing age.

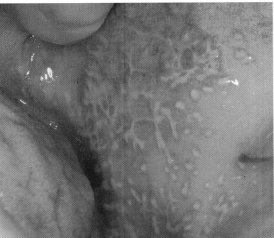 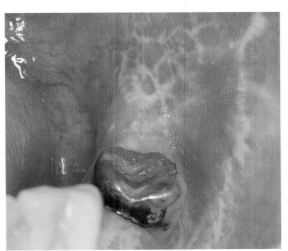

202   Oral lichen planus
Left: Papular and reticular lichen of the left cheek mucosa.

Right: Reticular lichen with its classical localization and classical clinical appearance. The old, extensive amalgam restoration aids in the differential diagnosis between lichen planus and lichenoid reaction.

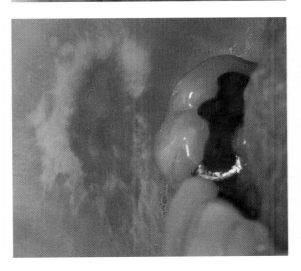 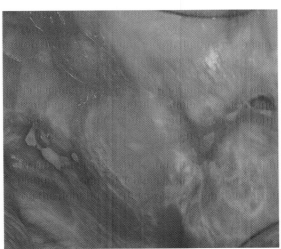

203   Oral lichen planus, erosive type
Left: In the vestibulum and on the buccal mucosa one can observe an ulceration and erosion, surrounded by a white epithelial reaction. Erosions and ulcerations lead to severe discomfort for the patient.

Right: Reticular atrophic and erosive expressions of lichen planus on the right buccal mucosa.

In addition to pathological conditions such as Plummer–Vinson syndrome, oral submucous fibrosis, syphilis, discoid lupus erythematosus, xeroderma pigmentosum and epidermolysis bullosa, lichen planus must be viewed as a *precancerous condition*. It is generally accepted that lichen planus, especially the erosive and ulcerative forms, undergo malignant transformation in 0.5–2% of cases in a time span of five to seven years. In one study from Germany, the transformation rate was 1.8% (Herrmann 1992).

The *treatment* of lichen planus is purely symptomatic. To date, steroids, retinoids, and cyclosporine are the medications that have been most comprehensively studied. Any

superinfection with *Candida albicans* must be treated using antimycotics.

Patients must be regularly checked for any change of the clinical picture, at least every six months. The classical *histologic characteristics* are saw-tooth profile of the rete pegs, degeneration of the basal cell layer (also know as basal cell liquefaction) and bands of lymphohistiocytic infiltrate.

Lichen planus—histology

204   Reticular type of oral lichen
This low-power histologic view depicts a Wickham's stria cut in cross section (arrow). There is a pronounced hyperplasia of the epithelium with hyperorthokeratosis and a dense subepithelial lymphocytic infiltrate (H & E, x 60).

Right: The subepithelial region contains a dense infiltrate of T-lymphocytes, primarily cytotoxic CD8 cells (H & E, x 200).

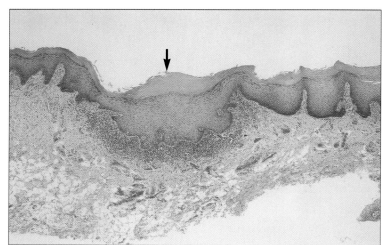
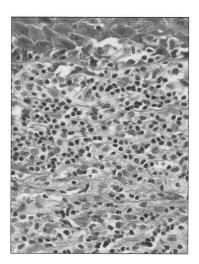

205   Wickham's striae
Histologic longitudinal section through a Wickham's stria (H & E, x 60).

Right: In a biopsy, reticular striae may be viewed as cross sections (Fig. 204) or longitudinally cut sections (Fig. 205) in the histologic picture.

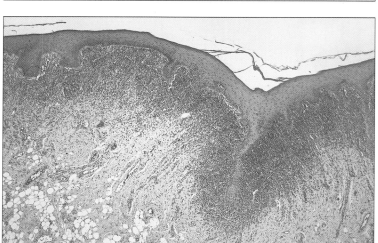
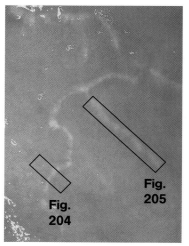

Fig. 204

Fig. 205

206   Bullous type lichen
The bullous type of lichen planus is relatively rare. Histologically one notes a subepithelial separation at the basement membrane resulting in bulla formation. The epithelium exhibits parakeratosis as well as massive subepithelial and sub-bullous T-cell infiltrates (H & E, x 100).

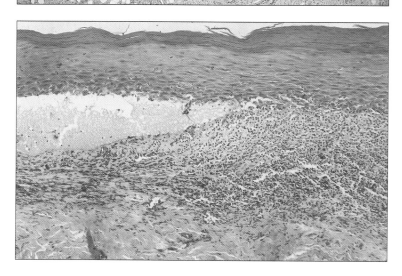

Lupus Erythematosus

Lupus erythematosus is a mesenchymal autoimmune disease that occurs in two primary forms: the systemic form (Jonsson 1983) and the discoid form. Genetic, hormonal and exogenous factors, such as deletion of T-cell receptors, estrogens, UV-light, and various medicaments are acknowledged pathogenic elements. Ultimately, however, the etiology involves disturbances in regulation of cellular and humoral immunity, with increased B-cell hyperreactivity elicited by antibody formation against host tissue structures (autoantigens). Antinuclear antibodies can be detected in over 95% of patients, especially those suffering from systemic lupus erythematosus.

Oral manifestations occur in 50% of cases of systemic lupus erythematosus, and in 15–20% of discoid lupus cases (Hornstein 1996). The typical oral lesions are white, frequently with striations in connection with ulcerated or eroded areas of mucosa. Lesions occur on the cheeks, as well as on the palate (Meyer et al. 1997).

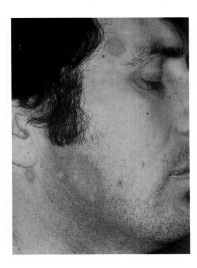
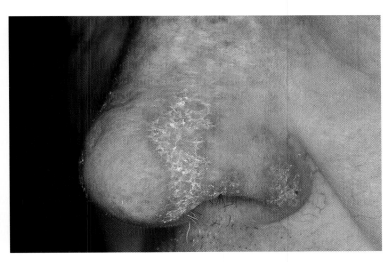

Lupus erythematosus

207   Lesions on the facial skin
The discoid or dermal lupus erythematosus exhibits discoid, reddish areas of inflammation with whitish desquamation. On the facial skin, the "butterfly erythema" is an acknowledged symptom.

Left: Note the multiple discoid lesions in the region of the forehead and the mandible. The lips exhibit a scaling cheilitis.

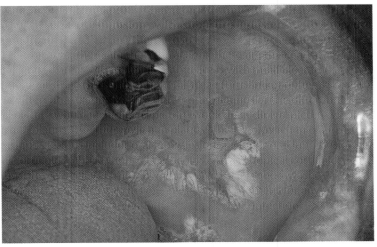

208   Characteristic mucosal lesions with subacute lupus erythematosus
In the central area, there are small ulcerated areas with radiating peripheral striae (brush-like). For the differential diagnosis, this clinical picture would include erosive lichen planus. The therapy for oral lupus lesions includes topical corticoids, antiseptic mouthwashes as well as treatment for any secondary Candida infection.

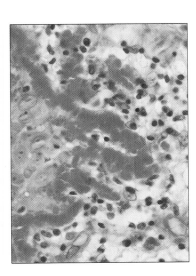
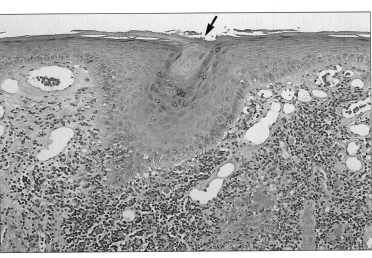

209   Histology
The epithelium exhibits atrophy alternating with areas of acanthosis. The diagnostic signs are the keratin plugs (arrow) in the epithelial surface. A massive infiltrate is obvious in the subepithelial region (H & E, x 100).

Left: PAS-positive material beneath the basement membrane, which corresponds to immunoglobulins and C3-complement (PAS, x200).

Benign Tumors

"Fibroma" and Adenoma

The so-called *fibroma* of the buccal mucosa is not a true tumor in the sense of neoplasia, but rather is a non-neoplastic connective tissue hyperplasia that occurs as a result of chronic trauma. For this reason, such lesions are often observed near the occlusal/incisal plane. Most of the tissue proliferations localized to this area can be classified as hyperplasia, although tumors of neurogenic or myogenic origin can also occur on the buccal mucosa. The treatment consists of simple excision, and histopathologic evaluation is always required. Recurrence is seldom. Oral benign salivary gland tumors *(adenoma)* consist of several types, such as cystadenolymphoma (70%) and salivary duct adenoma (20%). Rarer forms also exist, such as oncocytoma, myoepithelioma, or basal cell adenoma. The small mucous glands of the buccal mucosa are only seldom affected (Seifert 1997).

210 "Fibroma"
Opposite the premolars one can observe a new growth of redundant tissue covered by smooth oral mucosa. Upon palpation, the lesion exhibited a certain firmness. This lesion was without symptoms.
Right: Large connective tissue hyperplasia of the left buccal mucosa. Trauma has elicited a whitish alteration (frictional keratosis) and fissuring of the epithelial surface. Surgical excision is normally without difficulties even with lesions of this size.

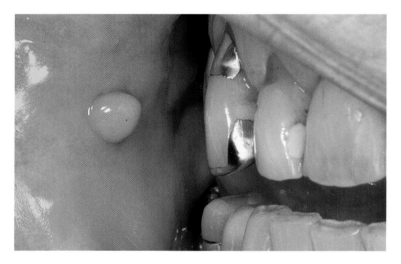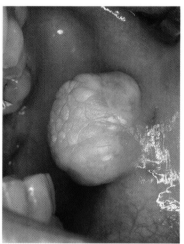

211 "Fibroma"
On the right buccal mucosa one can observe an indurated tissue hyperplasia at the level of the occlusal plane.

Right: Low-power histologic view of a fibroma from the buccal mucosa. The epithelium exhibits hyperplasia as well as hyperorthokeratosis. The connective tissue component is characterized by minimal cellularity (H & E, x 30).

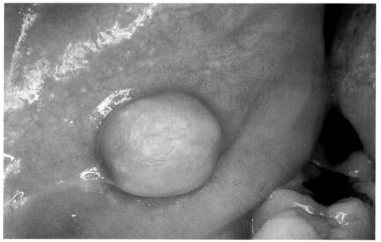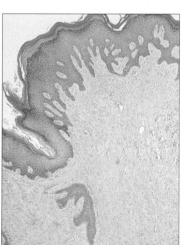

212 Adenoma
This redundant tissue was detected on the left buccal mucosa; clinically it was not possible to distinguish it from a fibroma. Upon palpation, it was mildly indurated. The lesion was asymptomatic.

Right: The biopsy exhibits an adenoma of the trabecular type. Note the reticular arrangement of cuboidal epithelial cells (H & E, x 80).

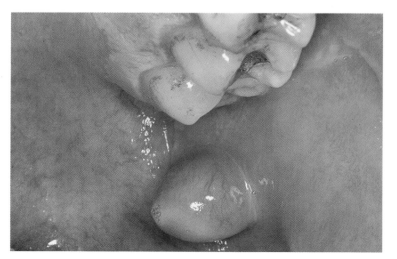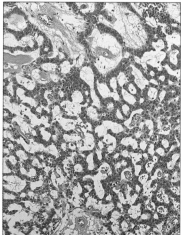

Hemangioma

Congenital vascular nevi of the skin may be isolated or may appear as a manifestation of the Sturge–Weber syndrome. The latter consists of an angiomatosis following the distribution of the trigeminal nerve and the leptomeninges of the ipsilateral side, which is associated with epilepsy, hemiparesis, and mental retardation. A less pronounced form consists of a vascular nevus of the face and the subjacent oral tissues, including the gingiva.

This form of the lesion usually exhibits a sharp demarcation ventrally and toward the midline. These nevi are develop-

mentally caused anomalies of the vasculature and consist of grossly widened vessels. A genetic component also plays an etiologic role.

Acquired hemangiomas appear later in life and are localized vascular ectases. Both clinically and histologically, there are no differences between congenital and acquired hemangiomas.

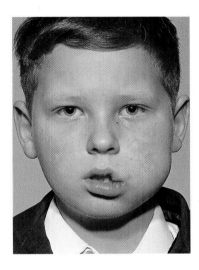
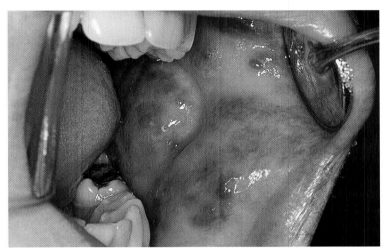
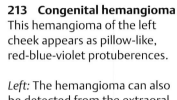

213 Congenital hemangioma
This hemangioma of the left cheek appears as pillow-like, red-blue-violet protuberences.

Left: The hemangioma can also be detected from the extraoral view. The left upper and lower lips appear also to be involved. Hemangioma of this size must be examined by angiography in order to localize the vascular source. Embolization and subsequent surgical intervention can improve the esthetics.

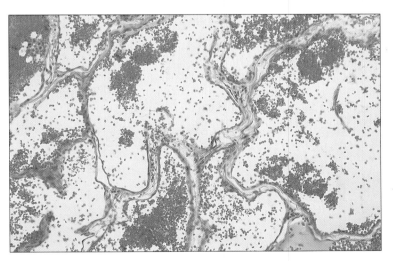

214 Congenital cavernous hemangioma
The histologic section reveals a cavernous hemangioma with large, dilated, blood-filled cavities lined with endothelium. Cavernous hemangiomas are often poorly demarcated (H & E, x 80).

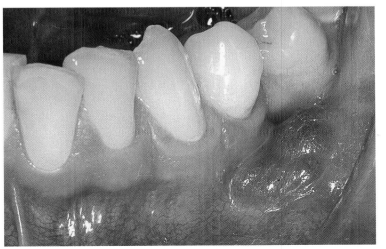

215 Acquired hemangioma
In the region of the labial vestibule one can see a circumscribed cavernous hemangioma. The medical history of this 35-year-old female revealed that this lesion had developed within a six-month period. A biopsy is not indicated to establish the diagnosis.

Other Lesions

Crohn's Disease, Reiter's Disease, and "Mucosal Peeling"

Crohn's disease, or regional enteritis, is a chronic recurring inflammatory disorder, part of which involves oral granulomatosis. It exhibits characteristic oral manifestations, primarily in the area of the buccal vestibule.

Reiter's disease encompasses urethritis, arthritis and conjunctivitis. The cause is unknown; many patients have a medical history of infectious enteritis involving Gram-nega-

tive bacteria. With these facts in mind, Reiter's disease would appear to be a post-infectious reaction with association to the HLA-B-27. Males aged 20 to 40 years are most often affected. In 20% of cases, oral manifestations will be observed.

"Mucosal peeling" is a superficial epitheliolysis which is caused by several toothpastes that contain high amounts of lauryl sulfate or pyrophosphates (Gagari and Kabani 1995, Rubright et al. 1978, Kowitz et al. 1973).

216 Crohn's disease
Left: In the left mandibular buccal sulcus, one observes multiple ulcerations and tissue proliferations (see p. 124).

Right: Histologic picture of Crohn's disease. Within the granuloma there are two large multinucleated giant cells (arrows). The caseous necrosis that is typical for tuberculosis is not observed and there is no evidence of mycobacteria (H & E, x 120).

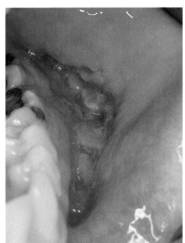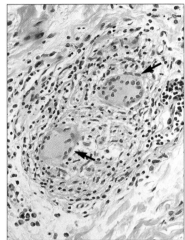

217 Reiter's disease
The buccal mucosa exhibits a whitish-red lesion with several white peripheral lines and areas. Oral manifestations can be herpetiform or plaque-like and have also been described as circinate stomatitis. The lesions may be found on the palate as well as on the mucosa of the cheeks and lips. The lesions are usually relatively sharply demarcated and arcuate in form and may also exhibit areas of erosion.

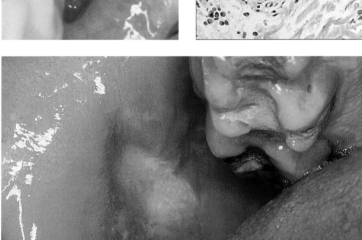

218 "Mucosal peeling"
Left: Areas of epithelium can be easily lifted from the buccal mucosa. No erosions are noted. This epitheliolysis is "toxic" in nature and is not an allergic reaction.

Right: The forceps holds a section of the removed epithelium. The problem regresses spontaneously if the patient ceases to use the toothpaste responsible for the reaction.

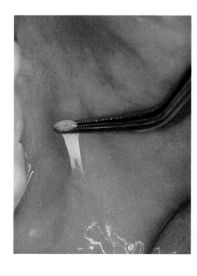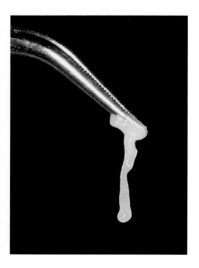

Mucositis Caused by Radiation and Cytostatic Therapy

Radiation mucositis is characterized primarily by erythema and edema, and later by pseudomembranous erosions. After healing, the mucosa becomes fibrotic and atrophic. Because radiotherapy often causes xerostomia, there is often secondary infection with *Candida albicans* (Ramirez-Amador et al. 1997).

Oral ulcerations caused by cytostatic medications are associated with erythema, epithelial desquamation, and erosion. Such lesions are particularly frequently observed after the use of methotrexate; the lesions are very painful (Rutkauskas and Davis 1993).

Graft Versus Host Reaction

Graft versus host reaction (GVHR) occurs mainly following bone marrow transplantation. The acute form is characterized by skin and mucosal manifestations, but also by hepatitis and diarrhea (Barrett and Bilous 1984). A chronic form of GVHR can ensue. The oral manifestations appear as lichenoid keratosis or ulcerations (Hiroki et al. 1994).

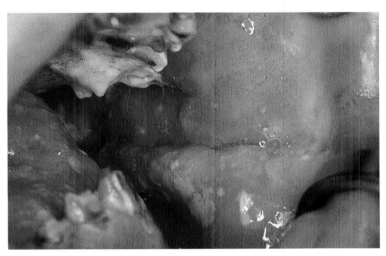

219 Radiation mucositis
The buccal mucosa exhibits edema and erythema with a whitish coating. This indicates a superinfection with *Candida albicans*. The tongue is also affected. The teeth exhibit the typical picture of radiation caries; they are as soft as rubber and serve as an entrance area for the feared osteoradionecrosis. Radiation mucositis can be treated with antimycotics and disinfectant mouth rinses. The most important concern is the prevention of all radiation-elicited side effects.

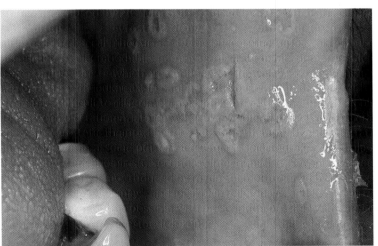

220 Mucositis caused by cytostatic drugs
The surface of the buccal mucosa exhibits numerous ulcerations, which are confluent in some areas. In patients with leukemia, it is sometimes difficult to differentiate between ulcerations caused by the cytostatic therapy and primary leukemia-associated ulcers. Secondary infections can be reduced by means of mouth rinses, and local pain relief may be possible with prescription of anesthetic lozenges.

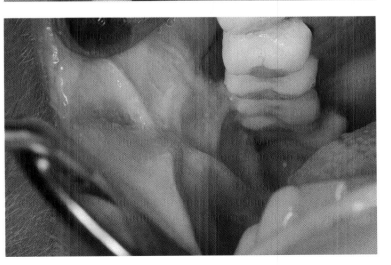

221 Graft versus host reaction
On the right buccal mucosa, this patient exhibits a massive epitheliolysis and apparent swelling of the entire oral mucosa. Other regions of the oral cavity are also involved. Graft versus host reaction is a life-threatening complication which, as with Lyell's syndrome (see pp. 58 and 59), can only be combated by means of massive therapeutic measures using immunosuppressive medications.

Tongue

Definition—Anatomy

The tongue is divided into the dorsum, the base, the lateral borders, the tip, and the ventral surface. The *dorsum* consists of a triangular region distal to the tip; it extends to the terminal sulcus and to the left and right borders of the tongue. The *base* is a rectangular area posterior to the terminal sulcus and between the two anterior tonsillar pillars. The *tip* is a circular area with a radius of 1 cm, whose center is at the tip of the tongue. Each of the lateral borders (left and right) consists of a rectangular area starting 1 cm posterior to the tip of the tongue, extending back to the anterior tonsillar pillar and covering 1 cm of the dorsal and ventral edge of the tongue. The *ventral surface* comprises a triangular area to the tip of the tongue and following the midline to 1 cm posterior to the tip of the tongue and following an imaginary line lying 1 cm from the borders of the tongue. The floor of the mouth is covered by the ventral surface of the tongue (Kramer et al. 1980).

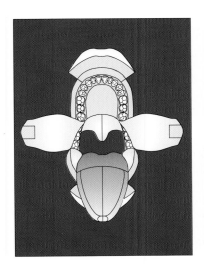

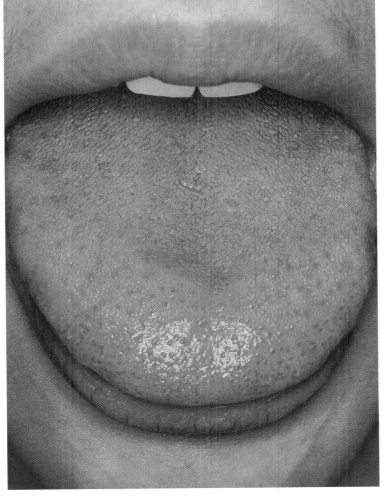

222 The human tongue viewed from a dorsal-anterior aspect
The anterior two-thirds of the tongue including the tip of the tongue are covered by filiform papillae and larger, rounded fungiform papillae. Further posterior, one finds the V-shaped arrangement of the circumvalate papillae. On the posterior margin of the tongue is a small anterior-posterior line of foliate papillae (also known as *folia linguae*).

Left: Schematic diagram outlining the different areas of the dorsum of the tongue.

Anomalies

Lingua Plicata, Hypertrophic Folia Linguae and Tetralogy of Fallot

Lingua plicata ("scrotal tongue") is a developmental anomaly. The prevalence varies between 2 and 16%, but can be much higher in patients with mental retardation. Clinically one observes a broad spectrum of fissure variations; usually there is a pronounced sagittal fissure.

The *enlarged folia linguae*, or hypertrophy of the foliate papillae, usually results from chronic irritation. The foliate papillae consist of lymphatic tissue, which can become hypertrophic. Patients who experience this condition may develop "cancerophobia."

The *tetralogy of Fallot* is a congenital malformation of the heart, which leads to cyanosis that is often obvious in the orofacial region.

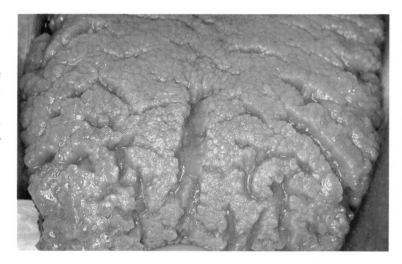
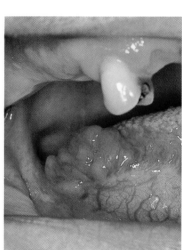

223   Scrotal tongue and hypertrophic folia linguae
Fissured tongue was obvious in this 25-year-old patient with Down's syndrome. The pattern of the fissures is irregular, exhibiting almost a cerebriform character. Residues of food may accumulate in the depths of the fissures, leading to inflammation.

Right: Hypertrophy of the right folia linguae. This tumor-like hypertrophy is, in fact, harmless and must not be confused with a lingual carcinoma.

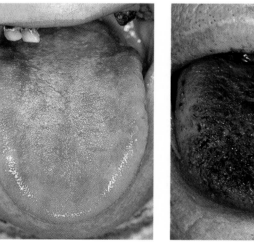
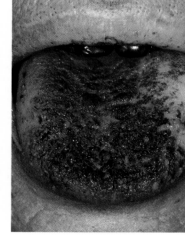

224   Pigmentation
This Caucasian female presented with melanoplakia of the dorsum of the tongue. It was not possible to establish a definitive cause, so this pigmentation was documented as idiopathic.

Right: Exogenous pigmentation in a betel quid chewer. The brown-red discoloration of the tongue derives from the constituents of the betel quid (areca nut, betel leaves, tobacco and slaked lime).

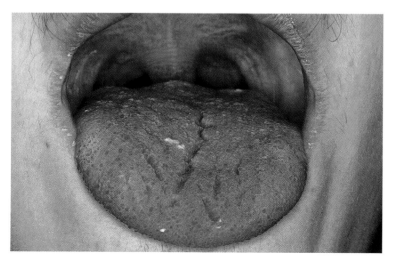
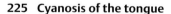

225   Cyanosis of the tongue
The tetralogy of Fallot includes pulmonary stenosis, ventricular septal defect, and an aorta that overrides both the right and left ventricles, as well as hypertrophy of the right ventricle. The cyanosis depicted in this young patient had been present since birth and was especially pronounced on the tongue and oral soft tissues.

Soft Tissue Cysts

Lymphoepithelial Cyst

The lymphoepithelial cyst is an epithelium-lined soft tissue cyst, which contains lymphoid tissue. This lesion is also referred to as "oral tonsil." It develops by proliferation of epithelium that became entrapped developmentally within lymph nodes or lymphoid tissues. Most lymphoepithelial cysts are localized in the floor of the mouth, followed by the tongue as the next most common location. The color of these cysts is generally yellow or yellowish-white. The cyst if often asymptomatic. Its diameter seldom exceeds 1.5 cm.

It is most often diagnosed in patients between the ages of 20 and 40 years (Chaudhry et al. 1984).

If the lymphoepithelial cyst presents on the border of the tongue, the differential diagnosis will include hypertrophic foliate papillae, and the differentiation is sometimes difficult. Carcinoma of the lateral border of the tongue, especially in the dorsal third of the tongue, must also be included in a differential diagnosis. The treatment, should it be necessary, consists of simple local excision.

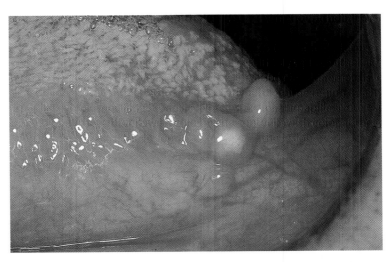

Lymphoepithelial cyst

226 Clinical picture
The lymphoepithelial cyst in this 60-year-old female is localized in the same region as a hypertrophic foliate papilla. Note especially the yellowish color at the center of the lesion.

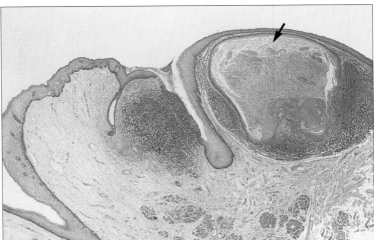

227 Histology
The protruding, mucosa-covered lobules contain aggregates of lymphocytes arranged in a follicular pattern. On the right (arrow) one can see an orthokeratinized epithelial cyst, which is depicted at higher magnification in Fig. 228 (H & E, x 40).

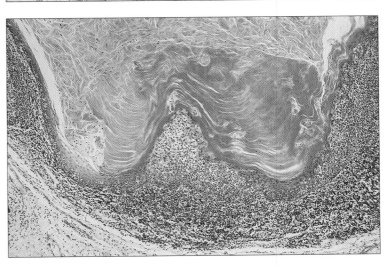

228 Histology
Higher magnification of the orthokeratinized epithelial cyst from Fig. 227. The lumen of the cyst is filled with keratinized material that derives from the epithelial lining. This keratin gives the surface of the lesion a yellow color. Subjacent to the cystic epithelium one observes lymphoid tissue (H & E, x 120).

Other Lesions

Geographic Tongue

Geographic tongue is also referred to as *exfoliatio areata linguae* or migrating glossitis. It is common and occurs in all age groups (Axéll 1976). The lesion is characterized by desquamation of filiform papillae in several irregularly formed but clearly demarcated areas. The desquamated regions are red, with an elevated white or yellow border. The fungiform papillae appear raised because the filiform papillae have been lost. The zones of desquamation change over the course of days and weeks. In 60% of cases, scrotal tongue is also observed in patients with geographic tongue.

The etiology is unknown. Patients with psoriasis often exhibit lesions that are indistinguishable from geographic tongue. In rare cases, other oral mucosal regions may also be affected, a condition known as geographic stomatitis.

229 Geographic tongue
A white border surrounds the erythematous areas caused by loss of the filiform papillae. Other than an occasional burning sensation, symptoms are rare.

Right: Histologic picture of geographic tongue. The epithelium is moderately hyperplastic. In the upper layer of the stratum spinosum, one notes several focal aggregations of inflammatory cells. A pronounced inflammatory infiltrate is present in the subepithelial region (H & E, x 100).

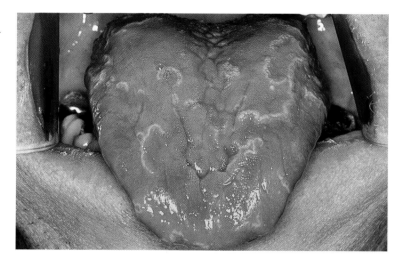
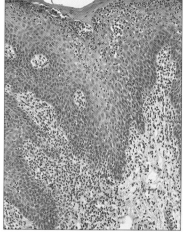

230 Geographic stomatitis
The ventral surface of the tongue in this 40-year-old female exhibits a typical lesion of geographic stomatitis. The dorsum of the tongue did not exhibit similar lesions.

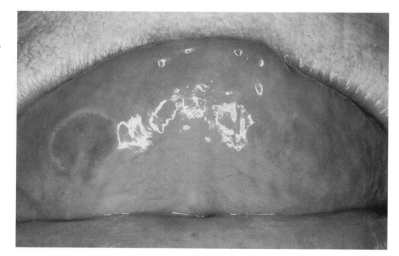

231 Geographic stomatitis
Note the characteristic lesion of geographic stomatitis on the lower lip and the labial vestibulum. These relatively rare manifestations were discovered by chance. Patients who worry excessively about cancer should be calmed and should be informed in detail about the harmless nature of such superficial lesions.

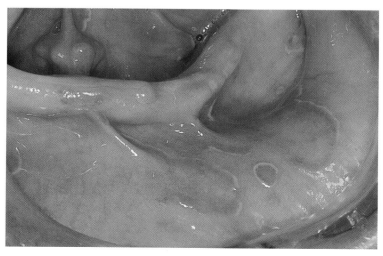

Infections—Bacterial

Syphilis and Tuberculosis

Syphilis elicits numerous oral manifestations. The primary ulceration, also known as a chancre, is usually accompanied by painless swelling of the regional lymph nodes. Five percent of the primary ulcers are localized on the oral mucosa, whereby the lower lip is most often affected, followed by the tongue and the gingiva. The typical chancre is painless, dark red, with a raised border, ulcerated and indurated, ranging in size from 2–3 cm. Secondary syphilis appears six to eight weeks or up to two years after the primary infection.

Tuberculosis (TB) of the oral mucosa is rare. According to the literature, the frequency of occurrence varies from 0.5 to 1.4%. Oral tuberculosis usually occurs secondarily, following a primary pulmonary tuberculosis. The most common localization is on the dorsum of the tongue, followed by the lips. The ulceration is characterized by an irregular border, with a crater-like center (Eng et al. 1996).

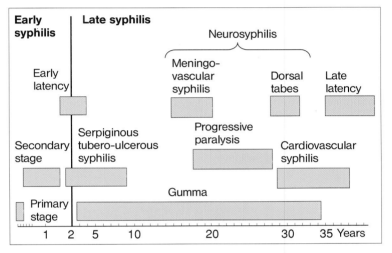

232 Manifestations of syphilis
This diagram depicts the various phases and courses of untreated syphilis. The secondary stage begins after the short primary stage. Late stage syphilis is characterized by various organ system manifestations, above all cardiovascular and neurogenic.

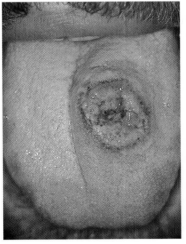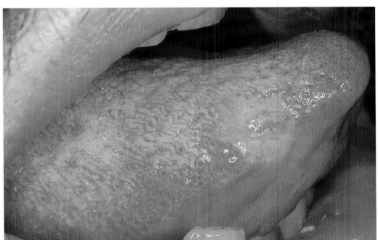

233 Secondary syphilis
On the right lateral border of the tongue of this HIV-seropositive patient there is a whitish lesion that corresponds to the *plaque muqueuse* of second stage syphilis.

Left: Primary ulcer on the dorsum of the tongue. The typical picture is not usually observed in the oral milieu, where secondary infection often occurs. For this reason, the ulceration appears smeared with a coating rather than red and indurated, which is how such lesions appear on the skin.

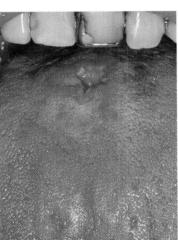

	Infected population		
Region	**(in millions)**	**New cases**	**Fatal cases**
Africa	171	1 400 000	660 000
America*	117	560 000	220 000
Eastern Mediterranean Area	52	594 000	160 000
Southeast Asia[1]	426	2 480 000	940 000
Western Pacific	574	2 560 000	890 000
Europe and other industrialized countries[2]	382	410 000	40 000
Total	1 722	8 004 000	2 910 000

* except United States and Canada
[1] except Japan, Australia and New Zealand
[2] United States, Japan, Australia, New Zealand

234 Tuberculosis
The table presents data about tuberculosis (TB) in various regions of the world (WHO 1991). Most persons who suffer from TB are found in Africa, Southeast Asia and in the Western Pacific regions. The WHO estimates that 1.7 billion people are infected worldwide. Of critical importance is the increase in TB cases that are resistant to therapy.
Left: TB ulceration with undermined borders. This 40-year-old female had pulmonary TB. The lingual lesion was painless.

Infections—Mycotic

Candidiasis, Median Rhomboid Glossitis

Like any other oral mucosal region, the dorsum of the tongue can be the site of infection with Candida microorganisms. A chronic form of lingual candidiasis, which is usually referred to as median rhomboid glossitis, appears as an erythematous, rhomboid or oval lesion on the dorsum of the tongue, in the midline, immediately anterior to the terminal sulcus. The affected region is usually well-circumscribed and is devoid of papillae. This area of the tongue is viewed as a predilection site because vascularity is reduced in this region; this enhances the development of inflammatory and infectious processes.

In earlier times, median rhomboid glossitis was believed to be a developmental anomaly and was referred to as a persisting *Tuberculum impar.* Patients with median rhomboid glossitis often exhibit lesions on the palate.

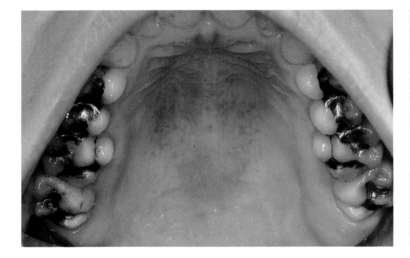

235 Candidiasis
Erythematous candidiasis on the palate of a 31-year-old, HIV-seropositive patient, whose tongue is depicted in Fig. 236. The candidiasis infection usually develops on the tongue first and then later on the palate due to direct contact. The palatal erythema has been referred to as a "kissing lesion."

Right: Chronic median rhomboid glossitis that is well demarcated; note the initial white hairy tongue.

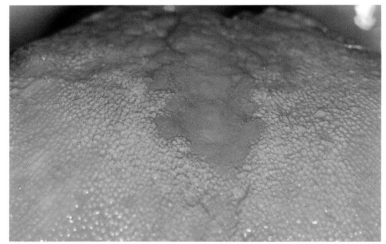

236 Median rhomboid glossitis
Chronic median rhomboid glossitis with less clearly demarcated margins. In the area of lingual erythema, lingual papillae can no longer be detected.
In immunocompetent patients, topical antimycotic therapy is usually effective, bringing the lesions under control quickly.

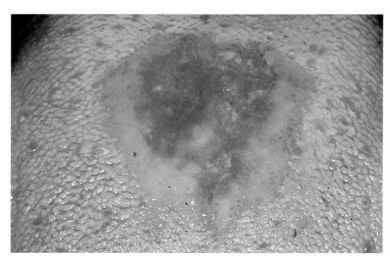

237 Ulcerating median rhomboid glossitis
Median rhomboid glossitis will occasionally ulcerate. Six days prior to this photograph, antimycotic treatment was initiated. Note that scar tissue has already begun to form at the borders of the lesion, but regeneration of the lingual papillae is not evident.

Candidiasis: Comparison between Immunocompetent and Immunodeficient Patients

Oral candidiasis in immunocompetent and immunodeficient patients exhibits similarities, but also differences. In individuals with a healthy immune system, oral candidiasis is most common in newborns and in elderly persons, or in patients who have taken antibiotics or antineoplastic medications over a long period of time. In contrast, in patients with AIDS or HIV infection, oral candidiasis occurs primarily in young males and females between the ages of 25 and 45. In this age group, oral candidiasis is almost never observed in immunocompetent individuals who do not otherwise have severe health problems.

The clinical picture of the various forms of candidiasis is similar in both immunocompetent and immunodeficient persons, but the individual lesions in immunodeficient patients can be more pronounced and more resistant to treatment. Arriving at a definitive diagnosis of erythematous candidiasis is difficult (Scully and El-Kabir 1994).

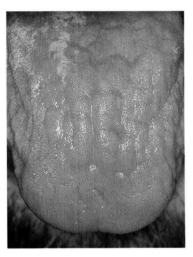 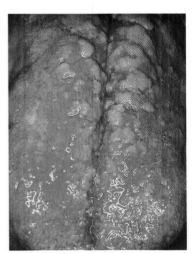

238　Candidiasis (HIV)

Left: Erythematous candidiasis in an AIDS patient. Almost the entire dorsum of the tongue exhibits loss of papillae. The lingual mucosa is dry as a result of the concomitant xerostomia.

Right: Pseudomembranous and erythematous candidiasis of the dorsum of the tongue in an AIDS patient. The brownish-yellow material consists of relatively rigidly anchored colonies of Candida.

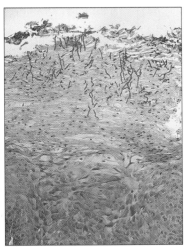 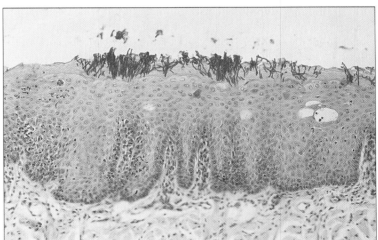

239　Candidiasis—histology

Histologic picture of pseudomembranous candidiasis. Colonies of PAS-positive Candida pseudohyphae can be observed within the stratum corneum of the lingual epithelium (PAS, x 100). Note that the pseudohyphae invade the epithelium perpendicularly to the surface.

Left: Hyphae and pseudohyphae in the superficial layer of the oral mucosal epithelium, which appears to be hyperparakeratotic (PAS, x 100).

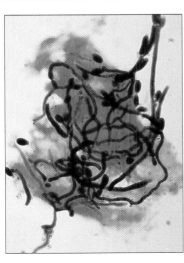 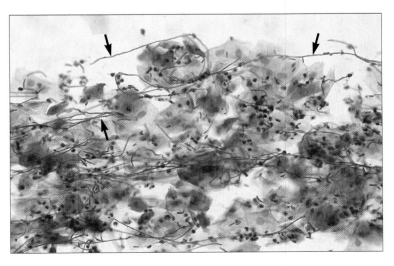

240　Candidiasis—cytologic smear

Smear of lingual pseudomembranous candidiasis. The cord-like organisms are pseudohyphae of *Candida albicans* (arrows). The cellular material represents desquamated epithelium and a few PMNs (PAS, x 150).

Left: Pseudohyphae and several ovoid blastospores in a cytologic smear of pseudomembranous candidiasis of the tongue (silver impregnation, x 300).

Infections—Viral

Gingivostomatitis (HSV-1)

Infection of the oral cavity with HSV-1 can lead to the development of herpetic gingivostomatitis. The most frequent vesicular eruption caused by HSV-1 is labial herpes. With the appearance of the HIV infection, it became clear that these patients were particularly affected by viruses of the herpes virus group. It is interesting that persistent ulcerations of the oral mucosa can be co-infected by various viruses from the herpes group (Langstädtler et al. 1996, Flaitz et al. 1996). In such cases, co-infection with herpes types 1 and 2 with the cytomegalovirus is particularly common. Most often affected are the buccal and labial mucosa (27%), tongue (25%) and gingiva (18%). In 47 individuals with persistent oral infections, 53% exhibited cytomegalovirus, 19% herpes simplex virus, and 28% a combination of cytomegalovirus and HSV. The drug Ganciclovir leads to healing of the lesions. Recurrence was noted in 23% of the cases. (See also pp. 46, 132, 152.)

241   Herpetic gingivostomatitis
This HIV-seropositive male exhibited an atypical, herpetic ulceration of the anterior dorsum of the tongue. Aciclovir-resistant HSV-1/2 infections of the oral cavity can occur.

Right: Herpetic stomatitis on the dorsum of the tongue in a 14-year-old immunocompetent female. The typical small, fibrin-coated aphthous lesions become confluent and are very painful.

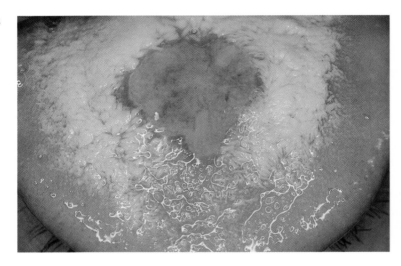
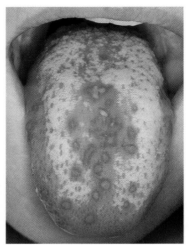

242   HSV-1/cytomegalovirus
This 35-year-old male with AIDS exhibited multiple, irregular, circumscribed ulcerations of the oral cavity and tip of the tongue. Persistent ulcerations were most evident on the palate and these did not subside despite high doses of Aciclovir. The definitive diagnosis requires culturing of the virus and especially a biopsy.

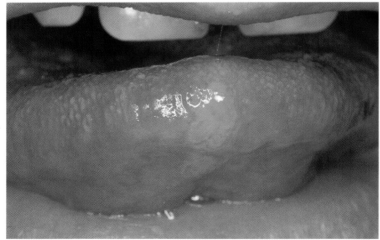

243   Proof of co-infection with HSV-1 and cytomegalovirus
A biopsy of the ulceration depicted in Fig. 242 revealed proof of a co-infection.
Left: Observe the immunohisto-chemically marked cells, which indicate an HSV-2 infection (APAAP, x 60).
Right: Cytomegalovirus infection in the region of the endothelium of small vessels (arrows). The orientation can be gleaned from the salivary gland duct (arrowhead), which can also be seen in the figure on the left (arrowhead) (APAAP, x 120).

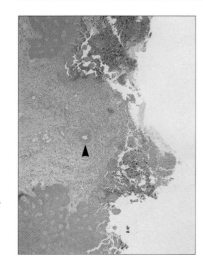
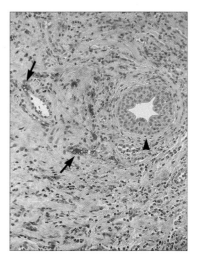

Hairy Leukoplakia

Oral hairy leukoplakia was first described in 1984 by Greenspan et al. The early suspicion was that this lesion of the lateral border of the tongue was characteristic for HIV-infected males; however, it was soon noted that oral hairy leukoplakia could also occur in patients who were otherwise immunocompromised; for example, organ transplant patients (Schmidt-Westhausen et al. 1990, 1993).

The *clinical picture* usually exhibits a bilateral, white, adherent lesion that follows the normal anatomy of the tongue. This often leads to a "zebra stripe" appearance with red and white stripes. About 30% of all HIV-infected patients exhibit oral hairy leukoplakia; females appear to be less often affected (7%; Schmidt-Westhausen et al. 1997). Other mucosal areas of the oral cavity are affected only in exceptional cases. The anogenital mucosae are not affected.

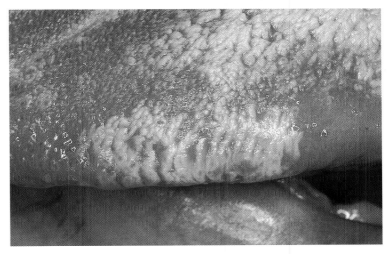

Hairy leukoplakia (HL)

244 Lesion on the left lateral border of the tongue
This 24-year-old, HIV-seropositive female presents a characteristic HL with intermittent red and white stripes. A similar lesion was present on the right side of the tongue. Areas of HL are sometimes only a few millimeters in size, but can become quite large, e.g., 3.5 x 2 cm. They are poorly demarcated and usually asymptomatic.

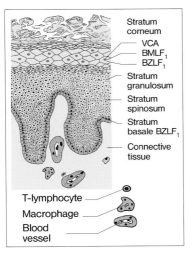

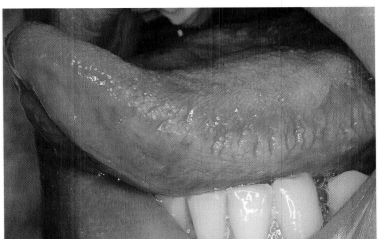

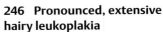

245 Lesion of the left lateral border of the tongue
This AIDS patient exhibits a less pronounced but nevertheless characteristic HL.
Left: Schematic diagram illustrating proof of the presence of the Epstein–Barr virus. It is easy to demonstrate the virus capsid antigens (VCA) by means of immunohistochemistry in the superficial epithelium. $BZLF_1$ and $BMLF_1$ represent "immediate early proteins" of EBV, which can be identified when they mature (adapted from Becker et al. 1991).

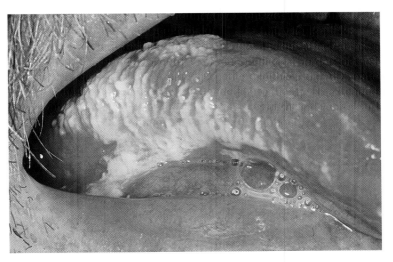

246 Pronounced, extensive hairy leukoplakia
Lesions affected the right and left lateral borders of the tongue in a 40-year-old AIDS patient. In this case, the HL extended onto the dorsal and ventral surfaces of the tongue.

The *etiology* of hairy leukoplakia is to be found in the Epstein–Barr virus (Cruchley et al. 1997, Raab-Traub and Webster-Cyriaque 1997). It is possible to demonstrate that the structure of the virus develops in parallel with epithelial differentiation; the maturation of the virus extends from the basal membrane by way of the so-called immediate early proteins (BZLF 1) up to the mucosal surface, where virus capsid antigens can be detected (Becker et al. 1991).

Oral hairy leukoplakia is asymptomatic and therefore no *treatment* is necessary. On the other hand, it has been reported that the use of various antiviral agents will cause remission of the lesions; however, when the medication is discontinued the lesions recur.

Oral hairy leukoplakia is not precancerous, although cases of oral cavity carcinoma in HIV and AIDS patients have been described (Langford et al. 1995, Flaitz et al. 1995).

The *histologic* picture of oral hairy leukoplakia is in no way characteristic, but does exhibit aspects of a viral infection.

Hairy leukoplakia (HL)

247   Low-power histologic view
This photomicrograph shows several keratin hair-like protrusion that have given oral HL its name (H & E, x 60).

Right: Higher magnification of a keratin process, showing parakeratotic epithelium and large, balloon-like cells in the epithelium (arrowheads) (H & E, x 120).

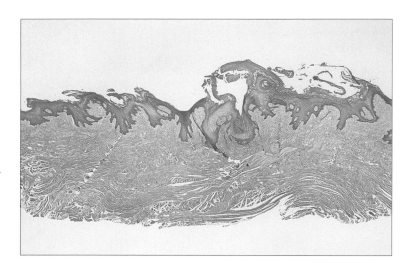
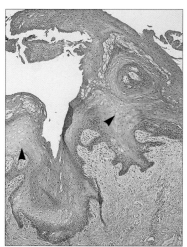

248   Histologic details
Parakeratotic epithelium with large, ballooned cells (arrow), which have also been referred to as koilocyte-like cells. Note the pyknotic nuclei and the perinuclear zone which, along with the inclusion bodies, indicates a viral infection (H & E, x 200).

Right: Note the Candida hyphae in the superficial epithelium. If the white lesion disappears after institution of antimycotic therapy, the diagnosis of oral hairy leukoplakia is probable (PAS, x 80).

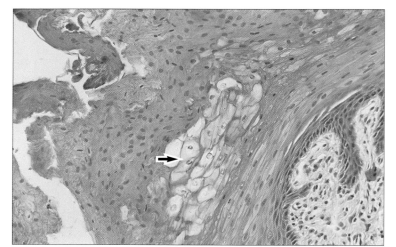
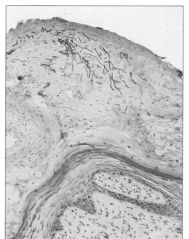

249   Immunohistochemistry
Following immunohistochemical staining, the superficial epithelium of HL is positive for the EBV virus capsid antigen VCA (APAAP, x 120).

Right: The EBV can also be depicted by means of electron microscopy. Multiple virus particles (arrows) are visible in the intercellular spaces; these derive from the herpes virus group (TEM, x 20 000).

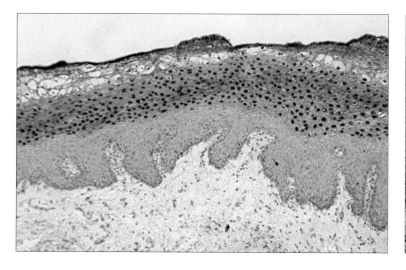
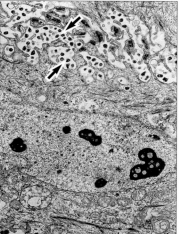

Focal Epithelial Hyperplasia, Verruca Vulgaris, Herpetic Gingivostomatitis

Focal epithelial hyperplasia (FEH) is a rare mucosal lesion exhibiting multiple, slightly raised, flat, broad, white nodules on the mucosa of the lower lip, cheek and dorsum of the tongue. The color of the individual lesions is whitish, or may maintain the color of the surrounding mucosa.

Immunohistochemical investigations have demonstrated human papilloma virus (HPV), types 13 and 32 (Syrjänen 1997). Spontaneous regression is frequent.

The *verruca vulgaris*, also known as a viral wart, occurs on the lips, the palate and the gingiva. Oral warts are usually small and exophytic. They occur in children who chew on their finger warts, thereby transferring HPV (types 2 and 4) onto the oral mucosa.

Herpetic gingivostomatitis is observed most frequently in children between the ages of two and four years.

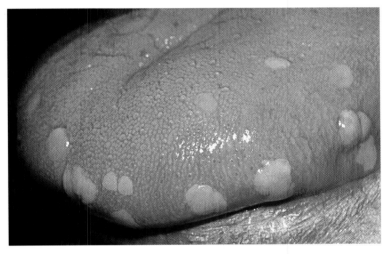

250 Focal epithelial hyperplasia
The tongue of this 35-year-old Greenland Eskimo exhibits multiple, slightly raised lesions that are characteristic for FEH. The tongue is affected in more than 50% of cases. FEH appears to be more common in Eskimos and Indians of North and South America than in other racial groups. It also occurs occasionally in HIV-infected individuals (see pp. 49 and 69).

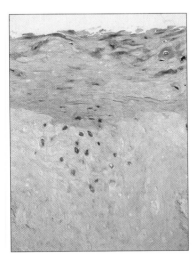
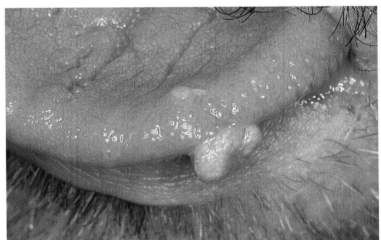

251 Verruca vulgaris
In the region of the left lateral border of the tongue in this HIV-infected young male, one can observe a proliferating lesion with a whitish surface. Note also the angular cheilitis. It is not always possible to differentiate clinically between verruca vulgaris and condyloma.

Left: Immunohistochemical identification of HPV antigens of virus types 2 and 4, which are typical for verruca vulgaris (APAAP, x 100).

252 Herpetic gingivostomatitis
On the lateral border of the tongue and beneath the tongue one can observe several aphthoid ulcerations. The vesicles burst shortly after they appear and then become covered with fibrin. The lesions are always surrounded by an erythematous zone. The individual lesions have a tendency toward confluence. Antiviral medications, such as Aciclovir, can be instituted therapeutically.

Disturbances of Keratinization

Leukoplakia

Oral leukoplakia has been defined as a primarily white lesion of the oral mucosa, which cannot be characterized as any other definable lesion. Some types of oral leukoplakia can become cancerous (Axéll et al. 1996). Leukoplakia can be divided into homogeneous and non-homogeneous forms. Lingual leukoplakia is localized on the lateral borders of the tongue, the dorsum or the ventral surface.

Five to ten percent of all leukoplakias occur on the tongue. If the dorsum of the tongue is affected, the lingual papillae disappear. Lingual leukoplakia may be diffuse or may appear as well-circumscribed, homogeneous spots, especially on the lateral lingual borders. Malignant transformation of leukoplakia on the lingual borders and on the ventral surface as well as the floor of the mouth occurs more frequently than in other regions. (Further information on leukoplakia can be found on pp. 11, 15, 52, 73, 117 and 154.)

Leukoplakia

253 Diffuse leukoplakia of the entire dorsum of the tongue
This 57-year-old male had never smoked, so this lesion was classified as idiopathic leukoplakia. The risk of malignant transformation is higher for idiopathic leukoplakia, especially in females. The patient exhibited scrotal tongue in addition to the diffuse leukoplakia.

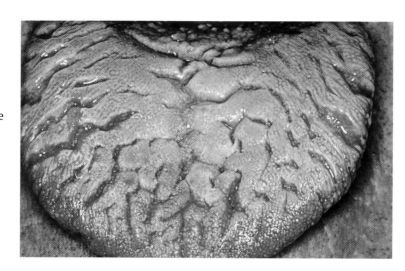

254 Homogeneous leukoplakia
Homogeneous leukoplakia of the left lateral border of the tongue and the ventral surface. This male patient smoked up to 35 cigarillos per day.
Right: Microscopic picture of the leukoplakia shown on the left. In addition to hyperparakeratosis, epithelial atrophy and basal cell hyperplasia, hyperchromatism of the basal cells is evident. All of these findings support the diagnosis of mild to moderate epithelial atypia (dysplasia) (H & E, x 120).

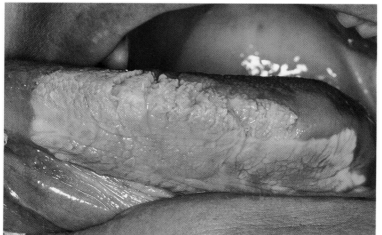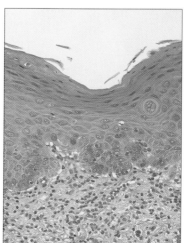

255 Idiopathic leukoplakia
Red and white striped lesion of the lateral border of the tongue and homogeneous leukoplakia of the floor of the mouth in a 70-year-old female who had never smoked. Note the similarity to oral hairy leukoplakia. The rest of the oral cavity also exhibited homogeneous leukoplakia; thus, the diagnosis was idiopathic leukoplakia. In such cases, the patient should be reexamined at three to six-month intervals.

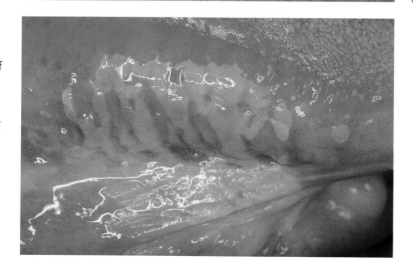

Dermatologic Manifestations

Lichen Planus

If the lingual mucosa is affected by lichen planus, it is usually the *plaque form* of this mucocutaneous disease. Clinically, white plaques of oral lichen are difficult to differentiate from homogeneous leukoplakia; this is especially true if patients with lichen planus are also smokers.

The tongue, however, may also be the site of *atrophic* and *erosive forms* of lichen planus, which in many cases are painful. Most important is the fact that both of these types of lichen planus can transform and become malignant. Recent literature indicates that the rate of transformation is 0.5–2.5% (Herrmann 1992, Markopoulos et al. 1997). For this reason, oral lichen planus is classified as a precancerous condition (Axéll et al. 1996). Whether this is justified or not has not yet been completely determined, although most specialists have adopted this view. (Further information about lichen planus can be found on pp. 80, 137, and 156.)

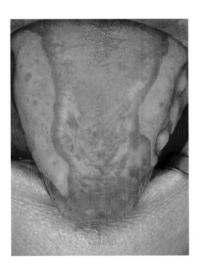
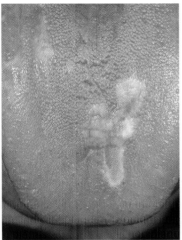
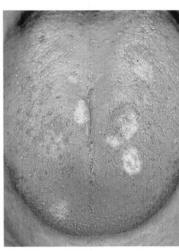

Lichen planus

256 Ulcerated and plaque-forming types

Left: Lichen planus of the dorsum of the tongue, with massive erosions of both lateral borders, leading to the diagnosis of erosive lichen planus.

Middle: Plaque-forming lichen planus, which must be differentiated from leukoplakia.

Right: Multiple white spots on the dorsum indicate plaque-forming lichen planus.

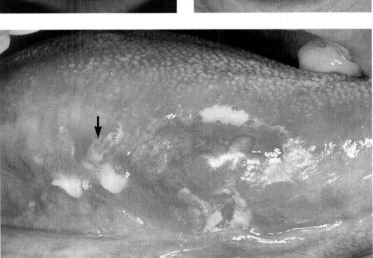

257 Mixed form

Lichen planus on the lateral border of the tongue with plaque-forming, atrophic and erosive ulcerating elements. The detection of Wickham's striae (arrow) sometimes facilitates the diagnosis.

Left: Microscopic picture of plaque-forming lichen. Parakeratosis, moderate epithelial hyperplasia, a zone of subepithelial liquefaction (arrow) as well as a band of subepithelial lymphocytic infiltration are evident (H & E, x 100).

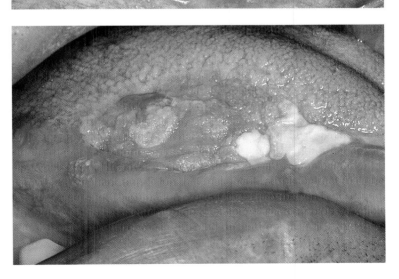

258 Suspicion of malignant transformation

This is the lateral border of the tongue of the patient in Fig. 257, two years later. The plaque-covered area has enlarged, the region that previously exhibited erosive lichen now shows nodule formations that are also noticeable upon palpation. This arouses suspicion that malignant transformation is occurring. The subsequent biopsy exhibited a carcinoma in situ, and the entire lesion was excised.

Physical, Chemical, Thermal and Other Causes

The tongue is subjected to numerous physical, chemical, thermal and other insults that can lead to *ulceration*. Acute trauma caused by tongue biting or the sharp edges of fractured teeth, dentures, clasps or denture margins can elicit chronic ulceration that can sometimes arouse suspicion of a carcinomatous ulcer. As is the case with pressure point lesions from dentures, the rule is to maintain a suspicion of malignancy regarding persisting ulcers until the opposite is proved, perhaps by a biopsy.

In rare cases of suicide attempts, corrosive fluids may be swallowed. If the patient survives, there is likely to be *scarring of the oral soft tissue* as well as esophageal strictures.

Post-irradiation ulceration may be accompanied by xerostomia and superinfection by *Candida albicans*.

259 Traumatic ulcer of the tongue
Ulcer on the right side of the tongue and floor of the mouth. The ulcer is surrounded by a whitish lesion of the oral mucosa. This female patient was a non-smoker. The following figure (Fig. 260) reveals the cause of this ulceration.

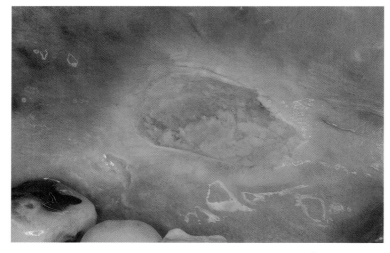

260 Traumatic ulcer of the tongue/lingual scar
The ulcer depicted in Fig. 259 was caused by a very jagged root fragment. With each movement of the tongue, the sharp root edge cut into the tongue. Following removal of the root, the ulceration healed spontaneously.

Right: Suicide attempt using acid. The entire margin of the tongue is scarred. The range of movement of the tongue was also compromised.

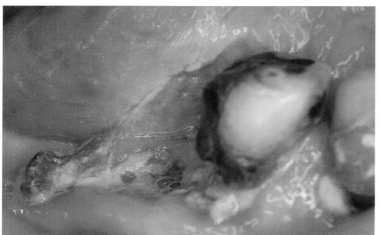
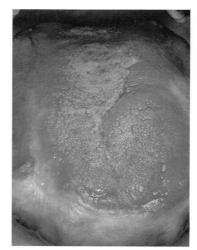

261 Post-irradiation Ulcer
The right border of the tongue exhibits a fibrin-coated ulcer associated with radiation mucositis and xerostomia. The ulcer was painful and persisted due to the sharp lingual surfaces of the mandibular premolars. Following remission of the radiation-associated lingual edema, treatment of the oral Candida superinfection and the reduction of secondary infection, such ulcerations will slowly heal.

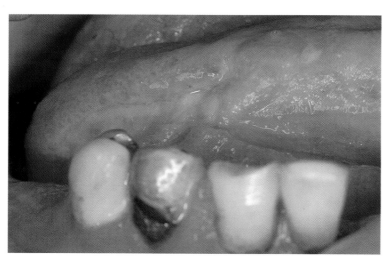

Ulceration of the Tongue Following Antineoplastic Therapy

Cytostatic medications and immunosuppressive agents are the most common causes of medication-related erosive or ulcerative stomatitis. The lesions are dosage-dependent, usually appear two to three weeks following initiation of therapy, and are related to toxic immunosuppression. Such reactions are particularly pronounced after use of methotrexate. The clinical picture consists of sharply demarcated and confluent areas of erythema and ulceration in all areas of the oral mucosa.

Burning Mouth Syndrome

Burning mouth syndrome (BMS) consists of a complex of symptoms and complaints related to the oral cavity (Tourne and Fricton 1992, Lamey 1996). In addition to a sensation of dry mouth and a loss of taste sensitivity, patients with BMS complain above all about a burning sensation of the tongue (glossopyrosis), which is usually bilateral and symmetrical. These symptoms are continuous and may persist over months or years. Clinically, it is often impossible to distinguish any lesions whatsoever. Cases of idiopathic BMS are very difficult to handle therapeutically.

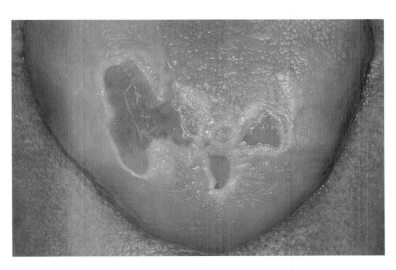

262   Lingual ulcer following cytostatic therapy
At the tip of the tongue one can observe several ulcerated areas with whitish margins; the latter indicate a tendency toward healing. It is important to avoid secondary infection of such oral ulcerations. Patients should rinse regularly with a chlorhexidine mouthwash.

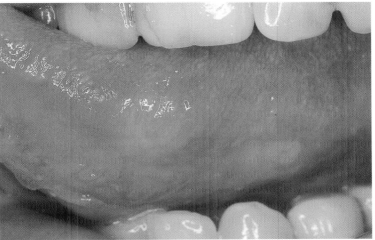

263   Ulceration following cytostatic therapy
On the lateral border of the tongue, one can see several small ulcerations that are aphthoid in appearance. These lesions appeared a short time after initiation of antineoplastic therapy and were also observed in the buccal mucosa and on the tongue as more or less pronounced manifestations. Functions that are regulated by the tongue, such as eating, drinking and speaking, are often severely compromised.

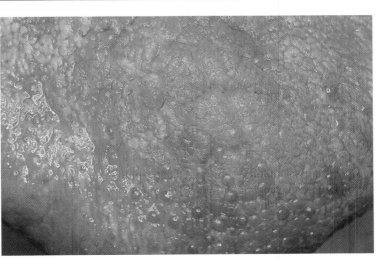

264   Burning mouth syndrome
It is important to note the localization of the area of burning sensation on the tongue. If the tip of the tongue of a dentulous patient is affected, the cause might be rubbing the tongue on the incisal edges of the mandibular anterior teeth. This leads to enlargement and erythema of the anterior lingual papillae. Surgery should be avoided. Psychotherapy may help.

Benign Tumors

"Fibroma"

The tongue is often the site of benign tumor development. Most common is the "fibroma," which is a benign connective tissue growth. The majority of so-called oral fibromas, irrespective of tumor location, are in fact hyperplastic, reactive proliferations of fibrous tissue. The lingual fibromas are usually caused by chronic irritation and trauma. The lesions are firm, well circumscribed, sessile or pedunculated. They are covered by normal mucosa. When subjected to local trauma, the surface of the lesion may appear white, which indicates hyperkeratosis (frictional keratosis).

Neurilemmoma

The intraoral neurilemmoma (Schwannoma) is rare and derives from Schwann cells; it is often located on the tip of the tongue. The tumor is well-demarcated and is of firm consistency. Chrysomali et al. (1997) recently described the immunohistochemical differentiation of benign neural tumors of the oral cavity.

265 "Fibroma" in the midline of the dorsum of the tongue
This lingual fibroma was noted in a 45-year-old female. Its localization in the middle of the tongue just anterior to the terminal sulcus is very uncommon. The fibroma developed over a 15-year period and had not caused the patient any problems. Simple surgical excision is the treatment of choice.

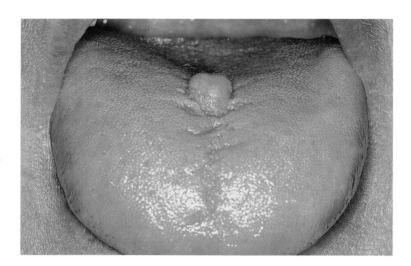

266 "Fibroma" of the tip of the tongue
Fibroma or fibromatous hyperplasia near the tip of the tongue, where such lesions are more common than in the midline of the tongue. The proximity of the incisal edges indicates the possibility of chronic trauma, which could play an important etiologic role. The surface of the fibroma does not exhibit any lingual papillae.

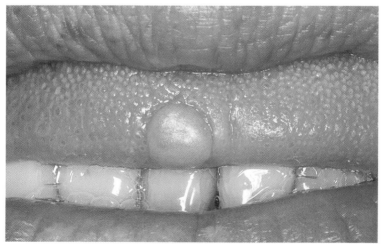

267 Neurilemmoma
Schwannoma on the tip of the tongue. Palpation revealed two circumscribed tumor nodules, which were not painful.

Right: Histologic picture of the typical architecture of Schwannoma. The nuclei of the Schwann cells are "shoulder to shoulder" in their arrangement (*), and form the so-called Verocay bodies (H & E, x 100).

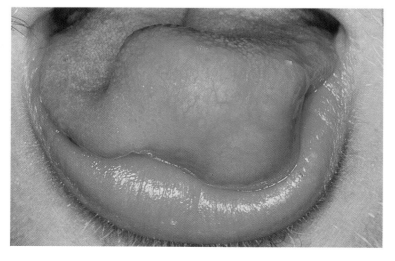
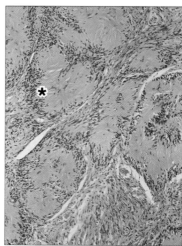

Neurofibromatosis

Generalized multiple neurofibromatosis (Recklinghausen's disease) is considered to be a developmental malformation which is hereditary in 40% of cases. This disease is characterized by melanin pigmentation in the skin (*café au lait* spots) and multiple neurofibromas of the skin, the gastrointestinal tract, and the skeleton. Oral manifestations comprise multiple neurofibromas with or without involvement of the jaw bones. The tongue is most frequently involved; macroglossia can occur (Baden et al. 1984, Keutel et al. 1997).

Granular Cell Tumor

The granular cell tumor, also known as the Abrikossoff's tumor or granular cell myoblastoma occurs on various visceral skin and mucosal surfaces. A third of such lesions occur on the tongue. The tumor is circumscribed, firm and symptom-free. Females are more often affected. Granular cell tumors appear to originate from neuroendocrine tissue (Williams and Williams 1997).

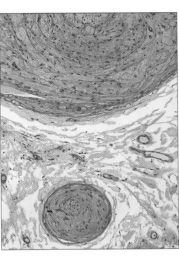
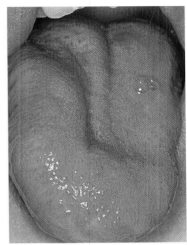
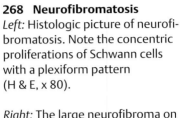

268 Neurofibromatosis
Left: Histologic picture of neurofibromatosis. Note the concentric proliferations of Schwann cells with a plexiform pattern (H & E, x 80).

Right: The large neurofibroma on the right border of the tongue is one component of Recklinghausen's disease. In this 23-year-old female, who exhibited numerous *café au lait* spots on her skin, unilateral macroglossia was also observed.

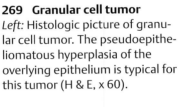

269 Granular cell tumor
Left: Histologic picture of granular cell tumor. The pseudoepitheliomatous hyperplasia of the overlying epithelium is typical for this tumor (H & E, x 60).

Right: A large tumor is obvious on the left side of the tongue. The overlying lingual mucosa exhibits normal filiform papillae and several hyperplastic fungiform papillae.

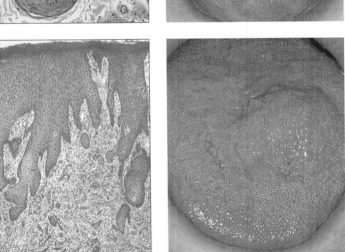
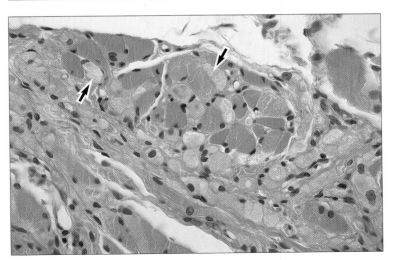

270 Granular cell tumor—histology
At this magnification, the granular cell tumor exhibits its characteristic architecture with enlarged, pale Schwann cells (arrows), which can achieve sizes of 50 μm or larger and which can infiltrate the musculature of the tongue (H & E, x 250).

Hemangioma

Next to fibromas, *angiomas* deriving from vascular tissue are the most common benign tumors of the oral cavity. Hemangiomas are tumors of blood vessels and there continues to be discussion about whether there is a true neoplastic component. For this reason, hemangiomas are considered to be hamartomas. Oral hemangiomas are reddish or blue in color and occur in all areas of the oral cavity.

The *congenital papillary type* of oral hemangioma is frequently encountered on the lips. If a hemangioma consists of large vascular spaces lined with endothelial cells, it is classified as a *cavernous hemangioma*. This form occurs either congenitally or in later life. Cavernous hemangiomas can also occur within the alveolar bone; severe hemorrhage following trauma or tooth extraction has been reported.

Small hemangiomas can be excised. A biopsy for diagnosis is usually not indicated.

271   Small hemangioma
A small hemangioma is localized just to the right of the tip of the tongue. In this location, hemangiomas are often traumatized, which can lead to severe hemorrhage. When pressure is applied to a hemangioma, it blanches, but fills immediately with blood when the pressure is released. This phenomenon does not occur with other lesions in the differential diagnosis, such as pigmentation or Kaposi's sarcoma.

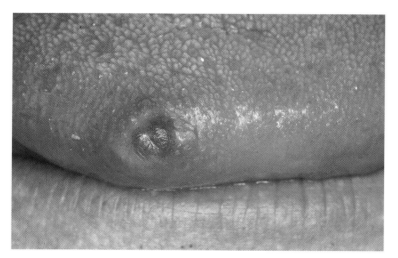

272   Large cavernous hemangioma of the right side of the tongue
This hemangioma had existed since birth and had become larger over the years. The patient's speech was mildly impaired.

Right: Histologic picture of cavernous hemangioma. The large, irregular vascular lumina are lined with endothelium and filled with accumulations of erythrocytes (H & E, x 60).

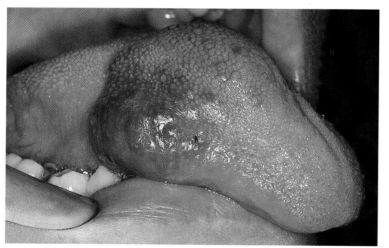
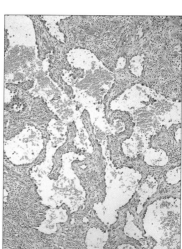

273   Cavernous hemangioma of the left side of the tongue
Before any surgical procedures are undertaken, the efferent vessels must be displayed by arteriography. Preoperative embolization of the hemangioma will reduce the risk of uncontrollable, massive hemorrhage.

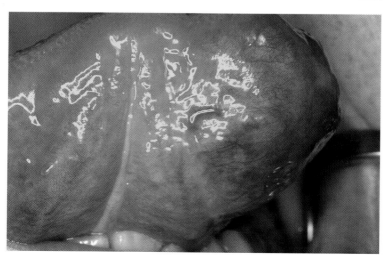

Benign/Malignant Tumors

Lymphangioma and Kaposi's Sarcoma

Lymphangiomas are tumor-like, hamartomatous lymphatic lesions that may occur in any area of the skin and mucosal tissues. They occur most frequently in patients under the age of 20. The oral cavity, especially the tip of the tongue, is particularly frequently affected. When localized superficially, lymphangiomas appear as colorless, soft, often pebbly swellings of the mucosa. If the lesion extends deeply, it can lead to a diffuse enlargement of the tongue (macroglossia).

This is especially apparent in the cervical, cystic hygroma, an infiltrating lymphangioma involving the neck and seen in children at birth.

The third most common localization of *Kaposi's sarcoma* is the middle of the dorsum of the tongue. In later stages, the lesions may become tumorous and may ulcerate. Intralesional cytostatic treatment or intraoral irradiation may elicit improvement of the condition (Epstein and Silverman 1992).

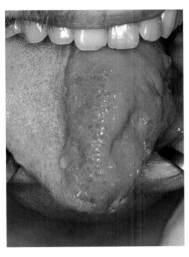
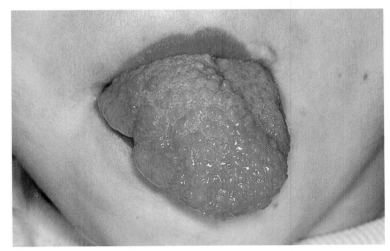

274 Lymphangioma
Superficial, diffuse, cavernous lymphangioma in an 8-year-old female. The tongue surface exhibits numerous nodular, soft protuberances that resemble large fungiform papillae.

Left: Unilateral, diffuse, cavernous lymphangioma of the left side of the tongue in a young male. The tumor is deeply situated and elicits the unilateral macroglossia.

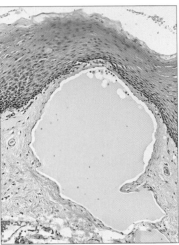
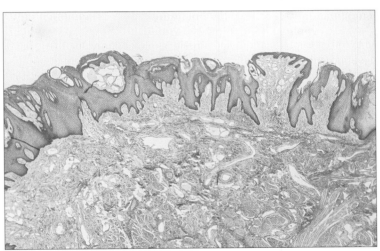

275 Lymphangioma —histology
Histologic picture of lymphangioma of the tongue. Numerous lymphatic vessels are evident within the connective tissue of the fungiform papillae (H & E, x 50).

Left: Biopsy from patient shown in Fig. 274 (right). Large, dilated lymphatic vessels are apparent; they are pushing the overlying mucosa and the epithelium upward (H & E, x 100).

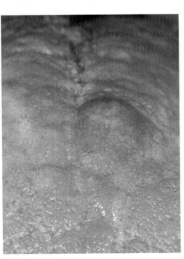
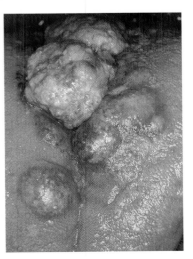

276 Kaposi's sarcoma
Left: Early, pale Kaposi's sarcoma just left of the midline on the dorsum of the tongue. The tumor is painless as long as it is not ulcerated.

Right: Multiple, tumorous Kaposi's sarcomas in the midline of the tongue, exhibiting partial ulceration. It is not yet known why the Kaposi's sarcoma is most often observed in the midline of the tongue (see also pp. 143 and 166).

Malignant Tumors

Lingual Carcinoma

The incidence of lingual carcinoma varies enormously from country to country. The annual, age-corrected incidence rate for German males is 4.9 per 100,000, in comparison to 24.0 for males in the Lower Rhine region of France. Lingual carcinoma is more common in males than in females. The highest incidence occurs in the sixth to eighth decades of life. If the carcinoma is located on the anterior two thirds of the tongue, usually on the lateral margins, there is often a painless swelling. On the other hand, if the posterior third of the tongue is affected, the tumor is often noticed only quite late by the patient and the pain is interpreted as neck pain. Carcinoma of the tongue is usually exophytic, in conjunction with ulcerations of varying depth. The tumor is surrounded by leukoplakia in 15–20% of cases (Scheifele and Reichart 1998). The risk of developing lingual carcinoma is dependent upon tobacco use and alcohol consumption (Zheng et al. 1997).

277 Epidemiology
Age-corrected incidence rates per 100,000 for cancer of the oral cavity from various European countries (Parkin et al. 1992). Recent data indicate a certain increase in carcinoma of the oral cavity in some countries, whereby especially young males are affected, even though there is no detectable risk factor.

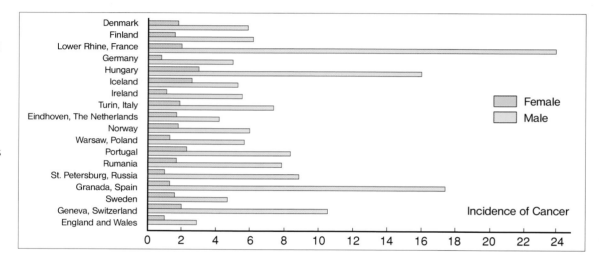

278 Etiology and clinical symptoms
The causative factors have been known for many years. Acknowledged risk factors are smoking and tobacco use in its various forms, the excessive consumption of alcohol as well as already existing, potential malignant lesions of the oral cavity and other diseases (Johnson 1997).

Right: Clinical symptoms of oral carcinoma.

Risk Factors
- Smoking
- Chewing tobacco/snuff
- Betel quid chewing, especially in combination with tobacco
- Alcohol in large quantities
- Already existing, potentially malignant lesions of the oral cavity or other diseases

Further Predisposing Factors
- Nutritional deficiency of vitamins A, C and E as well as of iron
- Familial or genetic predisposition
- Viral infection, especially with certain types of the human papilloma virus (HPV)
- Exposure to the sun (labial carcinoma)
- Candida albicans infection
- Immunodeficiency diseases or immunosuppression
- Anemia
- Environmental influences—pollution
- Chronic infections

- Pain
- Hemorrhage
- Swelling
- Sensory disturbances
- Tooth mobility
- Taste disturbances
- Weight loss

279 Life expectancies
This graph depicts the life expectancy following radical surgical operation alone versus preoperative radiochemotherapy and radical operation of advanced squamous epithelial carcinoma of the oral cavity or the oropharynx. Note the significant advantage of the combined therapy (adapted from Esser 1998).

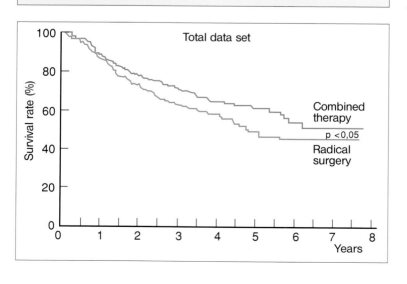

Cancer of the oral cavity comprises 4% of all carcinomas in males and 2% in females. These data are valid for Europe; in Southern and Southeast Asia, oral carcinoma may account for 40% of all carcinomas in the entire body. Such high incidence rates are due to smoking and chewing (betel quid) habits.

It is the nitrosamines derived from tobacco that are carcinogenic. Alcohol alters the barrier function of the oral mucosa so that the combination of smoking and alcohol consumption leads to a higher penetration rate of toxic substances. The carcinogenic pathway appears to progress from initiation in a single cell followed by promotion due to the influ-ences of additional carcinogenic or mutagenic agents which, over the long term, lead to the development of a malignant cell.

Traumatic ulcer of the tongue is an important differential diagnostic lesion when considering lingual carcinoma.

Carcinoma of the floor of the mouth can also involve the tongue completely or may infiltrate the tongue from below, so that occasional perforations occur in the lingual midline (Fig. 283). (See additional information about oral carcinoma on pp. 54, 79, 120, 70 and 198).

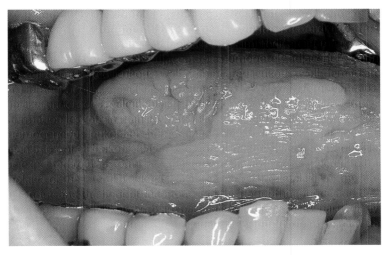

280 Carcinoma of the right lateral border of the tongue
The carcinoma resides immediately adjacent to a homogeneous, well-demarcated leukoplakia. Homogeneous leukoplakia undergoes malignant transformation less often than non-homogeneous leukoplakia. Between 5–6% of all leukoplakias can be expected to transform. Leukoplakia of the lateral borders of the tongue and the floor of the mouth are particularly likely to undergo malignant transformation.

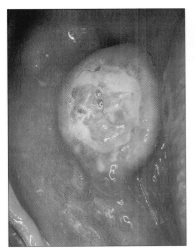
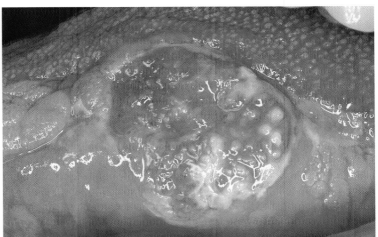

281 Exophytic, ulcerated carcinoma
Carcinoma of the lateral tongue border within a homogeneous leukoplakic area. The white nodules upon the erythematous background are primary signs of malignant transformation.

Left: Squamous cell carcinoma of the right vestibulum, immediately adjacent to the lingual border. Between 80–98% of all oral carcinomas are squamous cell carcinomas, the rest are verrucous carcinomas.

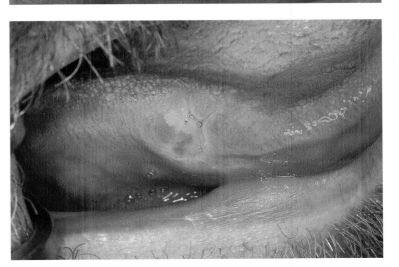

282 Traumatic ulcer
Traumatic ulcer of the lateral border of the tongue can usually be diagnosed based on the patient's medical history. Most important is the duration of the problems and symptoms. In the case of carcinoma, the symptoms usually persist for months, while symptoms from traumatic ulcers only last for days to weeks. If traumatic ulcers persist despite treatment, a biopsy is strongly indicated.

"TNM" Classification and Prognosis of Oral Carcinoma

Carcinoma of the lip and the oral cavity can be classified according to the TNM system (Pindborg et al. 1997), where T stands for tumor, N for lymph nodes, and M for metastasis.

The T in the classification pertains to the size of the tumor, and ranges from T_1 to T_4, wherein tumors of T_4 size have infiltrated adjacent structures. Size and extension of the infiltration determines the prognosis with regard to the five-year survival rate. While lingual carcinoma of T_1 size has a five-year survival rate of 70%, this is reduced to 30% in T_3 tumors (Pindborg 1982).

In determining the prognosis, the condition of the regional lymphnodes (N) is also important with respect to possible metastases (M). Distant metastases to other organ systems significantly impact the prognosis. Esser (1998) published data concerning the prognosis of oral cavity and oropharynx carcinoma vis-à-vis the radicality of the treatment.

283   Perforating lingual carcinoma
The midline of the dorsum of the tongue exhibits an ulceration with poorly demarcated borders. Using a blunt probe, it was possible to ascertain that the perforation continued several centimeters into the floor of the mouth.
Right: Histologic picture of a squamous cell carcinoma that is well differentiated. Some of the islands of malignant tissue exhibit keratinization. Note the presence of hyperchromatic nuclei of various sizes (H & E, x 100).

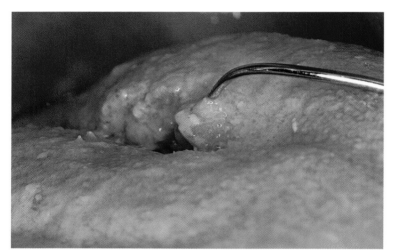
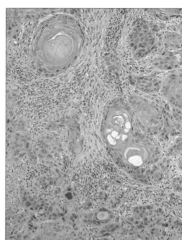

284   Sublingual area
Sublingual area of the patient depicted in Fig. 283. The tongue is essentially immobile and exhibits various ulcerations. Note also the incredibly poor oral hygiene.

Right: Histologic picture of squamous cell carcinoma, exhibiting moderate differentiation (H & E, x 80).

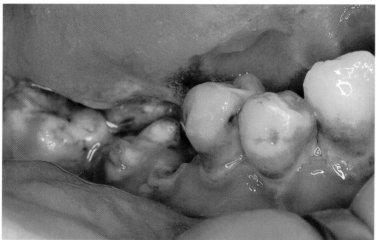
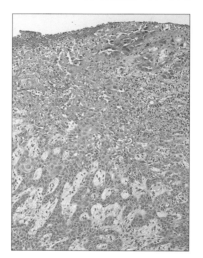

285   Formation of metastases
This is the same patient depicted in Figs. 283 and 284. Even macroscopically, it is evident that swelling has occurred bilaterally in the submandibular region. This can be interpreted as metastases to the regional, submandibular lymph nodes.

Right: Two small islands of poorly-differentiated squamous cell carcinoma within the connective tissue (H & E, x 100).

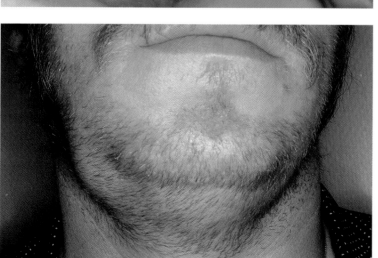
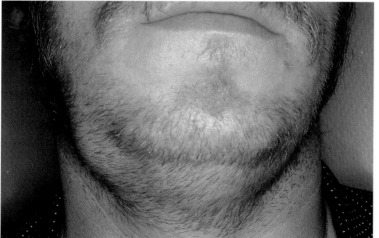

Other Lesions

Black Hairy Tongue

In patients with hairy tongue, the filiform papillae of the dorsum of the tongue are excessively long. This is due to a delay in the normal process of epithelial desquamation or an increase in epithelial keratin formation. Individual filiform papillae can become 15–20 mm long and 2 mm thick. The color of hairy tongue varies from white to yellow or from brown to black. The dark pigmentation results from an increase in the number of chromogenic microorganisms.

Anemia

Hematologic disorders, especially anemia, often lead to pathologic changes in the oral cavity. Anemia is characterized by reduced quantities of hemoglobin in the circulatory system because of a reduced erythrocyte volume and a reduction in the number of circulating erythrocytes. Iron deficiency, pernicious and hemolytic anemia are associated with more or less severe loss of tongue papillae.

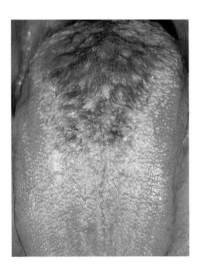
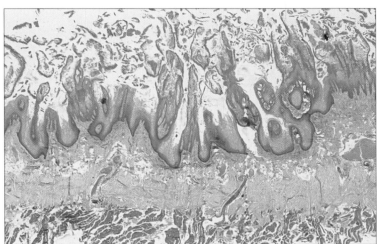

286 Hairy tongue
Histologic picture of hairy tongue, revealing elongated, keratinized filiform papillae (H & E, x 40).

Left: Brownish hairy tongue in a 36-year-old male who had been taking antibiotics over an extended period of time because of tonsillitis. The elongated papillae can be removed using a lingual spatula. Hairy tongue is harmless.

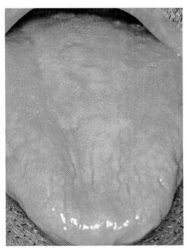
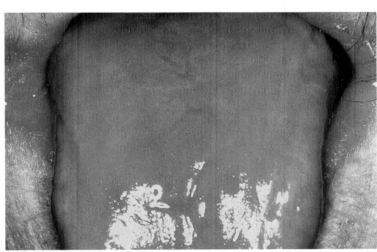

287 Iron deficiency anemia
This elderly female suffered from iron deficiency anemia. The dorsum of the tongue exhibits a pronounced atrophy of papillae. In addition, one notes bilateral angular cheilitis. The latter, as well as the lingual erythema, results from a secondary Candida infection.

Left: Atrophy of the lingual papillae and a pronounced pale appearance of the tongue in a case of iron deficiency anemia.

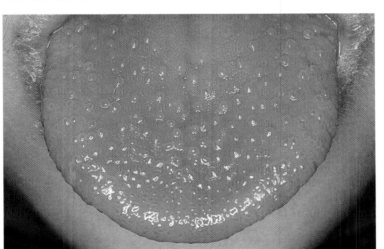

288 Pernicious anemia
Pernicious anemia with paresthesia of the tongue as well as burning and itching of the entire oral mucosa, with occasional xerostomia. There are almost no filiform papillae at all, which makes the fungiform papillae appears especially pronounced.
    In addition to basic medical treatment for the anemia, appropriate disinfectant mouth rinses should be used to prevent secondary infection in the oral cavity.

Sjögren's Syndrome

Sjögren's syndrome is an autoimmune disease of the exocrine glands and most often occurs in postmenopausal women. Patients suffer from oral and ocular symptoms, especially xerostomia with enlargement of the salivary glands, and keratoconjunctivitis sicca. In addition to a sensation of dry mouth, such patients have difficulty swallowing and they complain of a burning sensation of the oral mucosa, loss of taste sensation, and an inability to consume dry food. In addition, there are extraglandular manifestations, such as tiredness, muscle and joint pain.

The tongue often exhibits pronounced atrophy of the papillae; the lingual surface is smooth and lobulated. As a result of dryness in the oral cavity, dentulous patients often experience extensive dental caries.

The treatment of Sjögren's syndrome is difficult and is targeted toward reinstituting saliva production. Either sialagogues or saliva replacements are often employed (Stiller 1997). It is possible that patients with Sjögren's syndome will develop malignant lymphoma.

Sjögren's syndrome

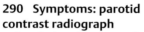

289 Bilateral enlargement of parotid glands
This elderly female exhibits the characteristic symptoms of Sjögren's syndrome.
   Verification of xerostomia is accomplished by sialometry. Radiographs of the parotid gland using contrast media as well as salivary gland szintigraphy is prudent. Immunoserological detection of autoantibodies (anti-SS-A or anti-SS-B) is positive.

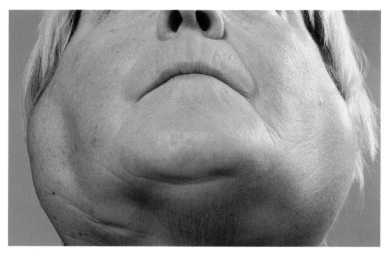

290 Symptoms: parotid contrast radiograph
Left: Lobulated and atrophic tongue; the patient also suffered from dry mouth.

Middle: Atrophy of lingual papillae and xerostomia.

Right: Radiograph of the parotid gland taken with a contrast medium reveals numerous small dilations of the ducts, giving the appearance of a "blossoming cherry tree."

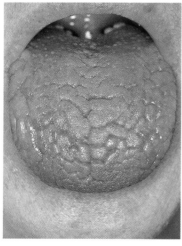
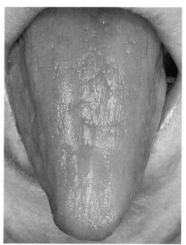
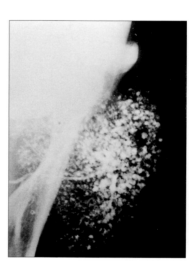

291 Cervical caries/autoantibodies
As a result of the Sjögren's syndrome and dry mouth, this patient developed multiple cervical carious lesions over the years.

Right: Immunofluorescent microscopic view of a small salivary duct in a labial gland, showing the reaction to an antinuclear antibody (IF, x 320).

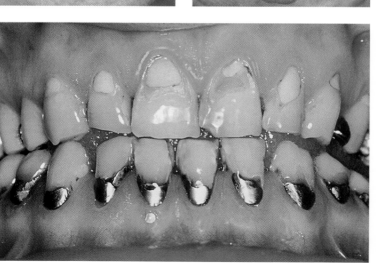
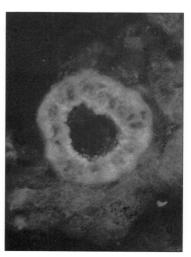

Amyloidosis

Primary, systemic amyloidosis must be distinguished from a secondary condition caused mainly by chronic inflammatory diseases. *Primary amyloidosis* is usually observed in connection with plasmacytoma, which is characterized by the deposition of circulating, monoclonal, light-chain immunoglobulins. On the basis of the variable types of proteins, various forms of the amyloid syndrome can be differentiated. The typical symptoms of primary amyloidosis include macroglossia with papule formation, infiltration, and ecchymoses. This form of macroglossia can occur as an early symptom of plasmacytoma and is pathognomonic.

Hyperpigmentation (HIV-Associated)

Oral hyperpigmentation occurs in 2–4.5% of all HIV-infected individuals (Langford et al. 1989). The clinical picture involves circumscribed, brown-black spots in the area of the buccal mucosa, the gingiva, the hard palate and the lateral borders of the tongue.

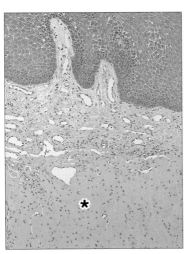

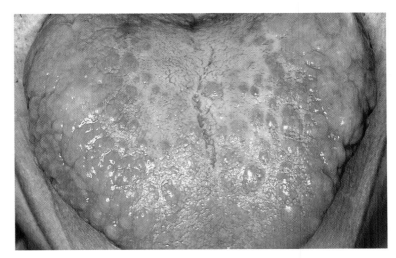

292 Primary amyloidosis
The tongue of this elderly patient with plasmacytoma exhibits the typical macroglossia with concurrent amyloidosis. The dorsum of the tongue and the lateral borders are virtually covered by large, glassy-appearing papules.

Left: The histologic picture reveals homogeneous deposition (*) of amyloid in the submucosal area. The amyloid can be easily made visible with special staining techniques, such as Congo red and thioflavin-T (H & E, x 100).

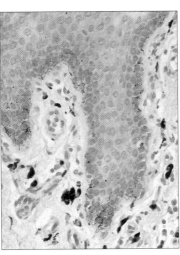

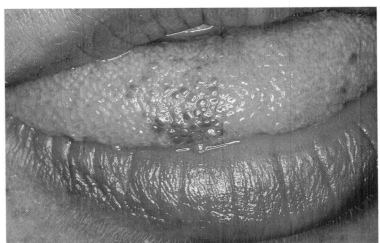

293 HIV-associated pigmentation
On the tip of the tongue of this HIV-infected patient one notes a circumscribed pigmentation of the papillae. Over the course of two years it involved large areas of the tongue and oral mucosa.

Left: Histologic picture of pigmentation. Multiple melanin granules are observed in the basal cells and in the subepithelial region; these appeared following ketoconazole therapy (silver impregnation, x 150).

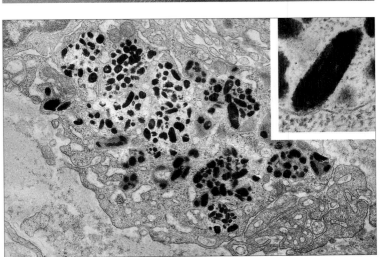

294 HIV-associated pigmentation
Electron microscopic picture with melanosomes, which are present in the cytoplasm. The upper right inset depicts a melanosome at higher magnification
(TEM, x 30 000).

Floor of the Mouth

Definition—Anatomy

The floor of the mouth is divided into one frontal and two lateral areas. The frontal region lies between two lines that extend from the distal surfaces of both canines to the lingual frenum and the anterior mandibular alveolar process lingually. The lateral regions comprise an area posterior to the frontal region between the lingual mucogingival vestibulum and the base of the tongue (Kramer et al. 1980).

From a diagnostic point of view, the floor of the mouth is an especially important region. It is easy to overlook this region during a clinical examination, especially when patients have no complaints. In the rest position, the tongue covers the floor of the mouth, so patients must be instructed to lift the tongue to permit examination of the ventral surface of the tongue and the floor of the mouth. Several especially serious, even life-threatening diseases occur on the floor of the mouth, and these must be detected at the earliest possible time.

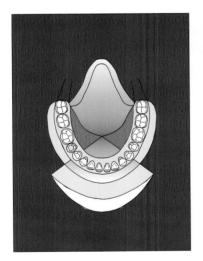 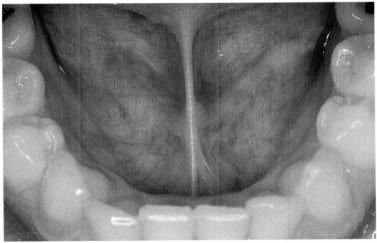

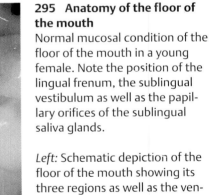

295 Anatomy of the floor of the mouth
Normal mucosal condition of the floor of the mouth in a young female. Note the position of the lingual frenum, the sublingual vestibulum as well as the papillary orifices of the sublingual saliva glands.

Left: Schematic depiction of the floor of the mouth showing its three regions as well as the ventral surface of the tongue.

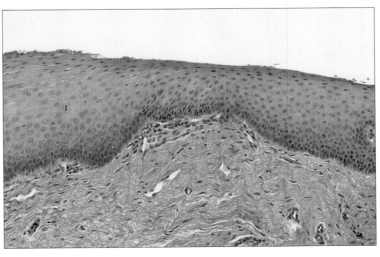

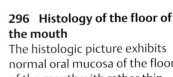

296 Histology of the floor of the mouth
The histologic picture exhibits normal oral mucosa of the floor of the mouth with rather thin epithelium. Note the presence of a focal parakeratosis and also the absence of rete pegs (H & E, x 80).

Anomalies

Ankyloglossia, Lingual Varicosities, Mandibular Torus

Ankyloglossia is a condition in which movement of the tongue is severely limited due to a short lingual frenum. The condition can be congenital or may be caused by trauma. The prevalence of the congenital form is 0.04–6.8%. Diastemata of the mandibular anterior teeth and gingival recession may be consequences of this condition.

The prevalence of *lingual varicosities*, or phlebectasias, is 68% in individuals over the age of 60 (Ettinger and Mander-

son 1974). The ventral surface of the tongue and the floor of the mouth exhibit small, round, violet-blue elevations that result from dilated veins. The most common location is near the salivary gland papillae.

The *mandibular torus* is an exostosis which occurs above the myohyoid line at the level of the premolars. The prevalence rate varies between 7 and 40%. Frequency and size both increase with increasing age.

297 Ankyloglossia ("tongue-tie")
The lingual frenum in this patient is broad, fibrosed and shortened. Surgical treatment can involve severing or lengthening the frenum, which permits greater lingual mobility. The occurrence of speech impediments due to ankyloglossia has probably been overestimated.

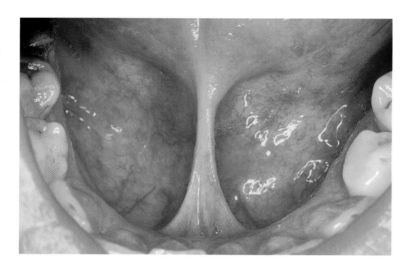

298 Lingual Varicosities
Left: On the left side of the ventral surface of the tongue one notes a distended vessel; this is often the initial event leading to lingual varicosities.

Right: Typical varices on the ventral surface of the tongue; the lesions appear in a row "like pearls on a string" (arrows). It is also referred to as "caviar tongue."

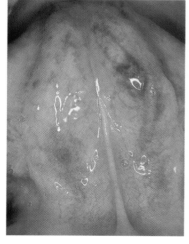
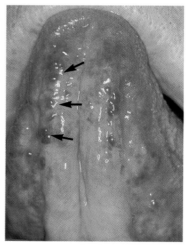

299 Mandibular Torus
Obvious in this clinical picture are the bilateral tori, which are of varying size and lobulation. The overlying mucosa is normal, and the superficial vasculature can be observed. This situation does not present an indication for surgical removal of the tori. In older patients who require a mandibular denture, surgical removal of the tori may be indicated. Among Caucasians, the prevalance is about 7%, while it is found in nearly 40% of the Eskimo population.

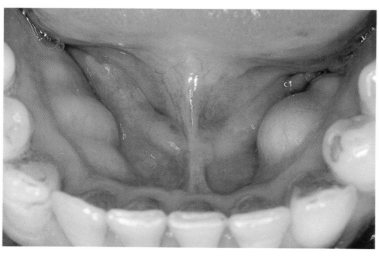

Disturbances of Keratinization

Leukoplakia

There is significant variation in incidence and prevalence of oral leukoplakia in various geographic regions. In a prospective, 10-year study in various regions in India with differing tobacco use habits, the annual, age-corrected incidence was 1.1 to 2.4 per 1000 inhabitants for males and 0.2 to 1.3 for females. The prevalence varied between 0.2 and 4.9% (van der Waal et al. 1997). In Sweden, the prevalence rate was 3.6%, and in Berlin it was 0.9% (Reichart et al. 1996). Leukoplakia occurs most often after the age of 30; the main inci-

dence, however, is in patients over 50 years old (van der Waal et al. 1997). There is significant variation in the gender distribution in the various studies: in India, males are most often affected, but for most Western countries, the male:female ratio is identical. Leukoplakia may appear as separate, localized lesions of the oral mucosa or as diffuse, often multiple forms. (Additional information about leukoplakia can be found on pp. 11, 15, 52, 73, 100, and 154).

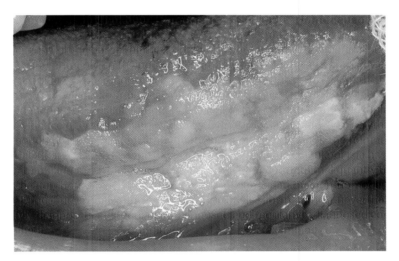

300 Homogeneous leukoplakia
On the right lateral border of the tongue and primarily on the ventral surface of the tongue, one can observe an extensive, homogeneous leukoplakia. There is no evidence of erythroplakia.

Although the homogeneous type of leukoplakia has less tendency to malignantly transform than the non-homogeneous form, it must nevertheless be carefully diagnosed and regularly examined.

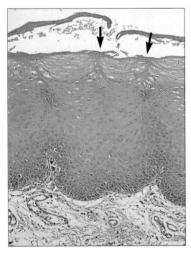

301 Homogeneous leukoplakia
This clinical picture reveals variably severe homogeneous leukoplakia of the ventral surface of the tongue and floor of the mouth. Some areas appear as leukoedema, others as thick, white spots.

Left: Histologic picture of homogeneous leukoplakia exhibiting hyperparakeratosis and the "Christmas tree" configuration (chevron-type of keratinization) (arrows) that is typical for patients who use tobacco (H & E, x 100).

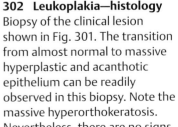

302 Leukoplakia—histology
Biopsy of the clinical lesion shown in Fig. 301. The transition from almost normal to massive hyperplastic and acanthotic epithelium can be readily observed in this biopsy. Note the massive hyperorthokeratosis. Nevertheless, there are no signs of epithelial dysplasia (H & E, x 60).

Leukoplakia of the floor of the mouth and the ventral surface of the tongue comprises 10–15% of all intraoral leukoplakia. Much of the homogeneous leukoplakia in this area exhibits a wavy appearance, like a beach at ebbing tide.

One interesting aspect of leukoplakia of the floor of the mouth is that females are affected in almost three-quarters of cases, while for other areas of the oral cavity female involvement is only one-third. In patients with leukoplakia of the floor of the mouth, the number of cigarillo smokers is significantly higher than those with other localizations of leukoplakia. Leukoplakia of the floor of the mouth is associated with a significantly higher risk of malignant transfor-

mation than is the case for lesions in other areas of the oral cavity.

Erythroplakia

Erythroplakia is a rare lesion of the floor of the mouth, which appears as a well-demarcated, red spot. Histopathologically, it appears as pronounced epithelial atrophy with dysplasia, and a carcinoma *in situ* or a squamous cell carcinoma is often already present.

303 Homogeneous leukoplakia
Homogeneous, well-demarcated leukoplakia of the floor of the mouth in a 57-year-old female who smoked 10–15 cigarillos per day. The mild folding is a typical sign of tobacco use. After cessation of smoking, lesions such as this leukoplakia may disappear completely within a few months.

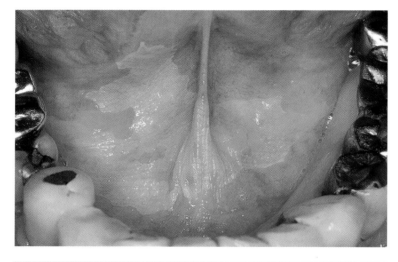

304 Non-homogeneous leukoplakia/erythroplakia
Non-homogeneous leukoplakia or erythroleukoplakia of the floor of the mouth. In the midline, note the area of small, white, noduleshaped formations against an erythematous background. This form of erythroleukoplakia is associated with a higher risk of malignant transformation.
Right: Erythroplakia of the floor of the mouth to the left of the lingual frenum. The probability of malignant transformation is particularly high.

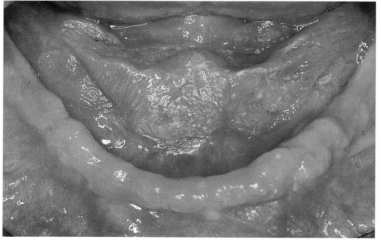
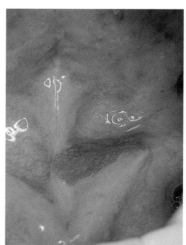

305 Leukoplakia—histology
The histologic picture shows an epithelial atrophy with mild to moderate atypia of the epithelium (H & E, x 160).

Right: Histologic picture of the clinical situation shown in Fig. 304 (left). The epithelium is atrophic as well as hyperplastic. In addition to moderate atypia, note the massive infiltrate of inflammatory cells (H & E, x 80).

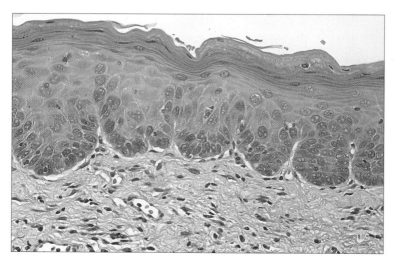
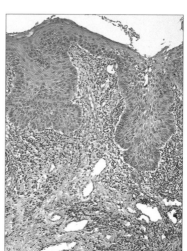
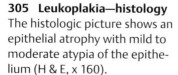

Benign Tumors

Lipoma and Verrucous Hyperplasia

The *lipoma* is a slowly-growing, painless, benign tumor of adipose tissue, which occurs primarily in the fourth and fifth decades of life. Apart from the buccal mucosa, the floor of the mouth is the most frequent location. The lipoma is well circumscribed, round or oval in shape, and may be broadly attached or pedunculated. The overlying mucosa appears smooth and unremarkable; the color is yellow. The differential diagnosis should include mucocele of the floor of the mouth.

Verrucous hyperplasia is similar in appearance to verrucous carcinoma (Ackerman's tumor). A similar lesion has been described as florid, oral papillomatosis. Hansen et al. (1985) reported a further similar form, which they called proliferative verrucous leukoplakia. Verrucous hyperplasia is usually diagnosed in patients over the age of 60. All areas of the oral cavity can be affected, primarily the gingiva, alveolar mucosa, tongue and floor of the mouth. Epithelial dysplasia is detected in 70% of cases.

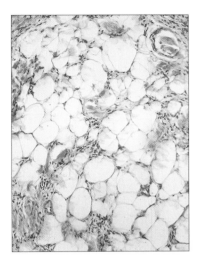

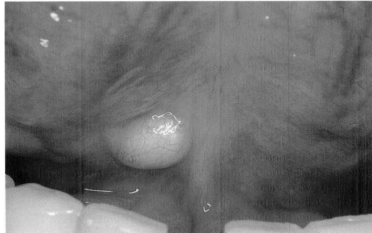

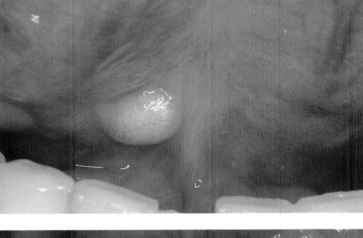

306 Lipoma
To the right of the lingual frenum, note a small lipoma that is yellow in color. The overlying mucosa reveals the vascular pattern. There were no clinical symptoms.

Left: The lipoma consists of normal fat cells with interstitial connective tissue. If the lesion contains a high content of connective tissue, the lesion is described as a fibrolipoma. The treatment consists of simple surgical excision (H & E, x 60).

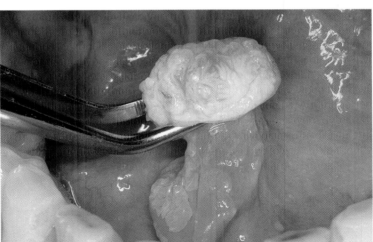

307 Verrucous hyperplasia
The floor of the mouth exhibits a homogeneous leukoplakia as well as an area of tissue hyperplasia that exhibits a white, wart-like surface when lifted with the forceps. Additional leukoplakia lesions were detected on the buccal mucosa and the alveolar mucosa. This patient was a heavy cigarette smoker.

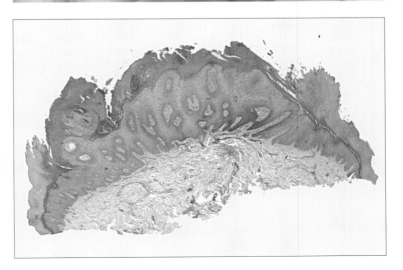

308 Verrucous hyperplasia— histology
The histologic picture of verrucous hyperplasia exhibits pointed, long, heavily keratinized, verrucous processes, or wide, flat, less heavily keratinized pegs. The epithelium is usually hyperplastic and orthokeratotic. It is often difficult to differentiate this lesion from verrucous carcinoma in the differential diagnosis (H & E, x 12).

Malignant Tumors

Carcinoma and Verrucous Carcinoma

Carcinoma of the floor of the mouth encompasses 10–15% of all cancers of the oral cavity in most Western countries. Such tumors are detected in middle-aged and elderly individuals, with the highest prevalence in the seventh decade of life. Invasion into adjacent structures, including the mandible, often occurs early on. The clinical picture is an ulcerated lesion with raised, indurated borders. Erythroplakia is a common component in carcinoma of the floor of the mouth.

From 2 to 20 percent of all carcinomas of the oral cavity are of the verrucous type (Ackerman's tumor). This type of oral cavity carcinoma is observed primarily in Southern and Southeast Asia. The buccal mucosa, the tongue and the floor of the mouth are often affected. Verrucous carcinoma is characterized by expansive growth, but relatively little invasion. The tumor appears as a white, papillomatous mass with deep folds and grooves. The prognosis is better than that of squamous cell carcinoma (Slootweg and Müller 1983). (See also pp. 54, 79, 108, 170, and 198.)

309 Squamous cell carcinoma
The squamous cell carcinoma (arrows) is located adjacent to less apparent leukoplakic alterations of the floor of the mouth (arrowheads). If the patient stops smoking, these unobtrusive areas of leukoplakia will disappear within a few weeks. The carcinoma, however, will persist.

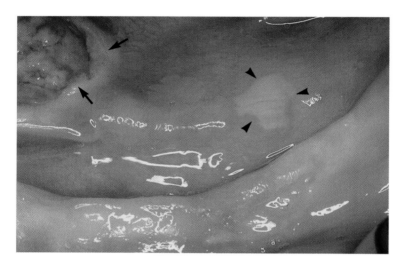

310 Ulcerated carcinoma of the floor of the mouth within an area of leukoplakia
The brown-black stains on the remaining teeth indicate long-term, intensive use of tobacco. The condition of the teeth is hopeless. Poor oral hygiene can elicit a certain premorbidity of the oral mucosa in the form of chronic inflammation. The significance of chronic trauma, for example, due to the sharp root fragments, may also be an accelerating factor.

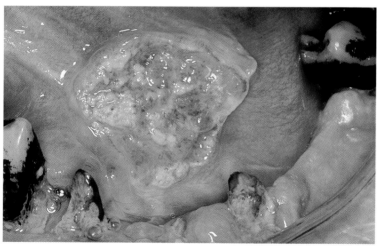

311 Verrucous carcinoma
A white lesion of varying thickness is observed in the anterior region of the floor of the mouth; leukoplakia is apparent. On the ventral surface of the tongue one can observe a papillomatous, sharply-demarcated tumor.
Right: The histologic picture reveals a verrucous carcinoma exhibiting hyperkeratotic and hyperplastic epithelium that is well differentiated, with an intact basement membrane. A severe inflammatory reaction is evident in the stroma (H & E, x 80).

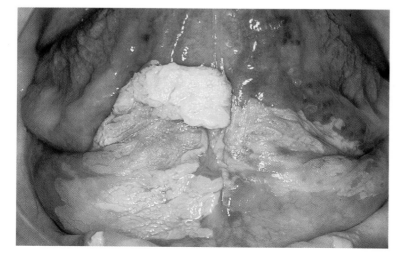
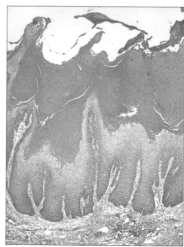

Other Lesions

Ranula

The term ranula describes a mucocele of the floor of the mouth. The ranula is usually a unilateral lesion, with a bluish, translucent appearance. The name "ranula" derives from the balloon-like appearance of these lesions, reminiscent of the distended belly of a frog. The ranula may be superficial or deep. The superficial variety derives from retention or extravasation, usually in connection with traumatization of one of the many orifices of the sublingual salivary glands.

Dermoid and Epidermoid Cysts

Dermoid or epidermoid cysts are most often observed between ages 15 and 35. The midline of the floor of the mouth is most often affected.

Dermoid cysts of the floor of the mouth are filled with skin and skin-related structures, such as hair follicles, sweat glands, sebaceous glands and occasionally even teeth (King et al. 1994).

Epidermoid cysts are lined exclusively with keratinized epidermis and do not exhibit accessory structures. Occa-

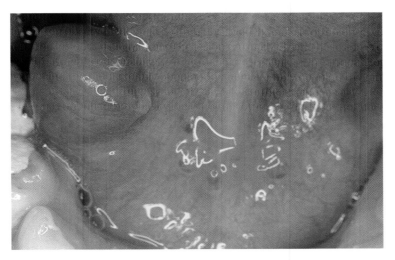

312 Ranula
Ranula is often observed in children. The lesion is usually painless. Treatment consists of simply opening the ranula to permit escape of saliva. Recurrence of the lesion is not uncommon.

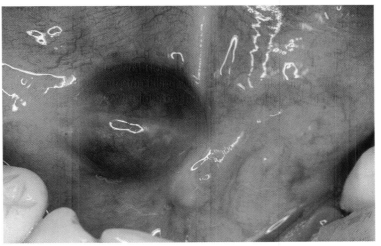

313 Ranula
Ranula in the region of the right, middle area of the floor of the mouth, with a bluish-gray coloration. The color is due to the lesion filling with saliva, mixed with internal hemorrhage.

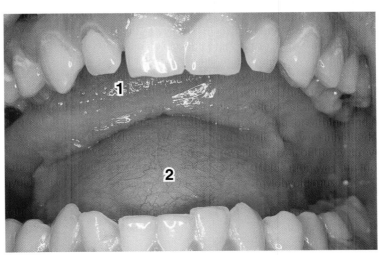

314 Epidermoid cyst
This 23-year-old male had been aware for several years of the presence of a sublingual swelling, which had slowly increased in size. The tongue was distinctly elevated. The patient's speech, eating, breathing and mouth closure were inhibited. Surgical removal of the cyst revealed that its location was superior to the mylohyoid muscle.

1 Tongue
2 Epidermoid Cyst

sionally, areas of pseudostratified epithelium may be found. The lumen is filled with masses of keratin.

Thyroglossal Duct Cyst

The primordium of the thyroid gland develops at about the fourth intrauterine week at the base of the tongue, a region that later becomes known as the foramen caecum. The thyroglossal duct disintegrates at about the tenth week of life. Remnants of this duct can lead to the development of cysts along the developmental pathway of the gland. These lesions are localized in the region of the hyoid bone, the floor of the mouth, or at the foramen caecum. Thyroglossal

cysts are found in the midline; they move upward when the patient swallows or protrudes the tongue. The histologic picture reveals a cyst lining composed of squamous epithelium as well as pseudostratified epithelium with cilia.

315   Incised epidermoid cyst
This epidermoid cyst derives from the patient in Fig. 314. The incised cyst exhibits the characteristic whitish-yellow keratin substance, which emits an acidic odor.

Right: Histologic picture of the epidermoid cyst, revealing an epithelial lining that is free of dermal structures. The lumen is filled with the typical, layered keratin material (H & E, x 60).

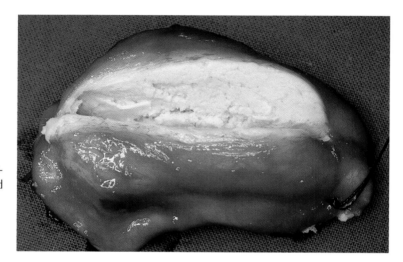
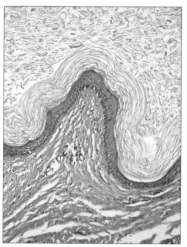

316   Thyroglossal duct cyst
The left side of the floor of the mouth is slightly elevated.

Right: In this female, one observes extraorally a swelling beneath the chin (left). The cyst is soft, mobile and not painful.

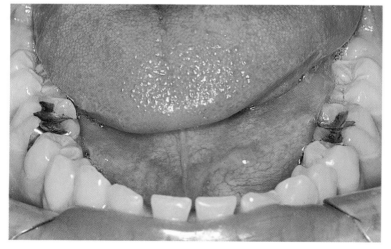
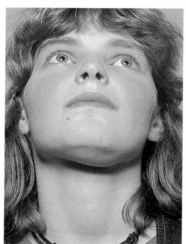

317   Thyroglossal duct cyst
Left: This young male exhibits a thyroglossal duct cyst in the midline at the level of the hyoid bone. The swelling had increased slowly over a period of years.

Right: Schematic depiction of a sagittal section through the head-neck region showing the various localizations of a thyroglossal duct cyst. The arrow points to the location of the cyst shown in the patient in the left photograph.

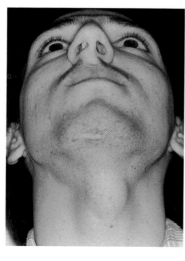
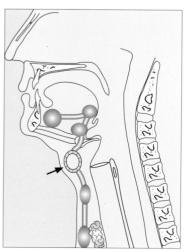

Sialolithiasis

The formation of sialoliths (salivary calculus) in the salivary ducts or in the salivary glands is almost always accompanied by inflammatory alterations of the gland. Sialadenitis with the accompanying sialolith formation occurs most often in middle age, with males being more often affected than females. Sialoliths occur primarily in the submandibular gland, followed by the parotid and the sublingual glands. Because of blockage of the saliva flow, the affected glands are enlarged and painful, especially before and during meals.

If sialoliths are present in the efferent ducts of the submandibular gland and adjacent to the inferior salivary papilla, the concrement can often be observed and palpated intraorally. Sialoliths can also be observed in radiographs. In rare cases, it may be necessary to perform salivary gland szintigraphy, computed tomography, or magnetic resonance imaging to achieve precise localization of the concrement.

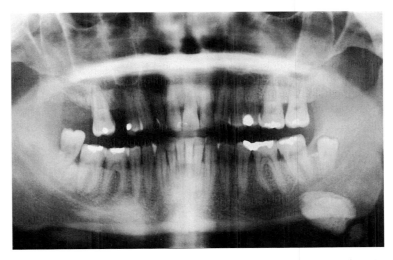

Sialolithiasis

318 Panoramic radiograph
This radiograph reveals a large sialolith in the region of the left submandibular gland. Calcifications within the cervical lymphnodes present a similar radiographic picture. Surgical removal of sialoliths within salivary ducts is accomplished by opening the duct. If sialoliths form within the gland proper, extirpation of the gland is indicated.

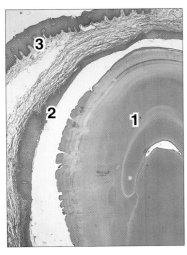

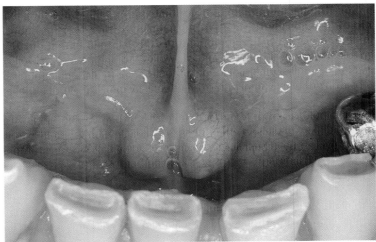

319 Sialoliths lodged immediately adjacent to the orifice of the left submandibular gland
The yellowish color might indicate a lipoma, but palpation revealed the firm consistency.

Left: Histologic picture of the sialolith, exhibiting the typical concentric layers of calcified material (H & E, x 20).

1 Sialolith
2 Ductal epithelium
3 Oral mucosal epithelium

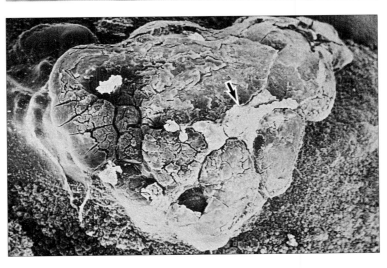

320 Sialolith
Scanning electron microscopic picture of a sialolith. The surface exhibits several soft tissue accumulations (arrow) as well as scale-like, partially granular, smooth or rough mineralized structures which exhibit layering (SEM, x 200).

Recurrent Aphthous Ulcers (RAU)

Recurrent aphthous ulcers (RAU) are characterized by recurring ulcerations in nonkeratinized oral mucosa. Although they are usually localized on the lips and cheeks, they may also occur on the floor of the mouth. The lesions exhibit a familial tendency and affect females more often than males. Smokers are less often affected than nonsmokers. It is possible to differentiate between major and minor aphthae. The causes encompass a broad spectrum: bacteria, viruses, immunologic and hormonal disturbances, foodstuffs, allergies, gastrointestinal disturbances, emotional stress. Infectious and immunologic mechanisms play the most impor-

tant role (Vicente et al. 1996). Most recently, a possible relationship with Epstein–Barr virus infections was described (Sun et al. 1998).

Crohn's Disease

As a form of regional enteritis, Crohn's disease encompasses granulomatous diseases of the entire gastrointestinal tract, including the oral cavity (Halme et al. 1993).

321 Recurrent aphthous ulcers—clinical findings
A fibrin-coated ulceration with a red halo is noted in the anterior region of the floor of the mouth. The patient had suffered for many years from the chronic appearance of such ulcerations. Since the cause of chronic recurrent aphthae has not yet been ascertained, the only possible treatment is purely symptomatic. The goal of therapy is to shorten the period of healing.

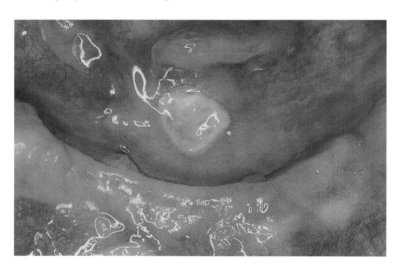

322 Recurrent aphthous ulcers—histology
The histologic picture of recurrent aphthae is nonspecific, appearing as an ulceration (H & E, x 100).

1 Atrophic oral mucosal epithelium
2 Fibrin-coated ulceration with polymorphonuclear leukocytes
3 Lamina propria exhibiting a massive inflammatory cell reaction

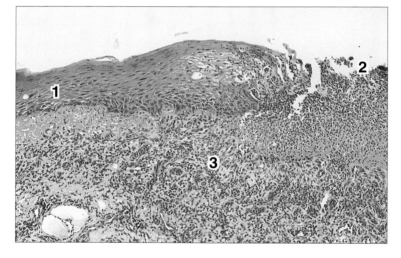

323 Crohn's disease
Adjacent to the alveolar process in the region of the sublingual plica, one notes a linear hyperplastic lesion with ulcerations. These lesions are typical and usually occur bilaterally.

Right: Hyperplasia and ulcerations are frequently also observed in the buccal vestibulum. Treatment for Crohn's disease must be left to the gastroenterologist.

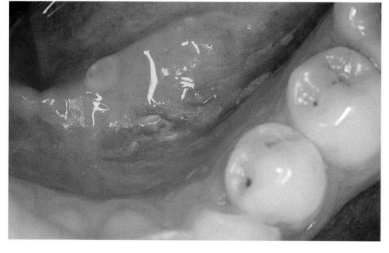
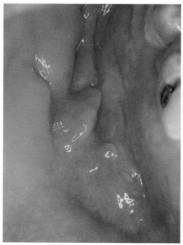

Granulomatous diseases such as Crohn's disease, Melkersson–Rosenthal syndrome, and sarcoidosis are today commonly referred to as "oral granulomatosis" (see also p. 86).

Scleroderma

Progressive systemic scleroderma is a collagen disease of unknown etiology. The disease is characterized by overproduction of collagen types I and III. Early symptoms in the perioral region include increasing microstomia. In addition, there is a thickening and shortening of the lingual frenum, with resultant reduction of lingual mobility. In 60–70% of patients, a widening of the periodontal ligament space can be observed radiographically (Eversole et al. 1984).

Amyloidosis

Amyloidosis primarily affects the tongue, but also the sublingual area and the floor of the mouth. Enlargement of the tongue with subsequent reduction of mobility is characteristic (Reinish et al. 1994).

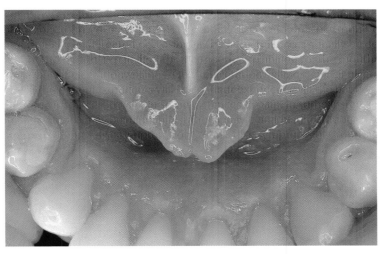

324 Crohn's disease
Symptoms of Crohn's disease may occasionally be detected on the floor of the mouth as painless swellings. Only if ulceration occurs will the patient experience pain. In some instances, these oral manifestations may be early symptoms of Crohn's disease.

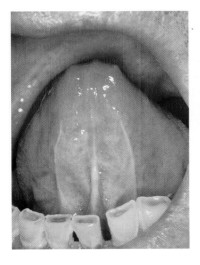
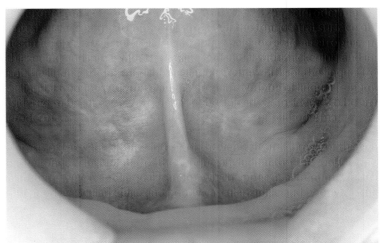

325 Scleroderma
The ventral surface of the tongue exhibits an atrophic, pale mucosa with thickening and initial shortening of the lingual frenum. This type of lingual frenum symptom is considered to be an early sign of scleroderma.

Left: Fibrosis of the ventral surface of the tongue, including the lingual frenum, which appears pale and poorly vascularized.

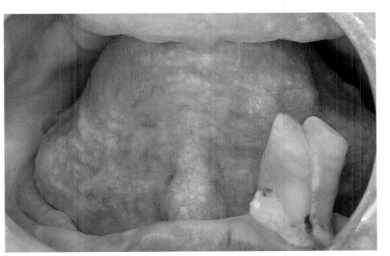

326 Amyloidosis
The ventral surface of the tongue, and especially the lingual frenum are expanded, and exhibit superficial nodular, white papules.
   Amyloidosis is a severe disturbance of protein metabolism and may appear as primary or secondary lesions. The prognosis is extraordinarily unfavorable and there are no special methods of oral treatment.

Palate

Definition—Anatomy

The palate is divided into the anterior hard palate and the posterior soft palate. The *hard palate* consists of right and left halves, each of which form a triangular area between the maxillary alveolar process palatally, the midline, and the junction of the hard and soft palates. The *soft palate* also consists of right and left halves, each of which forms a rectangular area posterior to the junction of the hard and soft palate, and between the anterior tonsillar pillar, and the midline, and including half of the uvula (Kramer et al. 1980). The mucous membrane of the hard palate is tightly affixed to the underlying periosteum and is, therefore, immobile. The epithelium is uniform in character throughout the hard palate, with a thick keratinized layer and numerous slender rete pegs. The soft palate is highly vascularized and of reddish color, noticeably differing from the pale color of the hard palate. The epithelium is nonkeratinized, with few and short rete pegs. The submucosa contains an almost continuous layer of accessory salivary mucous glands.

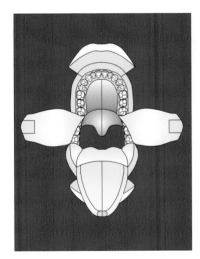

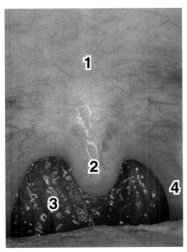

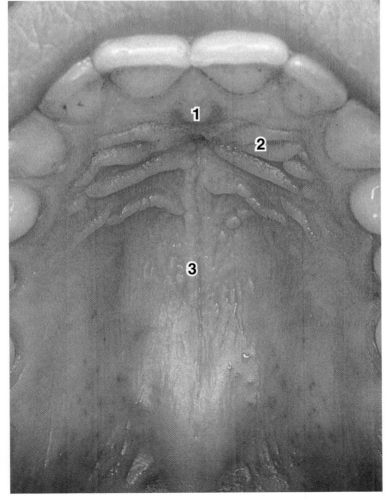

327 Palate—anatomy
Surface morphology of the normal mucosa of the hard palate.

1 Incisive papilla
2 Palatal rugae
3 Palatal raphe

Left, above: The schematic diagram depicts the palatal region with hard and soft palates.

Left, below: Portion of the midline area of the soft palate. The rich vascularization of the soft palate mucosa is obvious.

1 Palatal raphe
2 Uvula
3 Mucosa of the dorsal wall of the pharynx
4 Anterior tonsillar pillar

Anomalies

Palatal Torus and Bifid Uvula

The *palatal torus* is a flat, often spindle-shaped, and occasionally lobulated, symptomless exostosis in the midline of the hard palate. The etiology remains controversial; genetic and racial factors appear to play an important role. The prevalence in Caucasians is about 20%, but is significantly higher in Asians (Reichart et al. 1988).

The overlying mucosa is unremarkable, but may occasionally exhibit ulcerations after traumatization. Histologically, the palatal torus consists of a periphery of dense, compact bone with cancellous bone centrally.

The *bifid uvula* is a clinical micromanifestation of an isolated cleft palate. Various studies have shown the prevalence to range between 1.5 and 10%. It is a symptom of several chromosomal syndromes (e.g., trisomy). The lesion may possibly be genetically inherited. Bifid uvula is more common in males than in females.

328   Palatal torus
Dome-shaped palatal torus in a 45-year-old female; the overlying mucosa is pale and thin. Surgical removal is indicated only when a complete maxillary denture is planned.

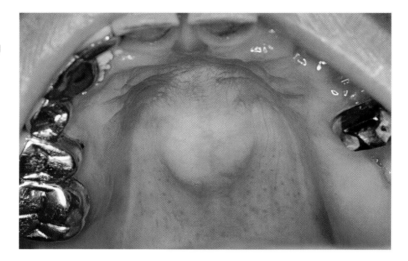

329   Palatal torus
Large, bifurcated palatal torus, exhibiting mucosal ulceration. The lesion is fibrin-covered, crater-like, and exhibits a white, hyperkeratotic border.

Right: Tomography of the same palatal torus. Both of the tori, the larger one on the left and the smaller one on the right, are clearly visible. The degree of opacity corresponds to the surrounding bone.

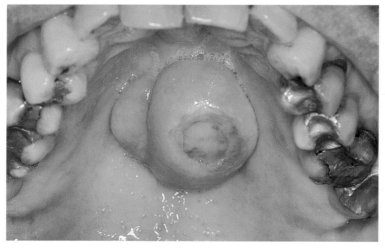
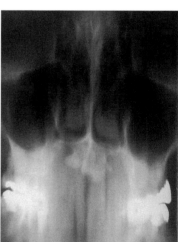

330   Age distribution of palatal torus/bifid uvula
The age distribution of palatal torus exhibits a broad peak between the third and sixth decades of life.

Right: Typical bifid uvula in a 12-year-old male. The diagnosis usually occurs by chance because bifid uvula is free of symptoms or discomfort. No treatment is necessary.

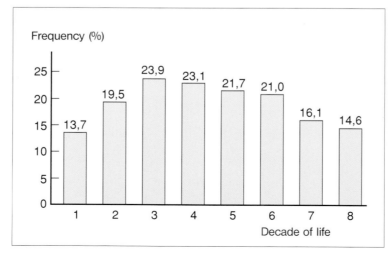
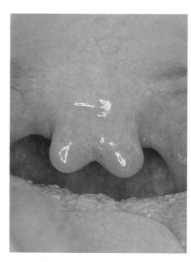

Frequency (%)

Decade	Frequency
1	13,7
2	19,5
3	23,9
4	23,1
5	21,7
6	21,0
7	16,1
8	14,6

Decade of life

Infections—Bacterial, Mycotic

Palatal Abscess and Pseudomembranous Candidiasis

Inflammatory lesions of the palatal area are not uncommon. Such lesions originate from the bone, especially the alveolar process, or from the palatal mucosa itself. An acute exacerbation of a periapical granuloma of a maxillary tooth or a secondarily infected cyst can cause subperiosteal or submucous *palatal abscesses*. The lateral incisors, the first premolars and the first molars of the maxilla are particularly predisposed to this condition, because their roots incline palatally.

Fungal infection of the palate, especially when caused by Candida microorganisms, is often observed in immunocompromised patients. The *pseudomembranous* form of *candidiasis* is often observed on the hard palate, and even more commonly on the soft palate, including the anterior tonsillar pillars in HIV-positive patients.

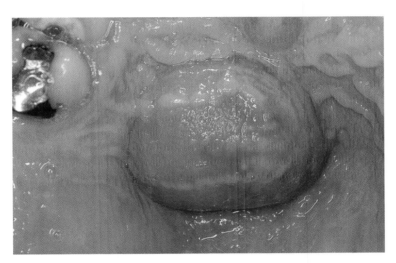

331 Palatal abscess of the anterior hard palate
This abscess derived from a granuloma of the palatal root of the right premolar. Fluctuation was noted, in addition to massive local pain. The clinical course is usually of short duration and, therefore, the differential diagnosis will not include palatal torus or tumor of a palatal salivary gland.

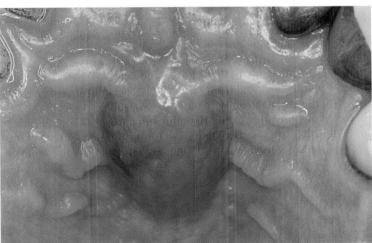

332 Palatal abscess immediately distal to the incisive papilla
This abscess derived from an infected nasopalatine cyst. Palatal abscesses must be incised, with the excision of some mucosa, otherwise the escape of pus from the lumen of the abscess cannot be guaranteed.

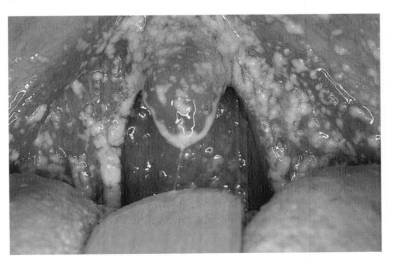

333 Pseudomembranous candidiasis
Acute pseudomembranous candidiasis in an HIV-infected patient; the yellowish-white spots were easily wiped away. These lesions consist of desquamated epithelium, necrotic tissues, inflammatory cells, bacteria and Candida hyphae. The adjacent palatal mucosa is severely erythematous. Difficulties in swallowing and taste disturbances are common in such patients.

Erythematous Candidiasis

As indicated by the clinical description "erythematous candidiasis," these lesions are red, partially due to epithelial atrophy and partially due to increased vascularization of the mucosa. If the lesion occurs on the palate, it is most often diffuse. Although erythematous candidiasis may occur as an isolated lesion on the palate, most often a corresponding lesion will be observed on the dorsum of the tongue. In such cases, it is reasonable to suspect that the palatal erythematous candidiasis was caused by direct contact (contact or kissing lesion), with the tongue being the primary focus of infection.

The differential diagnosis of palatal erythematous candidiasis must include denture stomatitis types I and II. These lesions may also occur in the oral cavity of dentulous patients who are immunocompromised. Symptoms are mild; patients may occasionally complain of a burning sensation in affected regions. (Further information concerning oral candidiasis can be found on pp. 45, 66, and 94.)

334 Poorly demarcated erythematous candidiasis
On the palatal vault one can see a pronounced but poorly demarcated erythematous candidiasis without any accompanying pseudomembranous candidiasis. The patient was HIV-positive.

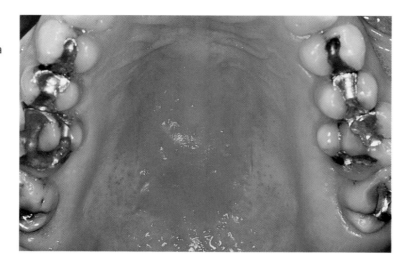

335 Localized erythematous candidiasis on the dorsum of the tongue
This is the same patient as in Fig. 334. The demarcation of this lingual lesion is more defined than in palatal erythematous candidiasis. This form of erythematous candidiasis is also referred to as median rhomboid glossitis.

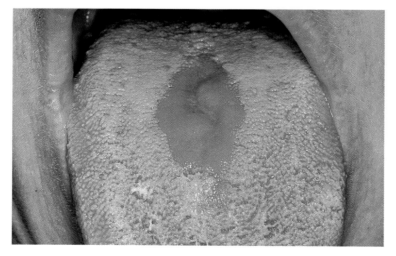

336 Erythematous candidiasis in an AIDS patient
Left: The accompanying xerostomia was particularly disturbing to this patient.

Middle: The palate of the same patient exhibits a diffuse erythematous candidiasis (contact lesion).

Right: The cytologic smear of erythematous candidiasis reveals blastospores. The arrow points to a leukocyte, and the arrowhead to an epithelial cell (PAS, x 360).

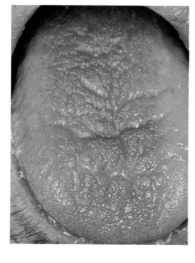
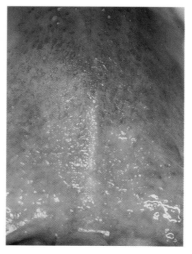
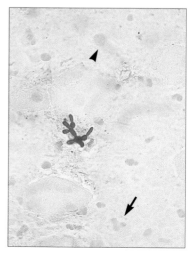

Denture Stomatitis

Inflammatory lesions of the mucosa beneath complete maxillary dentures have been described in various ways; "denture stomatitis" is a generally accepted term. It is subdivided into three types:

- Type 1 – Local inflammation with isolated red spots.
- Type 2 – Generalized inflammation with diffuse reddening of larger areas of the denture-bearing mucosa.
- Type 3 – Extensive inflammation exhibiting papillary or nodular patterns, usually located in the midline of the palate.

The prevalence of denture stomatitis is between 27 and 67%. Etiologic factors include chronic trauma resulting from ill-fitting dentures, bacterial and Candida infections as well as poor oral hygiene (Sakki et al. 1997). An additional important factor is a porous denture base, which enhances the accumulation of bacteria and fungi. Residual monomers in the acrylic base may also play a minor role.

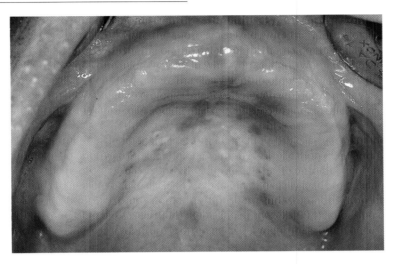

337 Denture stomatitis, type 1
Note the spotty, localized erythema on the palate of this elderly woman who wore a complete maxillary denture.
A cytologic smear was negative for Candida microorganisms in this case.
Topical treatment including application of an antimycotic paste onto the denture base usually leads to healing of denture stomatitis (Könsberg and Axéll 1994). Rebasing of the denture is often necessary.

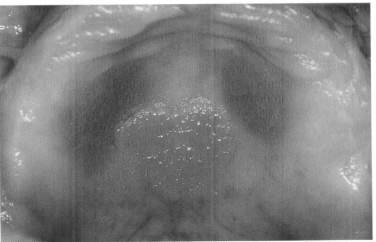

338 Denture stomatitis, types 2 and 3
Note the three large, erythematous, hyperemic regions; the lesion in the midline exhibits a granular, nodular surface. Type 3 denture stomatitis must be surgically removed by means of CO_2 laser surgery or electrosurgery. It is usually necessary to make a new denture. If the denture is not relined or renewed, recurrence of the lesions is to be expected.

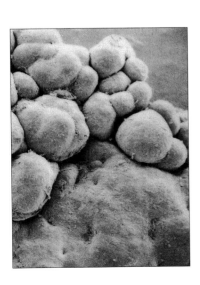
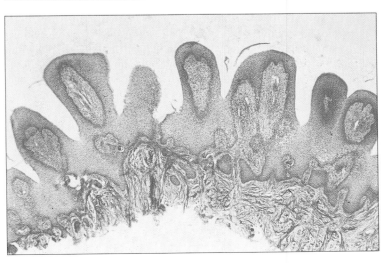

339 Denture stomatitis, type 3—histology
The epithelium is hyperplastic and the surface of the mucosa is irregular, exhibiting numerous rounded "pegs" (H & E, x 80).

Left: The scanning electron microscopic picture reveals the papillary or nodular surface with multiple nodules (SEM, x 50).

Infections—Viral

Herpes Virus Group

Of the more than 50 known viral types in the herpes group, only the following are pathogenic for humans (Scully 1996):

- Herpes simplex virus Type 1 (HSV-1, HHV-1 = human herpes virus 1)
- HSV-2 (HHV-2)
- Varicella zoster virus (VZV, HHV-3)
- Cytomegalovirus (CMV, HHV-4)
- Epstein–Barr virus (EBV, HHV-5)
- HHV-6
- HHV-8, Kaposi sarcoma herpes virus (Chang et al. 1994)

Over 90% of the population have been exposed to HSV-1, and about 50% to HSV-2. Herpes epidemics have not occured for two reasons: HSV-1 and its variants are genetically stable and the lifetime prevalence in people is very high. Herpes infections in the orofacial region are usually due to HSV-1. Less common are reactivations of VZV, CMV and EBV.

340 Herpes simplex virus (HSV-1)
The histologic picture reveals HSV-1-positive epithelium from an oral ulceration (APAAP, x 80). The diagnosis of an HHV infection or reactivation is based primarily on the clinical picture. Because the clinical picture may be atypical, additional methods for detecting the virus may be necessary, such as smears, biopsies or viral culture.

Right: Predisposing factors for reactivation of HSV-1 infections.

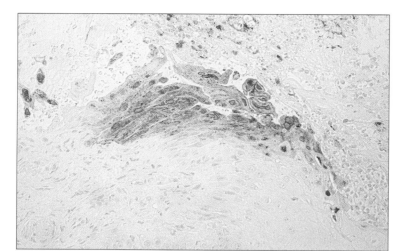

- Exposure to the sun (UV-light)
- Menstrual cycle
- Stress
- Pregnancy
- Gastrointestinal disorders
- Other infections
- Local trauma
- Eczema
- Immunodeficiency
- Food and medication intolerances

341 Herpes virus—ultrastructure
The fine structure of all herpes viruses is identical: ultrathin sections reveal the lipid capsule of the virion, with its glycoprotein spikes, and the isometric capsid that surrounds the viral nucleic acid in the center (TEM, x 150,000).

Courtesy H.-R. Gelderblom

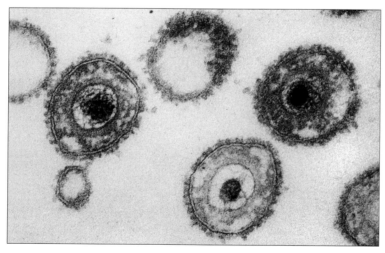

342 Herpes virus—ultrastructure
Sugihara et al. (1990) reported a detection method for EBV using electron microscopy and diagnostic negative staining. Smear preparations are observed directly in the electron microscope immediately after heavy metal salt contrast media. The isometric capsid can be recognized within the coating. Electron microscopy does not, however, permit conclusions about the type of herpes virus (TEM, x 90,000).

Courtesy of H.-R. Gelderblom

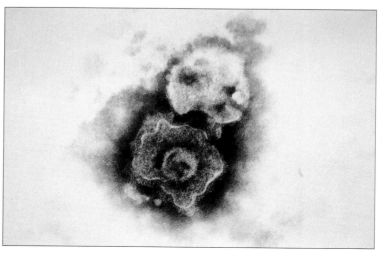
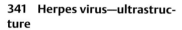

Herpetic Gingivostomatitis

Herpetic gingivostomatitis results from primary infection with HSV-1. However, in only 1% of cases does the complete picture of the disease appear. In 15–40% of individuals infected with HSV-1, recurrence can be expected, with reactivation later in life. (See also pp. 46, 96, and 152.)

Herpes Zoster

Herpes zoster (facial erysipelas) is most common beyond the age of 50. In most cases, it results from a reactivation of varicella zoster virus that has persisted in the Gasserian ganglion. One branch of the trigeminal nerve is usually affected; after a short-term period of blister formation, long-term scab formation on the skin ensues. Several effective antiviral medicaments are currently available (Aciclovir, Famciclovir, Valaciclovir, Foscarnet).

Cytomegalovirus Infection

Cytomegalovirus infection is rare in the oral cavity and is seen almost exclusively in immunodeficient patients (Langford et al. 1990).

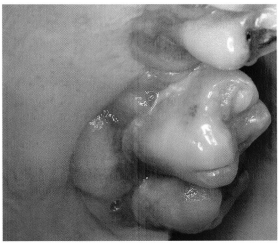
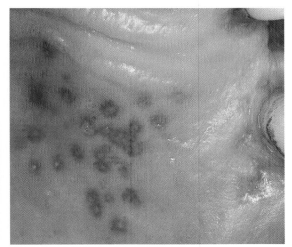

343 Herpes simplex virus 1
Left: Atypical HSV-1 infection in the region of the palatal gingiva of an HIV-infected patient. In such cases of recurrent HSV-1 infection, the clinical course frequently leads to extensive, therapy-resistant symptoms.

Right: A cluster of small ulcerations is observed on the palate as a result of a recurrent HSV-1 infection.

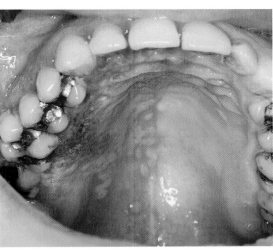
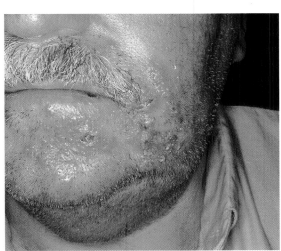

344 Varicella zoster virus
Left: Sharply demarcated, VZV-elicited infection of the second branch of the right trigeminal nerve, with blister formation and erosions.

Right: Blisters, erosion and crusting are apparent in the facial region served by the lower left branch of the trigeminal nerve. This condition is extremely painful. The patient was suspected of suffering from post-herpetic pain syndrome.

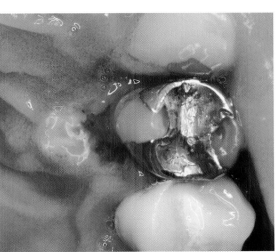
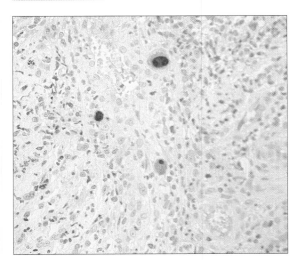

345 Cytomegalovirus
Left: This atypical ulceration on the palate of an HIV-infected patient had been present for a long time and could not immediately be diagnosed. A biopsy was performed.

Right: This high power histologic view reveals cells that are positive for CMV infection (APAAP, x 120). Treatment for these types of lesions must be referred to a specialist.

Verruca Vulgaris

The verruca vulgaris, or viral wart, is caused by the human papilloma virus types HPV-2 and HPV-4; it is observed on the lips, the palate and on the gingiva. The warts occur most often in children who also exhibit warts on their hands. If the child chews on these warts, the virus can be transferred to the oral mucosa. Viral warts are exophytic, whitish in color, with a papillomatous surface. The typical clinical appearance does not permit differentiation between verruca vulgaris and squamous papilloma.

Treatment for oral warts, including the condyloma (see also p. 151) consists of surgical excision, or possibly application of CO_2 laser therapy. Recurrence is rare, but can occur, especially in immunocompromised patients. (For further information about verruca vulgaris, see p. 151.)

Papillomas are, on the other hand, true benign tumors of the oral mucosal epithelium. Recent studies demonstrated HPV types 6 and 11 in 80% of all oral papillomas (Ward et al. 1995).

Verruca vulgaris

346   Localization at the transition zone between the hard and soft palates
This patient had not even noticed the small, exophytic, painless lesion, which exhibited white, finger-like projections. Both verruca vulgaris and papilloma are common in this transition zone. An immunohistochemical examination of this lesion did not reveal HPV-positive epithelial cells.

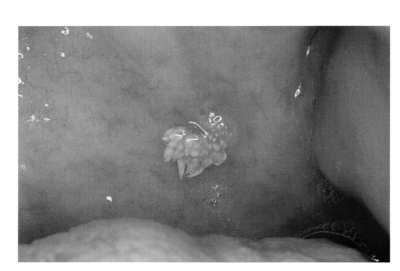

347   Further example with similar localization and histology
This patient presented with a pink-colored, cauliflower-like, pedunculated lesion at the transition zone on the palate.

Right: Histologic picture of a pedunculated oral wart, which exhibits numerous finger-like projections (H & E, x 15).

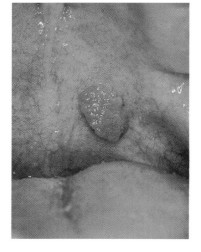
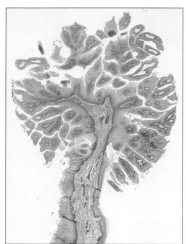

348   Histology
The histologic picture reveals a surface that is characterized by squamous epithelium and pronounced hyperkeratosis. This gives the intraoral wart its whitish appearance (H & E, x 80).

Right: Immunohistochemical depiction of HPV-2 in epithelial cells from an oral wart (APAAP, x 160).

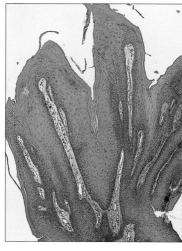
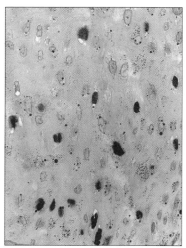

Chemical, Thermal and Mechanical Causes

Smoker's Palate

The frequently used term "palatal nicotinic leukokeratosis" is a misnomer, because nicotine is not a factor in the development of the hyperkeratosis that is characteristic of this lesion. Smoker's palate is a chemical-thermal reaction of the palatal mucosa, which is caused in most cases by pipe smoking. A similar appearing condition may also be observed in nonsmokers who routinely consume extremely hot drinks (Rossie and Guggenheimer 1990).

Following an initial phase that is characterized by palatal erythema, the palatal mucosa assumes a diffuse, grayish-white color. Grooves or folds on the palatal surface are also often observed. Subsequently, the mucosa becomes thickened and exhibits nodules with small red spots in the center. These represent the orifices of the secretory ducts of the minor palatal salivary glands. This form of leukokeratosis is not precancerous.

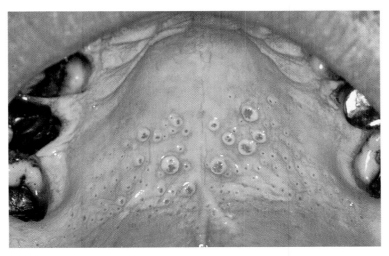

349 Smoker's palate
Typical picture of smoker's palate in an elderly woman who had used two or three packets (50 g each) of pipe tobacco per week over the course of many years. The entire palate is white due to the hyperkeratosis. The palatal salivary glands appear nodular, with reddened, crater-like central areas. These are especially obvious in the middle of the palate. After the patient stopped smoking, the palatal lesions regressed spontaneously.

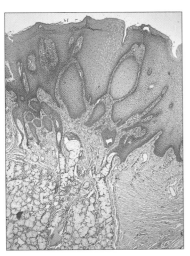
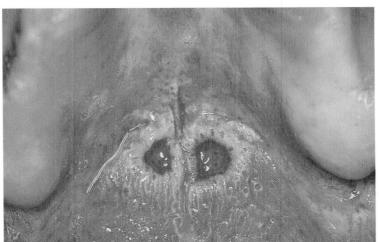

350 Ulcerated palatal foveolae
The palatal foveolae exhibit bilateral ulcerations that were caused by heavy pipe smoking. The lesions are surrounded by a whitish border and exhibit fine, whitish stripes extending toward the soft palate. The hard palate is not affected because it was protected by a complete maxillary denture (removed for this photograph).

Left: Massive epithelial hyperplasia with blockage of the salivary gland duct orifices (H & E, x 80).

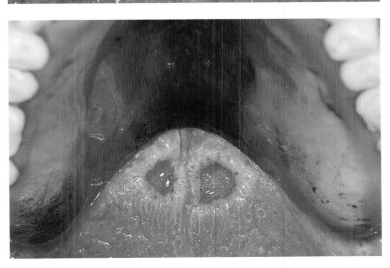

351 Smoker's palate with denture in place
This is the same patient as in Fig. 350, with the maxillary complete denture *in situ.* The palatal surface of the denture exhibits massive accumulations of tar. So-called "reversed smoking," in which the burning end of the cigar or cigarette is held inside the mouth, leads to similar lesions. The habit of reversed smoking is observed mainly in India.

Necrotizing Sialometaplasia

Necrotizing sialometaplasia is a non-neoplastic, spontaneously healing lesion of the salivary glands; the cause is inflammation. The palate is affected in 70% of cases. The age distribution exhibits a peak during the fourth decade of life, and there is an extreme difference in gender distribution, with males affected more often than females at a ratio of 18:1. The lesions are characterized by ulceration and pain. It has been suggested that the lesion evolves as a late stage of smoker's palate or as an infarction phenomenon (Seifert 1998).

Submucous Petechiae Following Fellatio

Mucosal lesions caused by orogenital contact (fellatio; Latin *fellare* = to suck) have rarely been published, even though this sexual technique is a relatively common practice today. The petechiae and ecchymoses result from the intraoral vacuum that is created by sucking.

352 Necrotizing sialometaplasia
Crater-like, punched out ulceration of the palatal mucosa. Following biopsy, the area healed spontaneously within ten days.

Right: The histologic picture of sialometaplasia exhibits pronounced hyperplasia and pseudoepitheliomatous changes of the surface epithelium. This must not be confused with squamous cell carcinoma (H & E, x 60).

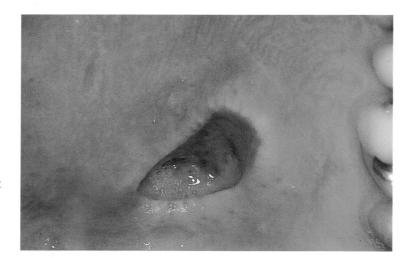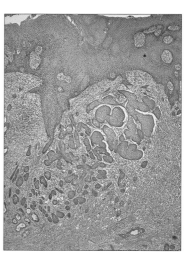

353 Necrotizing sialometaplasia—histology
Pseudoepitheliomatous hyperplasia of the palatal epithelium (arrow) and squamous epithelial hyperplasia of the salivary gland excretory ducts (arrowheads) (H & E, x 120).

Right: In addition to pseudoepitheliomatous hyperplasia (arrow) there is also epithelial metaplasia and dilation of the ducts (arrowhead) as well as necrosis of the acini (*) (H & E, x 60).

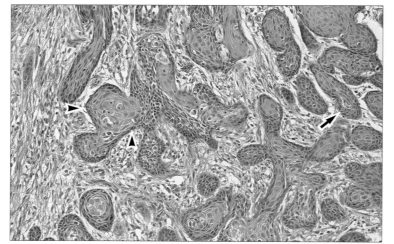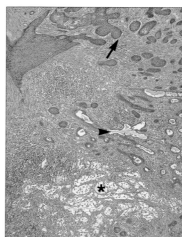

354 Intraoral submucosal hemorrhage following fellatio
Note the ecchymoses and petechiae on the soft palate and on the uvula of a young woman three days after orogenital contact. The patient was concerned about these reddened areas. The lesions disappeared spontaneously within five to six days. No treatment is necessary.

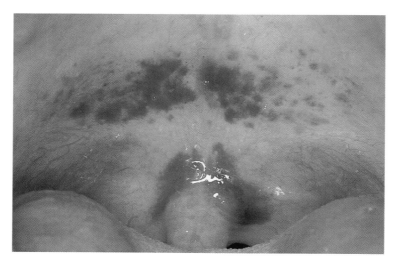

Dermatologic Manifestations

Psoriasis Vulgaris

Psoriasis has a prevalence rate of 2–3% in most surveys. It is a chronic recurring, inflammatory disease of the skin, an inherited regulation defect of the skin that is polygenic. It primarily affects the scalp, nails, elbows and knees; in contrast, the lips and oral mucosa are only rarely affected.

In cases of generalized pustular psoriasis, the pronounced exfoliation may mimic the clinical picture of geographic tongue.

Lichen Planus

Lichen planus is a common inflammatory disease of the skin, the cause of which has not yet been clarified (Becker 1992). Although lichen planus manifests primarily as a dermal lesion, 30–70% of affected individuals also exhibit various oral manifestations. The palate and the floor of the mouth are extremely rarely affected. (See also pp. 80, 101, 156.)

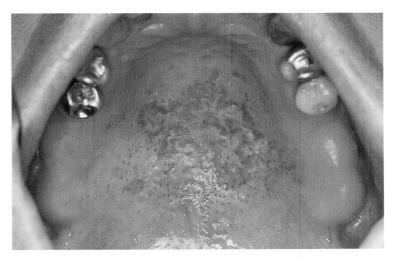

355 Psoriasis vulgaris of the palate
This elderly patient presented with psoriatic lesions on the hard palate. The lesions appear as white spots against an erythematous background. If the dentist suspects that such oral lesions are a manifestation of psoriasis, it is wise to inspect the typical predilection sites (elbows, scalp etc.) for signs of the typical scaly, silver-gray, exfoliative lesions.

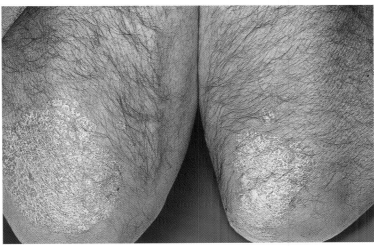

356 Psoriasis vulgaris of the elbows
This is the same patient as in Fig. 355. The elbows exhibit the typical extensive, scaly lesions that could also be observed on the knees, the buttocks, and the fingernails. The skin lesions of psoriasis are often symmetrical. Psoriasis is found especially on regions of the skin that are routinely exposed to increased pressures. The oral manifestation of psoriasis does not require any treatment.

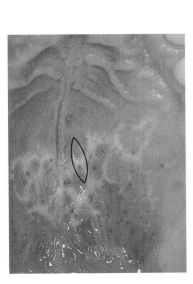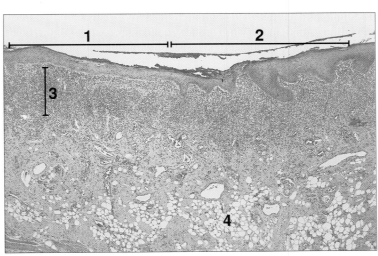

357 Lichen planus—histology
Right: Biopsy of the clinical lesions depicted on the left (H & E, x 60).

1 Epithelial atrophy
2 Epithelial hyperplasia with saw-tooth pattern of the rete pegs
3 Lymphocytic infiltration in the zone between epithelium and connective tissue
4 Fat cell–containing submucosal connective tissue

Left: Reticular lichen of the palate. The biopsy site is outlined.

Pemphigus Vulgaris

Pemphigus vulgaris is an autoimmune disease characterized by intraepithelial blisters of the skin and mucosa. The lesions result from autoantibodies against specific desmosomal proteins of the squamous epithelium (see p. 40). The circulating antibodies against keratinocyte surfaces lead to the loss of cell–cell adhesion. The disease usually appears between the fourth and sixth decades of life. In 60% of cases, oral lesions appear early on (Weinberg et al. 1997).

Pemphigoid

Pemphigoid lesions are caused by specific autoantibodies against various host antigens. Bullous pemphigoid must be differentiated from benign mucous membrane pemphigoid. Elderly females are more often affected. The ocular and oral scarring that occurs with benign mucous membrane pemphigoid is of special clinical significance (Mobini 1998). (See also p. 157).

358   Palatal ulcerations attributed to pemphigus vulgaris
The classical treatment for pemphigus vulgaris consists of corticosteroids combined with other immunosuppressants, such as cyclosporine, azathioprine, methotrexate or cyclophosphamide. Before the introduction of steroid therapy, the fatality rate for pemphigus vulgaris was 50%; today it is 5%.

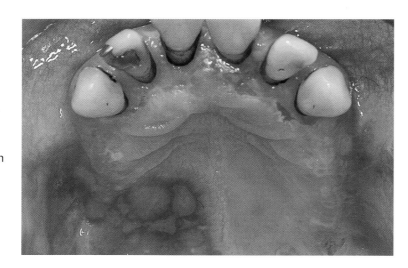

359   Pemphigus vulgaris—histology
The classic histologic picture consists of acantholysis with loss of cell–cell contacts within the epithelium. Intercellular edema occurs, with destruction of the intercellular bridges, expansion of the intercellular spaces and formation of suprabasal blisters. This histologic section depicts initial intraepithelial blister formation (*) (H & E, x 80).

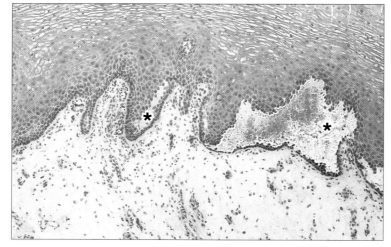

360   Bullous Pemphigoid
The typical oral lesions present as erosions of keratinized or non-keratinized mucosa, as well as the so-called desquamative gingivitis. The gingiva, buccal mucosa and palate are most often affected. In contrast to benign mucous membrane pemphigoid, bullous pemphigoid is not characterized by scars.

Right: Note the subepithelial separation between epithelium and lamina propria, with blister formation (H & E, x 60).

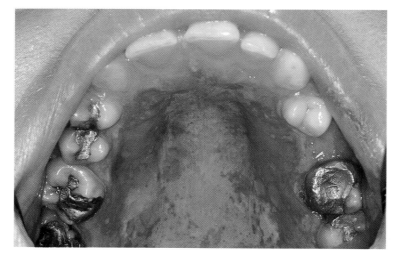
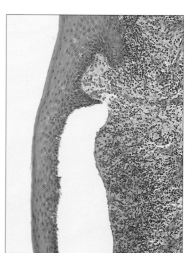

Benign Tumors

Benign tumors of the palate include the "fibroma", the vascular leiomyoma, the cavernous hemangioma, the intramucosal nevus, and the pleomorphic adenoma. These benign tumors of the palate cannot be distinguished clinically or histologically from identical tumors in other intraoral locations.

The *leiomyoma* is more commonly observed on the palate. It derives from the smooth muscle cells of the tunica media of the blood vessels ("angioleiomyoma").

Intramucosal Nevus

The intramucosal nevus is by far the most common of all oral nevi. In contrast to other pigmented lesions, which are almost exclusively at the level of the mucosa, the intramucosal nevus is raised. The differential diagnosis should include oral melanotic macula (Kaugars et al. 1993). Melanotic nevi are brown, bluish or gray; 15% are nonpigmented and reddish. For the differential diagnosis, the most important pigmented nevus is the malignant melanoma.

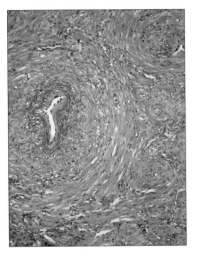 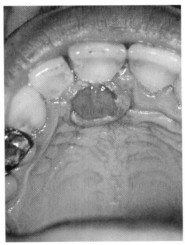 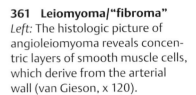

361 Leiomyoma/"fibroma"
Left: The histologic picture of angioleiomyoma reveals concentric layers of smooth muscle cells, which derive from the arterial wall (van Gieson, x 120).

Middle: Angioleiomyoma located palatal to the right central incisor. The clinical picture resembles a traumatized epulis.

Right: "Fibroma" of the anterior midline of the hard palate.

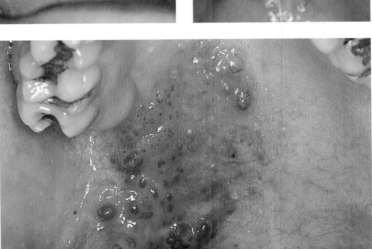

362 Cavernous hemangioma
Cavernous hemangioma of the right soft palate. The color and the nodular surface are characteristic, and are reminiscent of lymphangioma. The latter, however, is usually paler than the hemangioma depicted here. If numerous orofacial hemangiomas are observed, the differential diagnosis should include Sturge–Weber's syndrome.

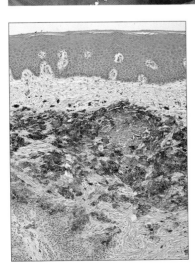 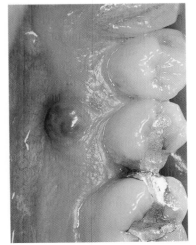

363 Intramucosal nevus
The raised, pigmented lesion appears palatal to the maxillary premolars. In contrast to the hemangioma, applying pressure to a nevus does not cause the region to blanch. Excision is indicated.

Left: Accumulation of melanin-filled nevus cells in the lamina propria. A zone of lamina propria free of nevus cells separates the nevus from the overlying epithelium (H & E, x 120).

Pleomorphic Adenoma

Two-thirds of all adenomas are pleomorphic adenomas, followed by cystadenolymphoma (22%), and basal cell adenoma (4%) (Seifert 1997). Intraoral pleomorphic adenoma is histologically identical to lesions of the major salivary glands. The great variations in tumor architecture derive from two principles of development:

- The varying stages of differentiation of ductal epithelium and modified myoepithelial cells,
- The amount and structure of the stroma.

The stroma-rich pleomorphic adenoma has a tendency to recur because tumor tissue is often implanted into adjacent tissues during surgical tumor extirpation. On the other hand, the cell-rich pleomorphic adenoma exhibits a tendency toward malignant transformation. The surgical technique plays an important role in determining the recurrence rate for pleomorphic adenoma. Following total tumor enucleation, the recurrence rate is below 10%; with subtotal lateral parotidectomy, below 5%; and with total parotidectomy, 0–3%.

Pleomorphic adenoma

364 Histopathologic classification of salivary gland adenoma
This table shows the frequency of the various adenomas of the salivary glands. The pleomorphic adenoma is most frequently diagnosed in the small accessory salivary glands, followed by adenoid cystic carcinoma (adapted from Seifert 1997).

Type of Tumor	n	%
Pleomorphic adenoma	2563	67,5
Warthin's tumor (adenolymphoma)	842	22,2
Basal cell adenoma	146	3,9
Cystadenoma	64	1,6
Oncocytoma	41	1,0
Myoepithelioma	21	0,6
Ductal papilloma	10	0,3
Canalicular adenoma	9	0,2
Sebaceous adenoma	7	0,2
Other adenomas	94	2,5
Total	**3797**	**100,0**

365 Pleomorphic adenoma of the right palate
The lesion was firm to palpation and the overlying mucosa was unremarkable.

Right: Small, spherical pleomorphic adenoma on the anterior third of the palate. This localization corresponds to the anterior zone in which palatal salivary glands are still found.

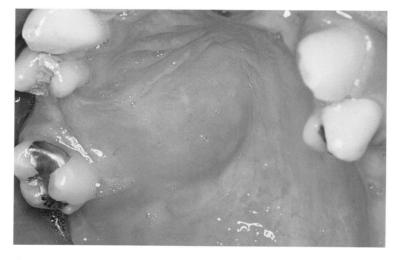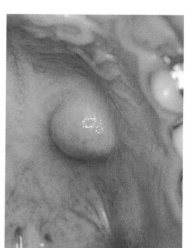

366 Surgical specimen from enucleation of a palatal pleomorphic adenoma
The surface is mildly nodular but well demarcated. It is not possible macroscopically to detect a perforation of the capsule.

Right: Pleomorphic adenoma on the alveolar process near the maxillary molars. Although there are no signs of inflammation, the differential diagnosis could include a palatal abscess.

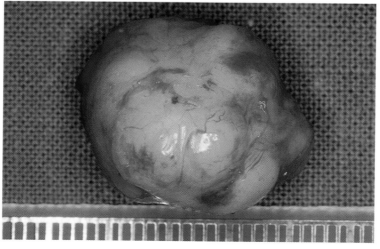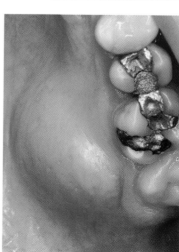

Little is known about the cause of salivary gland tumors in humans. The following have been discussed:

- Genetic influences
- Chromosomal aberrations
- Chemical noxious agents
- Ionizing radiation exposure
- Oncogenic viruses such as Epstein–Barr or the cytomegalovirus, which can remain latent in salivary gland tissues, especially in the epithelium.

From a histogenetic standpoint, the cells of the excretory ducts are involved in the formation of epithelial salivary gland tumors, because they represent pluripotent, regenerative transition zones between the duct system and the glandular acini. The large histologic variability derives from the pluripotent stem cells and their varying stages of differentiation.

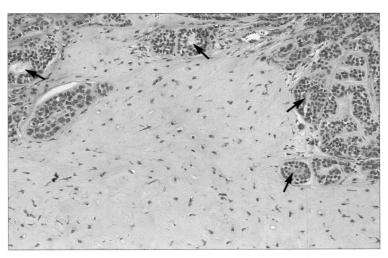

Pleomorphic adenoma

367 Histology
The histologic picture of this pleomorphic adenoma exhibits duct-like structures of epithelial components (arrows). The connective tissue stroma exhibits areas of myxoid degeneration (H & E, x 160).

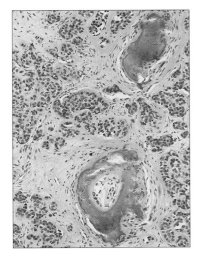

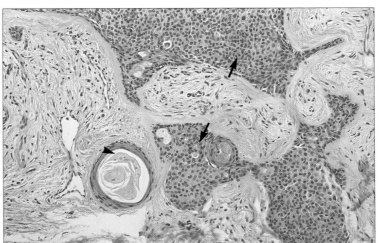

368 Histology
Islands of epithelial and myoepithelial cells predominate in this pleomorphic adenoma (arrows). Keratinized squamous epithelium (arrowhead) is also present (H & E, x 160).

Left: Metaplasia of the connective tissues, with formation of primitive osseous trabeculae (H & E, x 160).

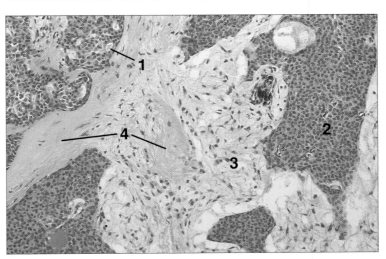

369 Histology
In this pleomorphic adenoma, the cellular spectrum of epithelial components is obvious (H & E, x 160):

1 Epithelial islands which mimic ductal structures
2 Epithelium and myoepithelium
3 Loose stroma
4 Fibrous stroma

Malignant Tumors

Adenoid Cystic Carcinoma

The most common intraoral malignant salivary gland tumor is the adenoid cystic carcinoma, which accounts for between 10% and 30% of all palatal salivary gland tumors. The infiltrative growth with perineural and perivascular expansion and the lack of a cellular stromal reaction at the invasive front are characteristic. The tumor consists of ductal epithelium and modified myoepithelial cells. Three subtypes have been described:

- Glandular–cribriform
- Tubular
- Solid-basaloid

Hematogenic metastases occur in 35–60% of cases, often years following the initial operation. The five-year recurrence and metastatic rate is 14% for the tubular, 36% for the glandular–cribriform, and 70% for the solid-basaloid subtypes (Seifert 1997).

Adenoid cystic carcinoma

370   Clinical findings
Left: A flat, slightly erythematous swelling is noted on the right side of the edentulous maxilla.
The lesion was symptom-free.

Right: In this elderly edentulous woman an erythematous swelling was detected on the palate; the lesion exhibited a dark central area. It is difficult to differentiate clinically between pleomorphic adenoma and adenoid cystic carcinoma of the palate.

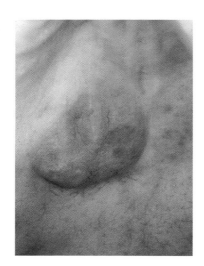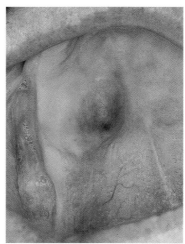

371   Histology
Adenoid cystic carcinoma of the tubular type. The ductal epithelial structures are surrounded by hyalinized, desmoplastic stroma. Residues of normal mucosal acini (*) can also be observed (H & E, x 80).

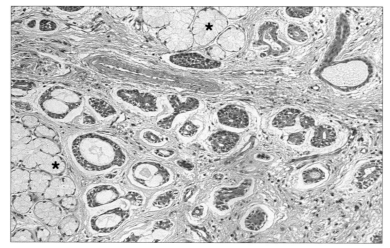

372   Histology
A mixed carcinoma consisting of tubular-solid and adenoid-cystic areas, exhibiting perineural and perivascular expansion (H & E, x 80).

1 Peripheral nerve
2 Vessel

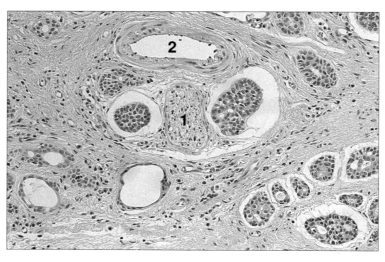

Kaposi's Sarcoma

The epidemic of Kaposi's sarcoma in AIDS patients has been regularly observed since 1981. Homosexual males are most often affected. The human herpes virus HHV8, discovered in 1994 and also known as the Kaposi's sarcoma herpes virus, plays a role in the pathogenesis.

Kaposi's sarcoma occurs as a disseminated mucocutaneous tumor, with lymph nodes and visceral organs frequently involved. Within the oral cavity, the hard and/or soft palates are most frequently affected, followed by the gingiva and the tongue (Reichart et al. 1993, Reichart 1996). It is easy to differentiate the initial, flat lesion from the later-stage tumorous Kaposi's sarcoma: The early lesion is red, violet or brownish-blue; the later tumorous form grows exophytically and often exhibits ulceration. The Kaposi's sarcoma is not classified as a true sarcoma, rather as a possibly reversible hyperplasia of endothelial cells (see also pp. 107 and 166).

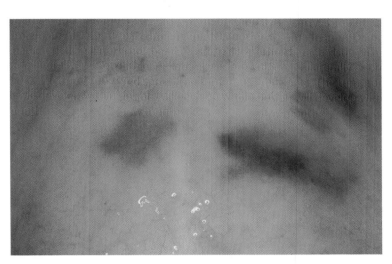

373 Early stage of Kaposi's sarcoma in an AIDS patient
The characteristic palatal lesions appear bilaterally as brownish-red spots. The tumorous type of lesion will develop within only a few months.

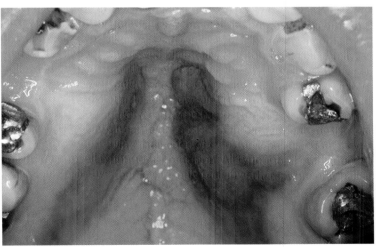

374 Advanced stage of Kaposi's sarcoma of the palate
Kaposi's sarcoma is typically observed bilaterally, as is the case here, following the course of the palatal vessels. On the left side, the lesions have already progressed into the tumorous stage. Treatment consists of intralesional injection of cytostatics or intraoral irradiation. All types of therapy are only palliative.

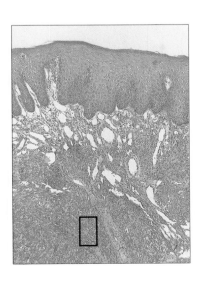
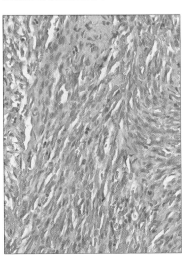
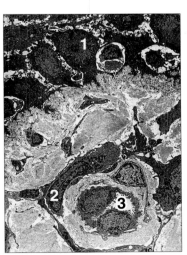

375 Kaposi's sarcoma—histology
Left: Note the numerous vessel lumina lined with endothelium, and spindle shaped tumor cells (marked area) (H & E, x 40).

Middle: Higher magnification of the marked area exhibiting typical spindle cells and extravascular erythrocytes (H & E, x 200).

Right: Electron microscopic picture reveals (**1**) basal cells of the overlying epithelium, (**2**) proliferating endothelial cells, and (**3**) capillary formation (TEM, x 15 000).

Non-Hodgkin's Lymphoma (HIV-Associated)

Apart from the epidemic Kaposi's sarcoma, the malignant non-Hodgkin's lymphoma is the most common tumor that develops during the course of an HIV infection. The prevalence is 8%. These rapidly growing tumors often mimic non-specific ulceration. A pathogenic correlation may exist with an Epstein–Barr virus infection. The morphological spectrum is broad; a new and frequent intraoral subtype has been described as a plasmoblastic lymphoma (Delecluse et al. 1997). A review article was published by Jordan and Speight (1996).

Leukemia

Oral manifestations are common in acute forms of leukemia. Gingival swelling or multiple mucosal nodes are indications of a leukemic infiltrate. The cardinal symptoms are ulceration and hemorrhage, in addition to generalized gingival hyperplasia. The oral mucosa and the facial skin are pale, which may be a further indicator of the underlying disease.

376 Non-Hodgkin's lymphoma
The panoramic radiograph of this AIDS patient exhibits, in the left maxilla, a diffuse radiolucency, which is an indication of a malignant tumor.

Right: Extensive, ulcerated malignant lymphoma that has progressed beyond the stage where cytostatic treatment could be beneficial.

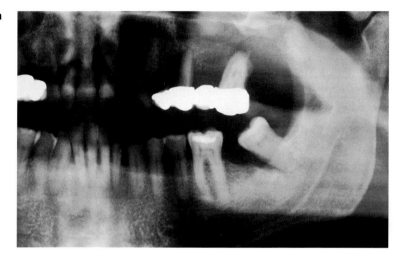
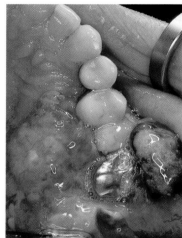

377 Non-Hodgkin's lymphoma—histology
Histologic view of the non-Hodgkin's lymphoma depicted above. Note the presence of lymphoid cells, which are interpreted as B-cells, as well as cytoplasmic inclusions. The histologic picture shown here is similar to that of the classic Burkitt's lymphoma (H & E, x 220).

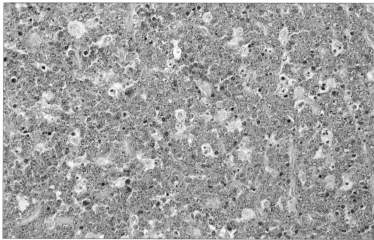

378 Leukemia
This elderly male suffered from an acute myeloid leukemia. The palatal mucosa is the site of multiple leukemic infiltrates, which appear in the form of brown-black nodules and non-specific ulcerations (arrow).

Right: The tongue of the same patient also exhibits multiple gray-black nodules. A pale appearing oral mucosa is often an additional finding in patients with leukemia.

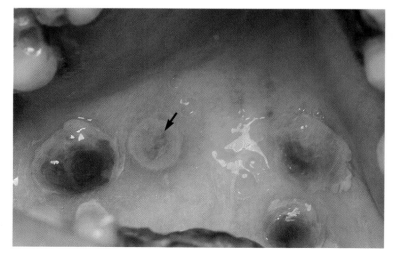
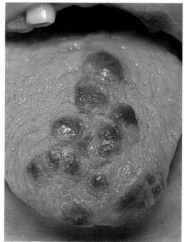

Verrucous Carcinoma

The verrucous carcinoma (Ackerman's tumor) is a squamous epithelial carcinoma whose growth is more expansive than infiltrative. Various epidemiologic studies have reported the frequency of verrucous carcinoma to be between 2% and 20%. It appears most frequently on the buccal mucosa, and with decreasing incidence on the tongue, alveolar process and labial mucosa.

Clinically, the verrucous carcinoma appears as a papillomatous, nodular tumor that is often preceded by leukoplakia. Those affected are usually heavy smokers.

Malignant Melanoma

The primary intraoral malignant melanoma is rare, but it is exceptionally dangerous. Only 0.5%–2.4% of all melanomas occur intraorally. The palate is the most frequently affected site. Malignant melanoma is painless, soft, and varies in color from brown to bluish-black. The lesion may be somewhat raised (Tanaka et al. 1994, 1998).

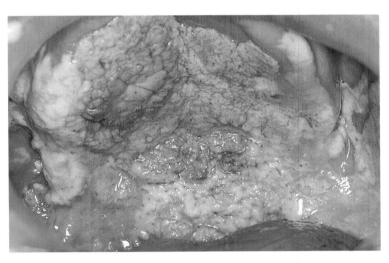

379 Verrucous carcinoma
Extensive verrucous carcinoma of the palate in an elderly male. The papillomatous surface has been stained a brown color in some areas due to tobacco use. This patient had not worn his maxillary full denture for six years.

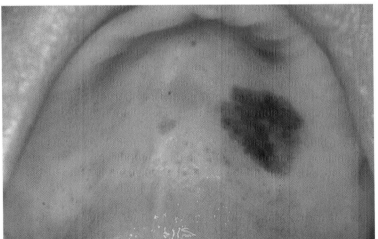

380 Suspicion of malignant melanoma
The heavily pigmented area on the left side of the palatal vault arouses suspicion of a malignant melanoma. The borders are indistinct. Treatment consists of radical surgery, but the prognosis is, nevertheless, unfavorable. Biopsy should *never* be performed if a malignant melanoma is suspected, because of the high danger of metastasis.

Courtesy I. van der Waal

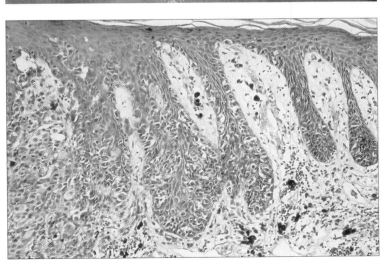

381 Malignant melanoma— histology
The superficial epithelium is partially hyperplastic and partially atrophic. Note the increased pigmentation of the basal cell layer as well as numerous typical and atypical melanocytes. Junctional activity is pronounced (H & E, x 200).

Courtesy I. van der Waal

Gingiva

Of the periodontal tissues, which comprise the gingiva, periodontal ligament, alveolar bone and root cementum, only the gingiva is visible upon clinical inspection. The gingiva consists of the free marginal gingiva, the attached gingiva and the interdental gingiva (interdental papillae). The *attached gingiva* extends from the free gingival groove to the mucogingival junction, where it meets the alveolar mucosa. The attached gingiva is firm in consistency and tightly affixed to the underlying periosteum. In contrast, the alveolar mucosa is mobile due to its loosely structured and highly vascularized connective tissue. This difference in tissue architecture also explains the pale, "salmon pink" color of the attached gingiva and the deeper red color of the alveolar mucosa. In addition to the common nonspecific, inflammatory diseases, numerous other pathologic conditions occur in the gingival area, including manifestations of systemic disease processes. The *Color Atlas of Periodontology* (Rateitschak, Wolf and Hassell 2001) provides an excellent contemporary resource for information about the anatomy and pathology of the periodontal structures.

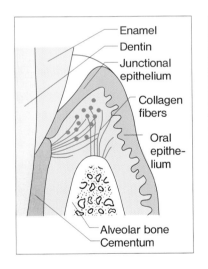

Enamel
Dentin
Junctional epithelium
Collagen fibers
Oral epithelium
Alveolar bone
Cementum

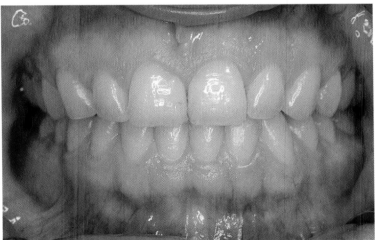

382 Healthy gingiva
Healthy gingiva exhibits neither erythema nor swelling. The surface appears mildly stippled. The papillae completely fill the interdental spaces.

Left: Schematic diagram of the periodontal structures.

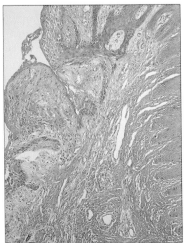

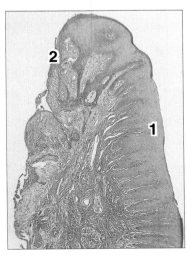

383 Healthy gingiva—histology
This low-power histologic picture of the gingiva demonstrates the gingival epithelium (**1**) as well as the junctional epithelium (**2**), which has been somewhat altered due to proliferation. This is an early characteristic of initial inflammation (H & E, x 20).

Left: Higher magnification of the proliferating junctional epithelium (left). The inflammatory reaction is relatively mild. No areas of hyperemia are apparent (H & E, x 50).

Anomalies and Physiologic Pigmentation

Mandibular Torus, Physiologic Pigmentation

Exostoses represent non-neoplastic osseous hyperplasia. Exostoses on the palatal midline distal to the rugae are known as palatal tori (see p. 128). Such tori are also often observed on the lingual aspect of the mandible. Tori grow slowly and painlessly; they are almost never observed in children. Tori are seen in all racial groups, but are much more common in Asians than in Caucasians (Reichart et al. 1988). The cause of tori is unknown, but there appears to be a genetic–racial component in the pathogenesis. Tori can become quite large; as such they are often associated with injury to the overlying mucosa. The surgical removal of tori is generally a preprosthetic measure.

Physiologic pigmentation, especially on the gingiva, is more common in Blacks and other darker-skinned individuals.

384 Exostoses of the maxillary alveolar process
The maxillary alveolar process exhibits several hard, spherical protuberances, covered by a thin mucosa. This patient exhibited similar exostoses in other areas of the jaws on both labial and lingual surfaces. The differential diagnosis should include osteoma, which has a somewhat less well-circumscribed growth pattern.

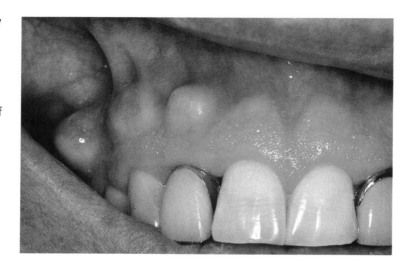

385 Mandibular tori
Mandibular tori are usually bilateral, located lingual to the first and second premolars. Multiple tori are common, and may grow to a considerable size. Surgical removal is achieved using an incision along the gingival margin and a mesial releasing incision. Care must be taken to avoid injury to the floor of the mouth when using rotating burs for the osteotomy procedure.

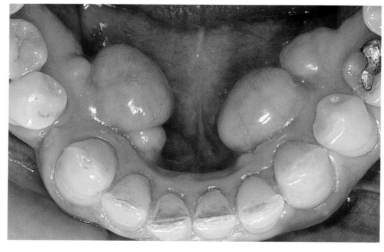

386 Physiologic pigmentation
Evident is the brownish-black coloration of the gingiva, especially several interdental papillae in both maxilla and mandible. Blacks often exhibit such pigmentation in other areas of the oral mucosa, for example, the cheek and tongue. No treatment is necessary. (Note also the massive accumulation of dental plaque and calculus.)

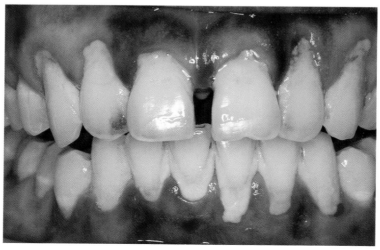

Infections—Bacterial

Gingivitis and Periodontitis

According to a classification by the European Union (EU) clearing house on oral problems relating to HIV infection and the WHO collaborating center on oral manifestations of the human immunodeficiency virus (1993), there are three forms of *HIV-associated gingivoperiodontitis*:

- Linear gingival erythema
- Necrotizing (ulcerative) periodontitis
- Necrotizing (ulcerative) gingivitis

Linear gingival erythema is described as a 1–3 mm wide band of inflammation in the region of the gingiva propria. The pathogenesis of linear gingival erythema remains under discussion. An association with *Candida albicans* has been described (Lamster et al. 1997), similar to erythematous candidiasis.

Necrotizing (*ulcerative*) *periodontitis* has a prevalence rate of 5% or less (Lamster et al. 1997). Severe forms of HIV-associated gingivoperiodontitis are usually associated with advanced stages of immunodeficiency (Johnson 1997).

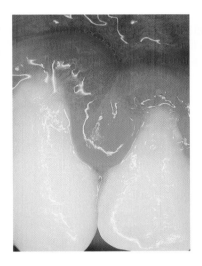
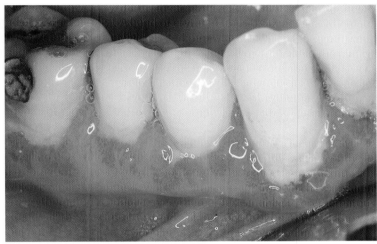
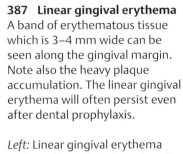

387 Linear gingival erythema
A band of erythematous tissue which is 3–4 mm wide can be seen along the gingival margin. Note also the heavy plaque accumulation. The linear gingival erythema will often persist even after dental prophylaxis.

Left: Linear gingival erythema with swelling of the interdental papilla. Sometimes this reddening, which is similar in appearance to erythematous candidiasis, extends all the way into the vestibulum.

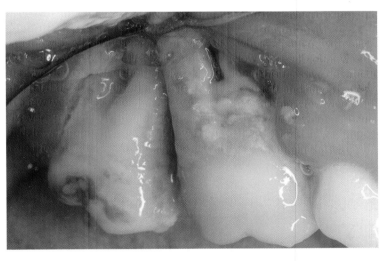

388 Necrotizing, ulcerative periodontitis
In a patient with AIDS whose CD4-cell count was below 10/ml, this massive destruction of both soft and hard tissues occurred within a few weeks. The molar regions were particularly severely affected. It was impossible to maintain these teeth.

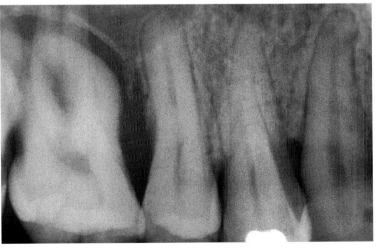

389 Radiograph of area shown in Fig. 388
The first molar area exhibits massive osseous destruction. In the early years of the HIV epidemic, the significance of gingival and periodontal lesions was overestimated. Factors such as lifestyle, professional dental care and the condition of the oral cavity before the HIV infection greatly influence the development and progression of gingivoperiodontal diseases following HIV infection.

In HIV-seronegative individuals, *acute necrotizing, ulcerative gingivitis* (ANUG) has become less and less common since the end of World War II, and the prevalence rate at present is 0.02–0.08%. However, since the appearance of HIV infection, ANUG is becoming much more common. It is observed in 5–11% of HIV-infected individuals (Pindborg and Reichart 1995).

There is no difference in the clinical appearance of necrotizing ulcerative gingivitis in seronegative and seropositive patients. In most cases, the first clinical symptom is pain.

Necrosis of the interdental papilla starts at the tip. Treatment consists of careful oral prophylaxis and instructions for proper oral hygiene.

Abscess—HIV-Associated

In patients with HIV, abscesses of the gingiva and periodontium are much less common than necrotizing gingivitis and periodontitis. When an abscess does occur, the inflammatory symptoms are frequently less pronounced as compared to an immunocompetent individual.

390 Necrotizing gingivitis
Note the crater-like ulceration between the mandibular canine and the first premolar. This is the initial lesion of necrotizing gingivitis. Halitosis is common, and the lesions are often quite painful.

Right: Electron microscopic picture of the microbial flora in necrotizing gingivitis. Spirochetes and Borrelia predominate in these infections (TEM, x 20 000).

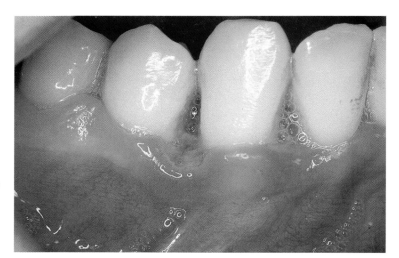 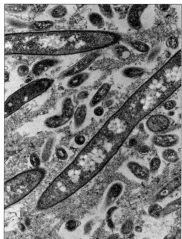

391 Necrotizing gingivitis
Note total loss of the interdental papilla between the mandibular central and lateral incisors. The yellowish-brown coating is an indication of earlier hemorrhage. Frequently, adjacent papillae become infected in a very short time. In rare cases, necrotizing gingivitis can transform into necrotizing stomatitis or into a noma-like clinical picture. This occurs not infrequently in patients with very low CD4-cell values.

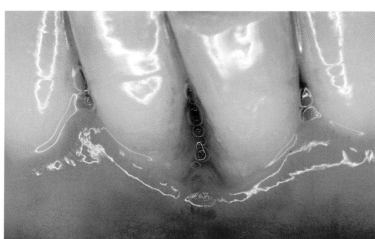

392 Submucosal abscess (HIV-associated)
A periodontal abscess developed between the mandibular canine and first premolar. Note that the symptoms of inflammation are relatively mild.

Right: Acute necrotizing ulcerative gingivitis in an HIV seronegative young male. The poor oral hygiene plays a clear role in the development of this condition.

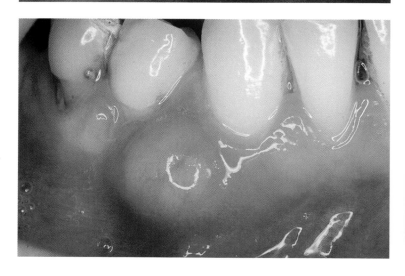 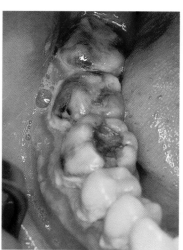

Infections—Viral

Verruca Vulgaris

Warts caused by the human papilloma virus are usually observed in children, but are also seen in HIV-infected adults. At present, 77 types of human papilloma virus (HPV) are recognized (Syrjänen 1997). Verruca vulgaris warts are caused by HPV types 2 and 4. The clinical picture is characterized by white, cauliflower-like or finger-like projections on the mucosal surface (see also p. 134).

Condylomata Acuminatum

Condylomata acuminata (genital warts) are sexually transmitted. The lesions are often found on the anogenital skin and mucosa, first as small nodules that subsequently coalesce. The resulting soft, papillary lesions are then observed on the mucosal surface, either pedunculated or closely adherent. There is a tendency for recurrence following surgical removal, especially in HIV patients. In HIV patients, unusual HPV types may be observed (Greenspan et al. 1988). HPV types 6 and 11 are usually associated with these lesions.

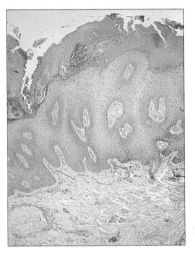
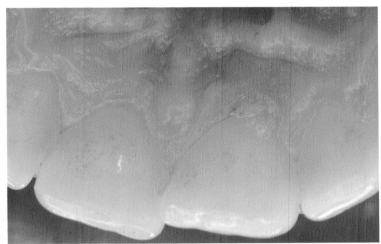

393 Verruca vulgaris
On the palatal aspect of the right central incisor there is a small papillary viral wart which would be easy to miss without careful inspection. This HIV-positive patient was not aware of the lesion.

Left: Histologic picture of verruca vulgaris. Note the pronounced hyperorthokeratosis and epithelial acanthosis. The subepithelial connective tissue exhibits no inflammatory infiltrate (H & E, x 40).

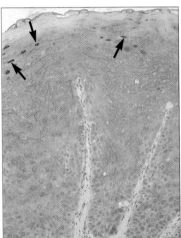
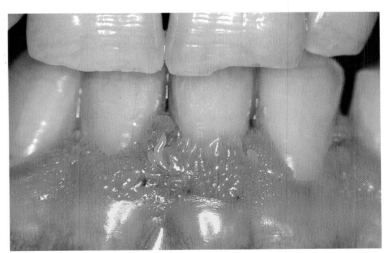

394 Verruca vulgaris
This HIV-positive male exhibits a verruca vulgaris on the mandibular anterior gingiva. Several finger-like projections can be seen emanating from the marginal epithelium.
Left: Immunohistochemistry has been used to depict positive reactions of several epithelial cells to HPV antigens (arrows). Since only a portion of the HPV subtypes elicit oral manifestations (types 2, 4, 6, 11, 13, 32 and others), only these antigens are usually tested (APAAP, x 80).

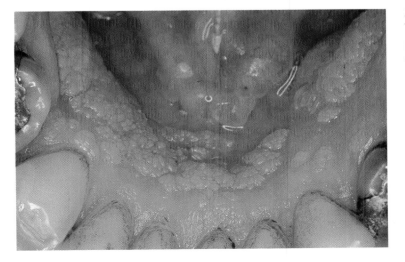

395 Condyloma acuminatum
The lingual gingiva in this HIV-positive patient exhibits flat, cauliflower-like lesions. HPV-induced oral lesions can be removed surgically or by laser, but recurrence is common, especially in patients who exhibit simultaneous occurrence of oral and genital HPV infection (Badaracco et al. 1998).

Infections—Viral and Bacterial

Herpetic Gingivostomatitis

Oral ulcerations can be caused by HSV-1 and/or HSV-2. HSV-1/2 ulcerations are observed in 0.6–9% of all HIV-infected individuals. In addition to labial herpes, intraoral gingivostomatitis may also occur. In HIV-infected patients, the course of the disease is often prolonged and severe. Identification of the virus is performed using immunofluorescence of oral smears, through virus cultures or a biopsy. (See also pp. 46, 96, 132).

Tuberculosis and Syphilis (Stage II)

Oral lesions are only seldom seen in cases of *tuberculosis*. However, in the USA and Southeast Asia, therapy-resistant tuberculosis is often associated with oral ulcerations. The lesions are characterized by a fibrin-coated ulcer with soft and indistinct borders.

Patients in the *secondary stage of syphilis* may exhibit the so-called "plaques muqueuses" in the oral cavity. These are highly contagious (see also p. 93).

396 Herpetic gingivostomatitis
Note the numerous small and large yellowish ulcerations against an erythematous background on the attached gingiva. Other regions of the oral cavity, especially the attached mucosa, were also affected.

Right: Numerous epithelial cells in the marginal area of the ulcer have stained red; this is a positive sign of HSV-1 (APAAP, x 100).

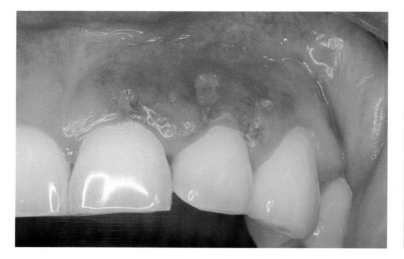 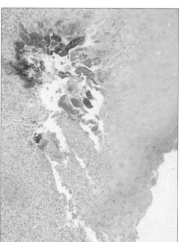

397 Tuberculosis
A large, crater-like ulceration surrounded by erythema is obvious on the left anterior tonsillar pillar in an AIDS patient from Thailand. The differential diagnosis should include atypical ulcerations, e.g., a major aphtha.

Right: The histologic picture reveals epithelioid cell granuloma with Langhans giant cells in a case of tuberculosis. The mycobacteria can be identified by means of specific stains (Ziehl–Neelsen) (H & E, x 120).

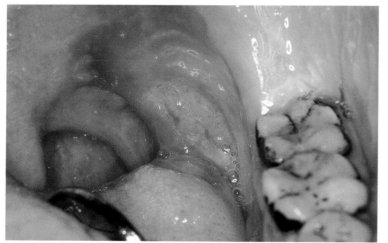 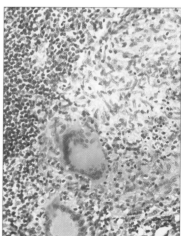

398 Secondary syphilis
In the region of the gingiva and the vestibulum, note the whitish, flat ulceration. This is a characteristic picture of secondary syphilis in the oral cavity. The danger of infection from such lesions is high, also for the dentist.

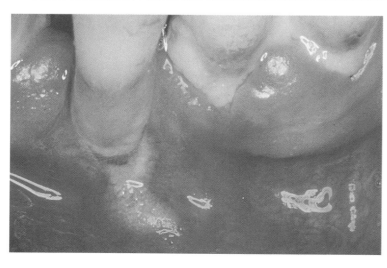

Hematologic Disorders—Non-neoplastic

Chronic Benign and Cyclic Neutropenia

Patients with agranulocytosis and neutropenia often present with a gingival condition resembling that of acute leukemia. One observes gingival hyperplasia, ulcerations and hemorrhage, with progressive alveolar bone loss. Various forms of neutropenia can be differentiated, whereby the *cyclic neutropenia* in addition to the chronic benign forms are occasionally associated with oral manifestations. While cyclic neutropenia is characterized by the temporary loss of peripheral neutrophilic granulocytes, the number of neutrophilic granulocytes in cases of *chronic benign neutropenia* is continually and severely reduced (Reichart and Dornow 1978). Treatment consists of impeccable oral hygiene, professional prophylaxis and short-interval recall. It is frequently impossible to avoid tooth loss.

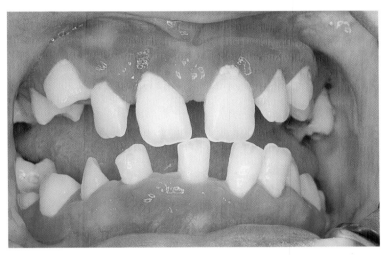

399 Neutropenia
This 12-year-old male had suffered from chronic and persistent gingivitis and periodontitis since age 5. He also had frequent infections of the respiratory tract and the skin. The gingiva exhibit a spotty erythema and teeth that are in the process of eruption, with irregular spacing. Some of the teeth were highly mobile.

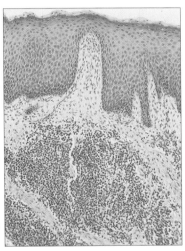
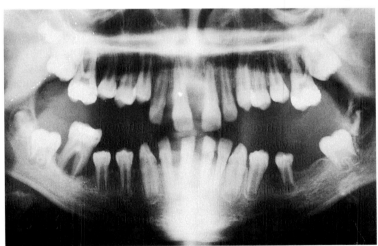

400 Panoramic radiograph and biopsy of the same patient
One notes massive periodontal destruction in all quadrants. In some areas, the alveolar bone loss has progressed all the way to the apex of the roots.

Left: Histologic picture from the gingival biopsy. Subjacent to the unremarkable gingival epithelium, one notes focal, dense infiltrates, consisting primarily of lymphocytic elements and plasma cells (H & E, x 80).

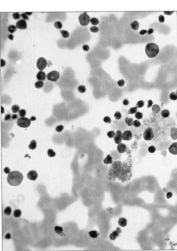
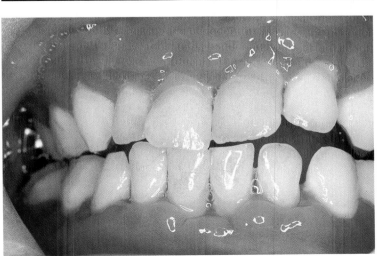

401 Cyclic neutropenia
Gingivitis and periodontitis in a 15-year-old female suffering from cyclic neutropenia. The gingiva exhibits an irregular erythema and areas of hyperplasia.

Left: This peripheral blood smear demonstrates the absence of neutrophilic granulocytes (Wright stain, x 200).

Disturbances of Keratinization

Frictional Keratosis

If a local etiology can be ascertained for white spots on the oral mucosa, the lesion should be appropriately classified and not simply documented as leukoplakia. Such lesions may be caused by friction, by "galvanic" reactions, cheek biting, and the white lesion of glass blowers (Pindborg et al. 1997, van der Waal et al. 1997). White lesions caused by friction are most commonly observed on the gingiva due to overzealous brushing of teeth. The chronic irritation leads to hyperkeratosis of the oral epithelium. When the cause is understood, it should be eliminated, in which case the lesions usually spontaneously regress within weeks or months. Old amalgam restorations at the cervical region may also elicit similar reactions; these were attributed historically to "galvanism."

Today, however, this phenomenon is attributed to a *lichenoid reaction* in which allergic reaction may play a role. Malignant transformation of keratosis caused by irritation or friction is highly unlikely.

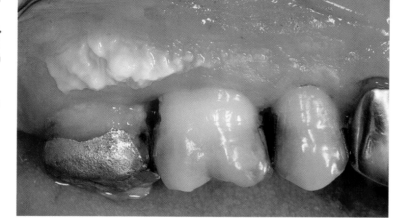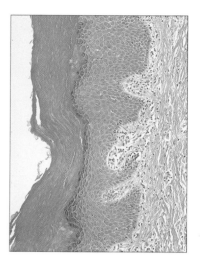

402 Frictional keratosis
The gingiva of the right maxilla in the molar and premolar areas exhibits a very thick, white lesion, especially adjacent to the second molar, which has an old amalgam restoration. The patient history included chronic toothbrush trauma, but it is possible that the amalgam restoration represents an additional irritation factor.
Right: Histologic picture of friction keratosis, exhibiting pronounced hyperorthokeratosis and minimal inflammatory reaction (H & E, x 80).

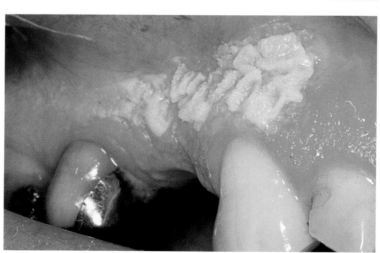

403 Frictional keratosis caused by toothbrushing
Clinical view of toothbrush-induced frictional keratosis on the right maxilla in the canine-premolar region, which is particularly frequently affected. The interdental papillae are often spared from these lesions because they are protected by the crowns of the teeth. The clinical picture is consistent with one of homogeneous leukoplakia. However, because the cause is known, leukoplakia is not a consideration in the final diagnosis.

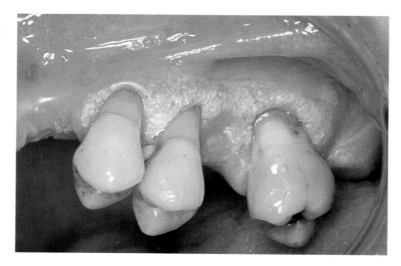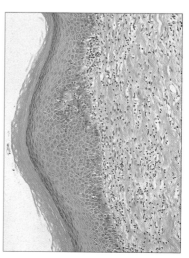

404 Frictional keratosis
This case of frictional keratosis on the left maxilla is similar in appearance to a case of homogeneous leukoplakia. The wedge-shape defects on the premolars and molars provide evidence of toothbrush trauma. In extreme cases, soft tissue ulcerations may also be observed.

Right: The histologic picture of frictional keratosis exhibits hyperorthokeratosis with unremarkable epithelium and a mild subepithelial infiltrate (H & E, x 80).

Leukoplakia

Localization of oral leukoplakia on the gingiva and the adjacent vestibulum with its mobile alveolar mucosa is less common. Especially in patients with no history of tobacco use or other causative factors, one occasionally observes a gingival localization of idiopathic leukoplakia. In such cases, however, other areas of the oral cavity are also affected, especially the borders and the ventral surface of the tongue. The clinical picture is almost always that of a homogeneous leukoplakia. (See also pp. 52, 73, 100, 117.)

Burns

Burns on the oral mucosa may occur unbeknownst to the patient or even intentionally, as in a suicide attempt. The most common is the so-called "aspirin burn" that is caused when patients with toothache apply an aspirin tablet topically in the oral cavity. The result is local disruption of the epithelium with subsequent ulcer formation. The disease picture can only be clarified by taking a precise medical history. No treatment is necessary. Such ulcerations heal spontaneously within eight to ten days.

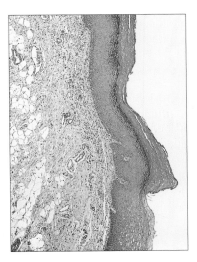
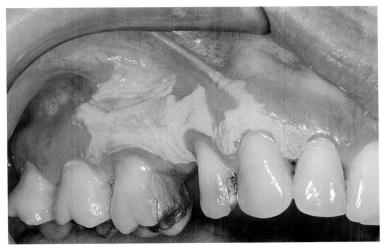

405 Leukoplakia
Homogeneous idiopathic leukoplakia in the region of the attached gingiva and adjacent alveolar mucosa.

Left: The histologic picture reveals the abrupt transition zone between the hyperorthokeratosis and the normal adjacent gingival mucosa. This zone is also clearly obvious in the clinical picture (H & E, x 60).

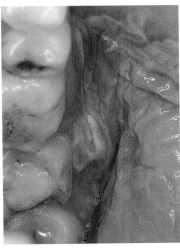
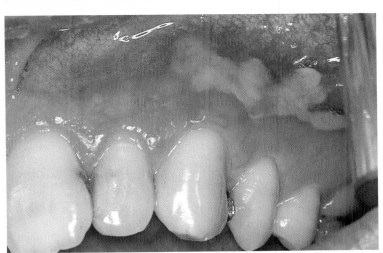

406 "Cotton roll stomatitis"/burn
The maxillary vestibulum exhibits an irregular ulceration extending from the canine to the first molar. The cause was traced to the application of a cotton roll during dental treatment.

Left: The left maxillary vestibulum exhibits a whitish-yellow discoloration and massive swelling. The cause in this case was an aspirin tablet that the patient had placed into the vestibulum in the region of the painful second molar.

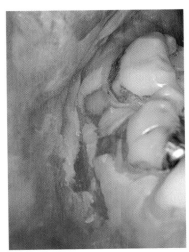
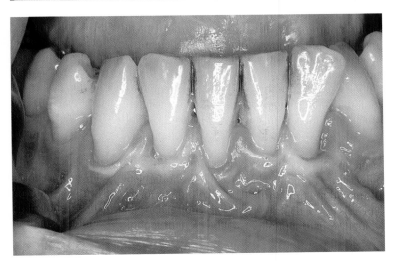

407 Burn
In an attempted suicide, this woman ingested a highly aggressive drain cleaner, which elicited massive tissue loss on the tongue, the vestibulum and the gingiva. The mandibular vestibulum exhibits the scars of the healing process.

Left: The "aspirin burn" exhibits ulcerations and a white (desquamating) epithelium. The history of such lesions is usually not longer than 24 hours.

Dermatologic Manifestations

Lichen Planus

Gingival manifestations of lichen planus are relatively rare and are characterized by a particular therapy resistance. The entire spectrum of clinical subforms of lichen planus may appear. If erosive forms are present, the clinician will note a high degree of similarity with gingival benign mucous membrane pemphigoid or desquamative gingivitis. The various clinical forms are characterized by different clinical courses. Papular lesions are generally observed in patients under 50 years of age, while atrophic lesions are more often detected in patients over 60. Ulcerative forms usually have a short clinical course (Thorn et al. 1988). Long-term studies have shown complete remission in 70% of patients with lichen planus. Treatment for the gingival lesion is especially difficult; frequently even high and long-term doses of steroids or cyclosporine have been shown to have no effect (Jungell and Malmström 1996). (See also pp. 80, 101 and 137.)

Lichen planus

408 Reticular/atrophic form
Left: Reticular form of lichen planus in the area of the premolars of the left maxilla. Such lesions may be confused with frictional keratosis.

Right: Atrophic form of lichen planus on the attached gingiva of the anterior maxilla. 60% of all affected patients complain of a burning sensation of the gingiva.

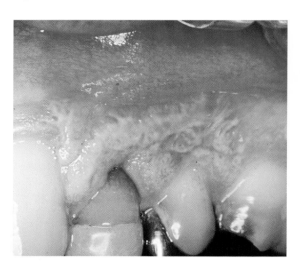
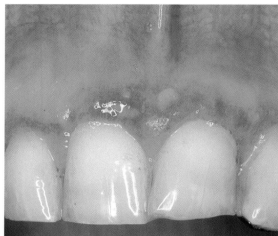

409 Atrophic form
Left: Atrophic form of lichen planus with minimal clinical symptoms. One can observe only small, erythematous lesions of the interdental papilla and the marginal gingival.

Right: Atrophic lichen planus of the gingiva in the right maxilla. If there is a suspicion of gingival lichen planus, the entire oral cavity should be examined for signs of lichen, particularly Wickham's striae.

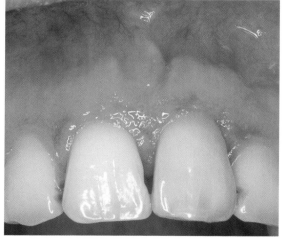
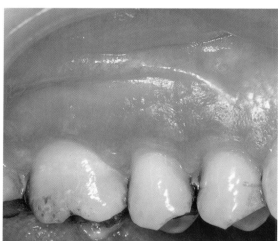

410 Atrophic erosive form
Left: Atrophic erosive lichen planus of the gingiva in the right maxilla. Crown margins and poor oral hygiene favor the formation of ulcerations and erosions.

Right: Atrophic erosive lichen planus in the right maxilla. The gingivae exhibit erythema and small ulcerations at the cervical region as well as whitish, plaque-like lesions in the molar area.

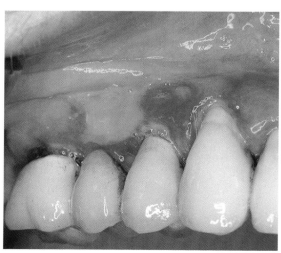
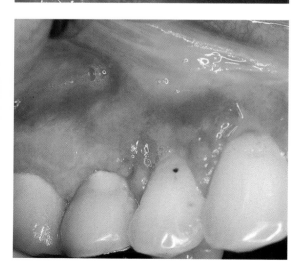

Pemphigus Vulgaris and Pemphigoid

Epithelial autoimmune diseases such as pemphigus and pemphigoid are observed mainly in middle-aged and elderly individuals. Intradermal blistering is characteristic of pemphigus, while subepidermal blistering is often observed in pemphigoid.

In cases of *pemphigus vulgaris*, the oral mucosa is almost always initially affected. One observes extensive areas of epithelial lysis, in which a suprabasal epithelial split is almost always present. Examination using direct immunofluorescence reveals suprabasal and interkeratino-cytic immunoglobulins of type IgG, as well as C3 complement. The autoantigen in pemphigus vulgaris is a 130-kd glycoprotein. (See pp. 40 and 60.)

The lesions of *benign mucous membrane pemphigoid* appear in many cases as desquamative gingivitis, wherein the vestibular gingiva is severely erythematous, exhibiting extensive areas of erosion. The mobile alveolar mucosa may also be affected, but the vestibulum is usually spared. Females near the menopause suffer more often from benign mucous membrane pemphigoid (Hornstein 1996).

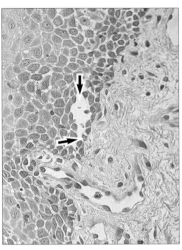
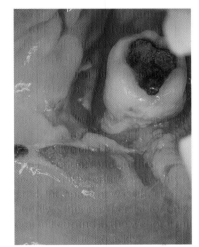

411 Pemphigus vulgaris
Left: Histologic picture of pemphigus vulgaris. The basal cells have retained their normal position, but the initial epithelial split (arrows) is suprabasal (H & E, x 120).

Right: In the region of the gingiva and the vestibulum of the right mandible there is extensive erosion and epithelial disruption. The entire oral cavity of this patient was affected. Intraoral blisters persist for only a short time in the wet oral milieu, and burst quickly.

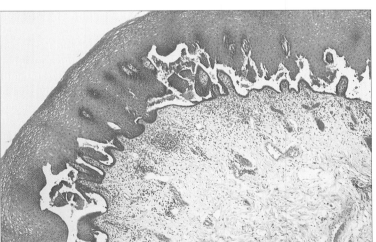

412 Pemphigus vulgaris—histology
This low-power histologic picture depicts the oral mucosa in a case of pemphigus vulgaris, exhibiting the classic suprabasal split as well as individual epithelial cell clusters within the blister, which appear as the so-called "Tzanck cells" in cytologic smear preparations (H & E, x 40).

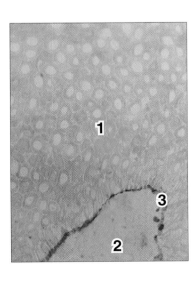
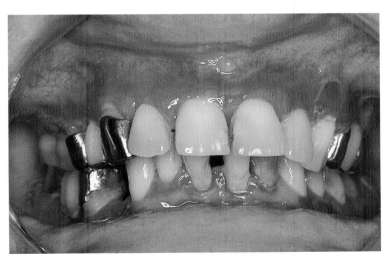

413 Pemphigoid
The upper and lower vestibular gingiva exhibit a massive, persistent erythema with several areas of erosion. This is a form of desquamative gingivitis, a variation of pemphigoid, which renders therapy particularly problematic.
Left: The immunohistochemical preparation reveals the C3-complement in a case of pemphigoid (PAP, x 200).

1 Gingival epithelium
2 Connective tissue papilla
3 Basement membrane

Bullous pemphigoid is observed less often on the oral mucosa than *benign mucous membrane (scarring or cicatricial) pemphigoid*; in addition to the oral cavity, the genital mucosa and the eyes (75%) are affected. Mucosal scarring and adhesions lead to corneal opaqueness and eventual blindness. As is also the case with bullous pemphigoid, benign mucosal pemphigoid is characterized by subepithelial blister formation.

Immunosuppressive therapy is the choice for treating bullous autoimmune diseases. Medications include corticosteroids, azathioprene, cyclophosphamide as well as cyclosporine.

Lichenoid Reaction

In earlier times, the lichenoid reaction was interpreted as a mucosal reaction caused by galvanism. The lesion is frequently observed near old, corroded amalgam restorations in the cervical areas of the teeth. Corrosion products, dental plaque, and also allergic reactions to amalgam and mercury have been considered as pathogenic factors.

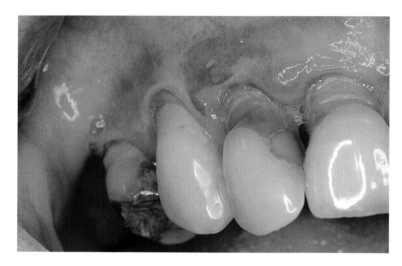 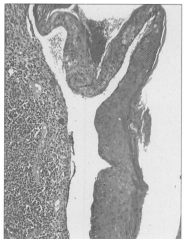

414 Bullous pemphigoid
The gingiva of the right maxilla exhibits whitish and erythematous areas. In affected patients, even toothbrushing leads to sloughing of the epithelium; it is for this reason that many affected patients exhibit poor oral hygiene.

Right: Histologic picture of bullous pemphigoid with split formation between the epithelium and connective tissue. Notice the intense inflammatory reaction in the lamina propria (H & E, x 80).

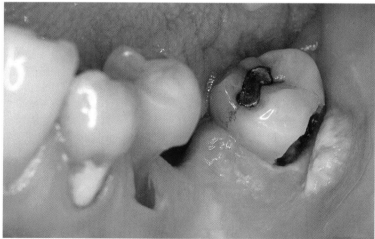

415 Lichenoid reaction
Immediately adjacent to the second molar in the mandible there is a white, sharply demarcated mucosal lesion. Such lesions are often observed near old amalgam restorations. Medicaments may also cause a lichenoid reaction. The lesions are harmless and disappear spontaneously after removal of the cause. Amalgam restorations can be replaced by ceramic inlays or glass ionomer cement restorations.

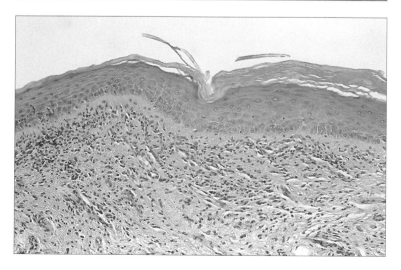

416 Lichenoid reaction—histology
The histologic picture reveals an epithelium devoid of rete pegs, with hyperorthokeratosis, which is particularly pronounced on the right. In the subepithelial area there is a diffuse infiltrate of immunocompetent cells, primarily lymphocytes (H & E, x 100).

Vulvo-vagino-gingival Syndrome

The vulvo-vagino-gingival syndrome is a rare disorder which usually affects young females. In this condition, a massive erythema of the gingiva as well as similar reactions of the mucosa of the vulva and vagina are observed (Pheiffer et al. 1988). The gingival erythema is clinically similar to desquamative gingivitis, a special form of benign mucous membrane pemphigoid (Williams 1989). In terms of the clinical and histologic pictures, the differential diagnosis should include atrophic lichen planus.

The lesions in the oral cavity are usually localized in the gingival area and normally precede the vulvo-vaginitis. Laboratory findings are uncharacteristic and do not contribute to a precise diagnosis. In order to rule out blister-forming disorders such as pemphigus vulgaris and pemphigoid, immunofluorescent microscopic examination of biopsies should be performed.

Treatment consists of topical application of corticosteroids, which usually leads to a significant improvement in the clinical situation.

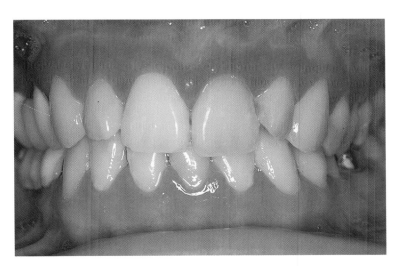

Vulvo-vagino-gingival syndrome

417 Gingival erythema
A clearly visible band of gingival erythema, several millimeters wide, is evident in both maxilla and mandible. Plaque accumulation does not play a major role.

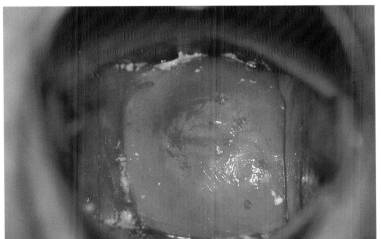

418 Vaginal erythema
Pronounced colpitis (vaginitis) with extensive erythema, similar to the clinical picture of gingivitis (from Pheiffer et al. 1988).

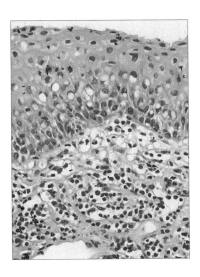
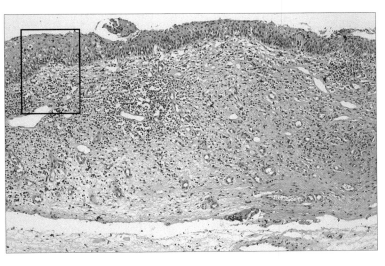

419 Histology
Histologic picture of vulvo-vaginitis, which corresponds to the findings in the gingiva. Primarily there is a dense, subepithelial infiltrate of immunocompetent cells (H & E, x 80).

Left: This magnified section depicts parakeratotic, normally layered epithelium, without atypia. In the subepithelial area there is a dense infiltrate of lymphocytes and plasma cells (H & E, x 200).

Figs. 417–419: Courtesy B. Hoffmeister

Non-neoplastic Lesions

"Fibroma", Hyperplasia of Maxillary Tuberosity, Familial Gingivofibromatosis

The *"fibroma"* is the most common tumor-like connective tissue hyperplasia in the oral cavity. "Low-grade trauma" has traditionally been the accepted cause, but the actual irritation is often not apparent. The lesions are covered by an unremarkable mucosa of normal color.

Hyperplasia of the maxillary tuberosity is a firm accumulation of connective tissue usually occurring bilaterally. The cause is not known. Treatment consists of simple excisional surgery. Recurrence is rare. Connective tissue hyperplasia should be differentiated from true fibromatosis (Fowler et al. 1994).

Familial gingivofibromatosis is an autosomal dominant trait; it is a generalized lesion wherein a few or all of the teeth are covered by connective tissue. The clinical picture may be one of pseudoanodontia. Despite the pseudopockets, the level of gingival inflammation is usually low.

420 Hyperplasia of maxillary tuberosity
Although hyperplasia in this area is usually a bilaterally symmetrical condition, this patient developed a pronounced hyperplasia that was limited to the left side only. In this case, the indication for surgical removal of the hyperplastic tissue was the patient's complaint of impairment of speech.

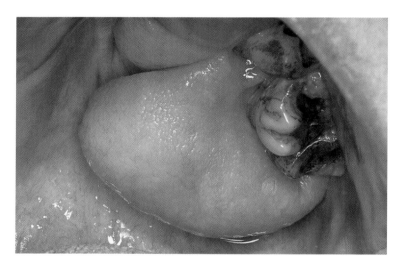

421 Hyperplasia of maxillary tuberosity
This case of typical, bilateral hyperplasia extends into the premolar region. Because the tissue accumulates very slowly, the redundant tissue does not bother most patients.

Right: Unilateral hyperplasia of maxillary tuberosity of the left maxilla. A surgical wedge excision of the tissue created a tuberosity suitable for the insertion of a denture.

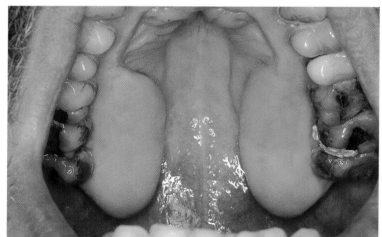
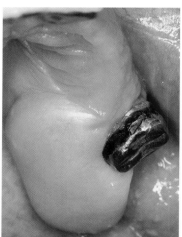

422 Familial gingivofibromatosis
In this patient, massive, localized fibromatosis was evident in both maxilla and mandible, primarily in the molar regions. This condition inhibited the eruption of some teeth (e.g., the molars in the maxillary right area).
The son of this patient exhibited an identical clinical picture, wherein all molars of the maxilla and mandible were completely covered by fibrous tissue.
Even if the tissue is resected, the teeth do not always erupt.

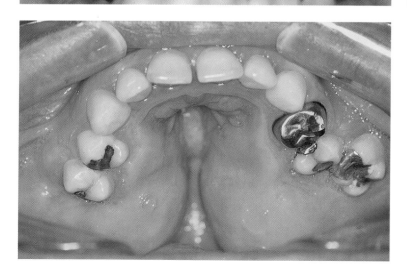

Gingival hyperplasia

Gingival hyperplasia (overgrowth, enlargement) results from an excessive proliferation of fibroblasts and an increase in collagen synthesis. Gingival overgrowth is often observed following chronic intake of drugs, such as antiepileptics (hydantoin), immunosuppressives (cyclosporine-A), antihypertensives (Nifedipine), as well as in patients with neurological brain stem syndromes. If no etiologic agent is apparent, the condition is classified as idiopathic hyperplasia. In patients with Trisomy 21 (Down's syndrome), gingival hyperplasia may occur due to chronic mouth breathing. Poor oral hygiene and other local irritat-ing factors enhance the development and severity of hyperplastic gingiva. The differential diagnosis of gingival hyperplasia should include agranulocytosis and leukemia.

Clinically, the anterior segments of the dentition are initially involved, and in some cases the entire crowns of the teeth may be covered by redundant gingival tissue. Due to the development of pseudopockets, other factors such as bacterial plaque and calculus may complicate the situation. The hyperplasia will often persist even after cessation of the medication.

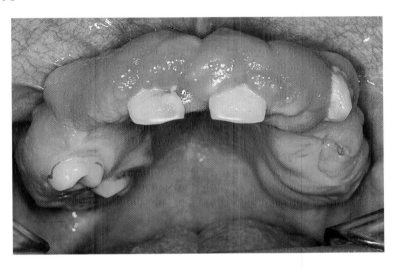

423 Gingival overgrowth in the maxilla
This young male with Trisomy 21 exhibits gingival overgrowth in the region of the entire maxilla and mandible (see Fig. 424). The gingiva is mildly erythematous and covers about half of the clinical crowns of the teeth. Other segments of the oral mucosa are unaffected. One possible contributory factor is dryness of the gingiva due to mouth breathing.

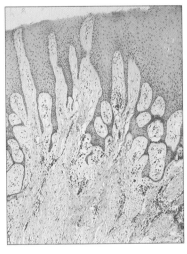

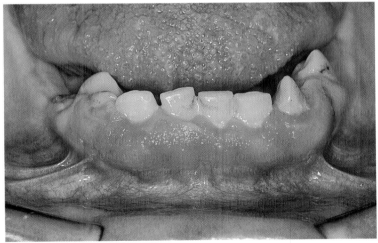

424 Gingival overgrowth in the mandible
The anterior segment of the mandible also exhibits enlarged gingiva with mild stippling and erythema. The obvious plaque accumulation enhances the hyperplastic condition.

Left: Histologic picture of gingival hyperplasia resulting from hydantoin medication. The tissue exhibits deeply penetrating epithelial rete. The lamina propria reveals fibroses (H & E, x 80).

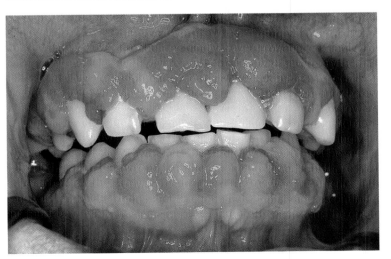

425 Hydantoin-induced gingival overgrowth
Pronounced gingival overgrowth with severe erythema in some segments, especially around the poorly contoured crowns. There was a tendency toward spontaneous gingival hemorrhage. Such massive gingival overgrowth must be surgically excised, but there is a tendency toward recurrence if the medication is not discontinued. Oral hygiene must be optimized.

Fibrous Epulis

The Greek term "epulis" translates as "situated upon the gingiva." Thus, literally, this term could be used to describe any and all lesions of the gingiva. However, in common professional parlance, the term is reserved for isolated gingival growths, such as the fibrous epulis, the peripheral giant cell granuloma as well as the pyogenic granuloma.

The fibrous epulis is usually located in the region of the interdental papilla. Adjacent teeth may be displaced, and there may be actual septal bone loss. Females and patients in the second decade of life are most often affected. Eighty percent of all epulis lesions occur in the anterior segments of the dentition.

The fibrous epulis is usually asymptomatic. Local irritation may lead to fibrous hyperplasia; the initial lesions are usually soft, vascular and erythematous, with fibrosis occurring later on.

Similar lesions have been noted in small animals, particularly in certain species of dogs (boxer) (Reichart et al. 1989). Despite the existence of histopathologically rare forms, the clinical and histologic characteristics exhibit similarities to fibrous epulis of humans.

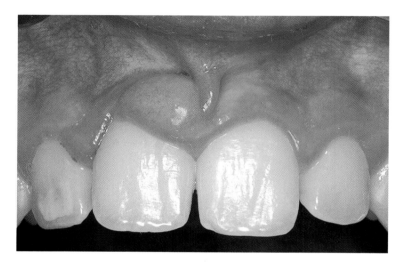

426   Fibrous epulis
The marginal gingiva adjacent to the right central incisor exhibits a small swelling, covered by normal-appearing mucosa, which has displaced the labial frenum. Palpation revealed that the lesion was firm and immobile. The radiograph showed no osseous destruction. Treatment consists of simple excision. This type of fibrous epulis does not tend to recur.

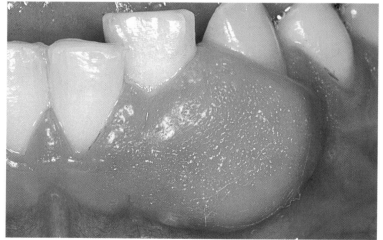
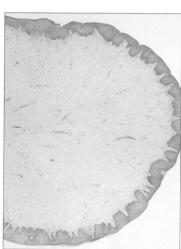

427   Fibrous epulis
On the left side of the mandible, a fibrous epulis developed between the lateral incisor and the canine and displaced these teeth. The lesion was asymptomatic; such lesions may increase in size slowly.

Right: Histologic picture of the fibrous epulis shows acanthotic epithelium, fiber-rich hyperplastic connective tissue, and very little vascularization (H & E, x 5).

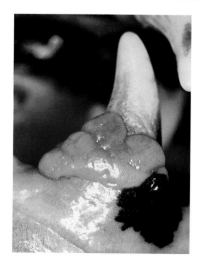
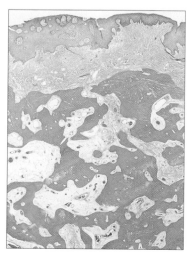

428   Epulis in a dog
Left: In the area of the mandibular canine of a boxer, one notes a fibrous epulis with inflammatory symptoms, which appear to be caused by plaque accumulation. Mesial to the canine there is an area of dark physiologic pigmentation, which is typical for the canine gingiva.

Right: This histologic picture of a canine epulis exhibits large areas of ossification; this picture is occasionally observed also in human epulis (H & E, x 10).

Pyogenic Granuloma

The pyogenic granuloma is a particular type of inflammatory hyperplasia. The granulomatous tissue, which is caused by local trauma, becomes contaminated by the flora of the oral cavity. The surface of the pyogenic granuloma is often covered by fibrin, which may mimic pus. However, suppuration is not a characteristic of the pyogenic granuloma.

The pyogenic granuloma is asymptomatic and appears as a soft, polyp-like tissue exuberance with a rough, ulcerated and necrotizing surface. Up to 70% of all pyogenic granulomas occur on the gingiva. The gingiva of the maxilla is most often affected. Sixty percent of all affected patients are between the age of 11 and 40. Females develop pyogenic granuloma more frequently than males.

The treatment of choice involves surgical excision, professional prophylaxis and scrupulous oral hygiene (Makek and Sailor 1985).

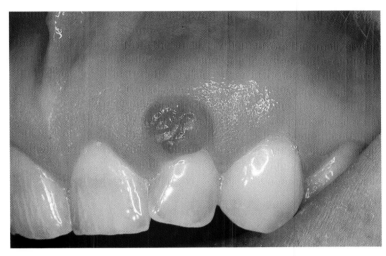

429 Small pyogenic granuloma
Note the small, erythematous lesion on the gingiva adjacent to the left maxillary lateral incisor. The adjacent gingiva exhibits no signs of pathologic involvement. Even minor local trauma can lead to granulomatous lesions. In cases exhibiting small, pyogenic granulomas, the use of antiseptic mouth rinses may lead to regression.

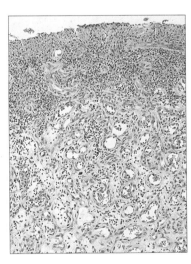
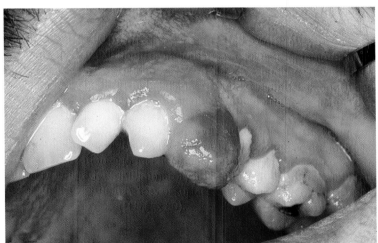

430 Large pyogenic granuloma
With time, an untreated pyogenic granuloma may exhibit a tendency toward fibrosis. The differential diagnosis should include peripheral giant cell granuloma.

Left: The histologic picture of a pyogenic granuloma exhibits pronounced vascularization and inflammatory infiltration. Notice the loss of surface epithelium (H & E, x 80).

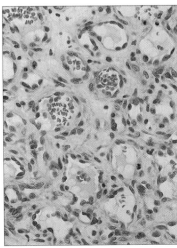
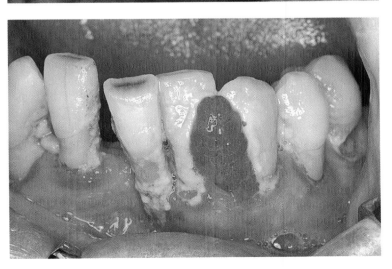

431 Pyogenic granuloma
As a result of the massive plaque accumulation, a hemorrhagic pyogenic granuloma developed in the papilla between the mandibular canine and lateral incisor.

Left: The histologic picture of a pyogenic granuloma is shown here at higher magnification. Multiple cross sections through vessels with unremarkable endothelium, pronounced hyperemia, and proliferation of young fibroblasts are characteristic features (H & E, x 50).

Peripheral Giant Cell Granuloma

The peripheral giant cell granuloma occurs as an exophytic lesion in the region of the gingiva or the edentulous alveolar mucosa (18%). Although the cause is unknown, local trauma appears to play a role. The clinical picture reveals a nodular mass that may be pedunculated or closely adherent to the surface. Upon palpation, one may note a lesion that is either soft or hard, depending upon the composition of collagen and/or inflammatory components.

Females are more often affected (male:female = 1:1.5), especially between 20 and 60 years of age. Radiographic evaluation often reveals osseous destruction. The frequency of peripheral giant cell granuloma in the maxilla versus the mandible is 1:2.4. Various epidemiologic studies have indicated a recurrence rate of 5.0–70.6% (average 9.9%) (Mighell et al. 1995). Histomorphologic studies have demonstrated that the peripheral giant cell granuloma consists primarily of mononuclear phagocytes and multinucleated giant cells (Carvalho et al. 1995).

Peripheral giant cell granuloma

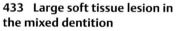

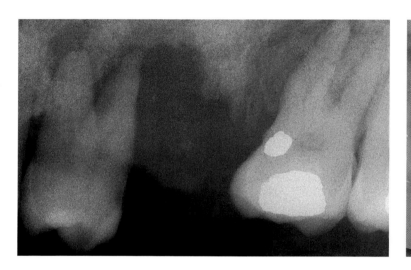

432 Radiograph and clinical picture
A massive area of osteolysis is evident in the left maxilla.

Right: Clinical appearance. Note the large, tumor-like mass of tissue expanding buccally and palatally and exhibiting a dark red color. The growth may expand quite rapidly. The differential diagnosis should include osteosarcoma.

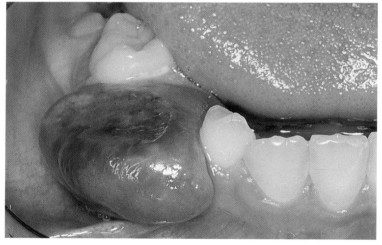

433 Large soft tissue lesion in the mixed dentition
This bluish-red lesion with its superficial ulceration is a classic illustration of a peripheral giant cell granuloma, in this case occurring in a 9-year-old girl.

434 Histology
Left: The microscopic view reveals multinucleated giant cells within the granulation tissue. Extravascular erythrocytes and hemosiderin granules are usually observed. (H & E, x 100).

Right: A higher magnification of the multinucleated giant cells (arrows), which may contain up to 300 nuclei (H & E, x 250).

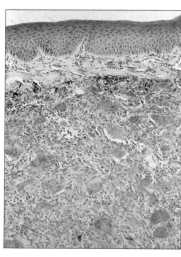

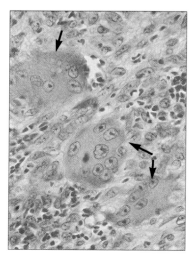

Gingival Hyperplasia—Medicament-Induced

Long-term medication with cyclosporine-A or calcium channel antagonists, for example, nifedipine (Thomason et al. 1987) is associated with gingival enlargement or overgrowth (Brown et al. 1991, Seymour et al. 1997). Both of these medications are routinely prescribed for organ transplant patients. Thirty percent of the dentulous patients who receive cyclosporine-A develop gingival lesions to an extent that requires surgical therapy. The combination of cyclosporine-A and nifedipine increases the prevalence rate of gingival overgrowth to 50%.

The enlargement is observed within three months after initiation of the medication, and it is the labial gingiva that is most often affected. Children are more likely to develop the lesions than adults.

The pathogenesis is multifactorial; the primary factor is the medicament, but additional factors include growth factors, activation of collagen synthesis, various subpopulations of fibroblasts, and other factors (Brown et al. 1991).

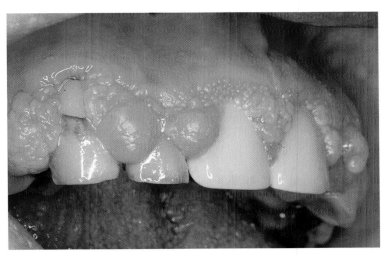

Cyclosporine-induced gingival overgrowth

435 Heart transplant patient
This patient has developed a pronounced cyclosporine-associated gingival overgrowth. The lesions are relatively free of inflammation, consisting primarily of small nodules on the surface of the gingiva, with primary lesions in the interdental areas. Improper restoration margins and poor crown margins enhance the hyperplasia.

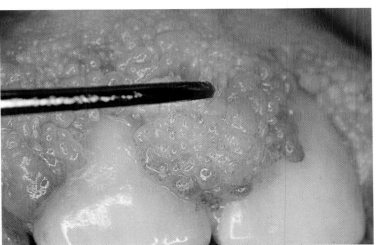

436 Recurrence following gingivectomy
Following periodontal surgery, this patient (shown in Fig. 435) developed new lesions within six months. The pressure exerted by the forceps illustrates the consistency of the fibrous tissue. Because it is rarely possible to change the medication or reduce the dosage, individual patients must endure recurrence of these gingival lesions.

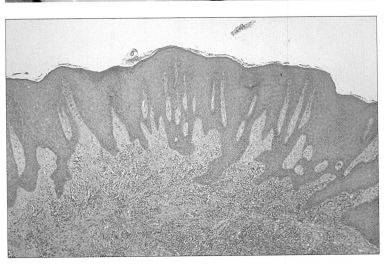

437 Histology
Similar to the picture of hydantoin-associated gingival hyperplasia (Fig. 424, left), the tissue exhibits a downgrowth of extensive epithelial rete deeply into the connective tissue. Note the heavy inflammatory infiltrate in the subepithelial area (H & E, x 100).

Malignant Tumors

Kaposi's Sarcoma

The epidemic, AIDS-associated Kaposi's sarcoma is observed primarily in homosexuals and less frequently in heterosexuals, i.v.-drug users, women and children. The median age of patients with Kaposi's sarcoma is 38 (Reichart et al. 1993). The palate is most often affected, followed by the gingiva and the tongue. The intraoral Kaposi's sarcoma appears clinically as a reddish-blue or violet spot, and in later stages it may appear as a tumor, often with ulceration.

The differential diagnosis should include hematoma, hemangioma, tattoo formation, and other neoplasias of vascular origin (Reichart 1996). (See also pp. 107 and 143.)

The pathogenesis of Kaposi's sarcoma is associated with numerous factors. The Kaposi's sarcoma herpes virus (KSHV; Chang et al. 1994) plays a significant role, in addition to various cytokines and growth factors.

438   Kaposi's sarcoma—etiology
A variety of possible causes, primarily the HI-virus, but also other viruses from the herpes virus group and human papilloma virus are considered as possible factors, in addition to various behavioral risk factors. The endothelial cells of the vessels represent the end organs of paracrine and autocrine processes, which are determined by growth factors and cytokines.

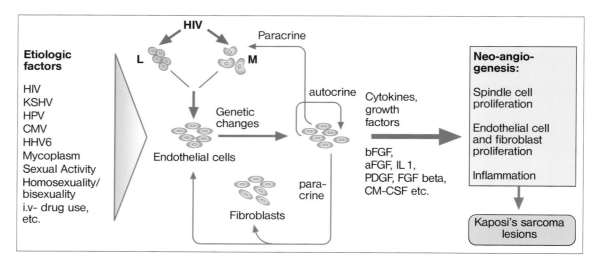

439   Kaposi's sarcoma
The violet tumor mass is similar in appearance to a peripheral giant cell granuloma. If other Kaposi's sarcomas are present, it is usually not necessary to harvest a biopsy.

Right: Immunohistochemical picture of Kaposi's sarcoma with the clearly delineated basement membrane (NC1) of the sinusoidal vascular space. A vascular origin of the Kaposi's sarcoma is likely (IF, x 200).

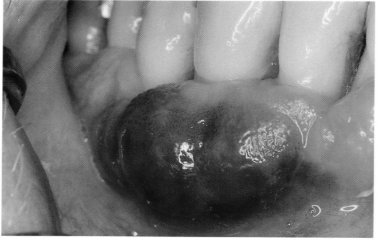
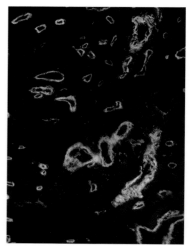

440   Ulcerated Kaposi's sarcoma
Clearly evident is the ulcerated Kaposi's sarcoma on the gingiva in the anterior segment of the mandible. The typical dark coloration is lacking. There have been reports of Kaposi's sarcoma without pigmentation (Reichart and Schiødt 1989).

Right: Electron microscopic picture. The intracytoplasmic tubular structures (arrows) are typical. The evidence of Weibel–Palade bodies offers clues of a vascular origin (TEM, x 30 000).

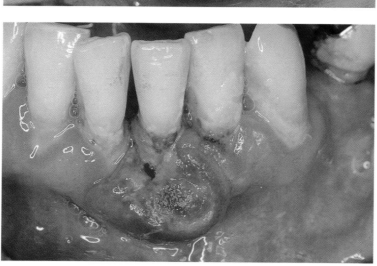
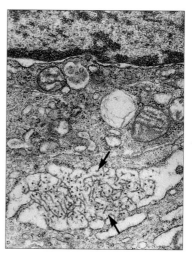

Keratoacanthoma

The keratoacanthoma ("self-healing carcinoma") is a benign tumor. It is relatively common on the skin and the lower lip, but less common in the oral cavity. Males are more often affected. The keratoacanthoma appears between the ages of 12 and 80 years. It appears clinically as a painless, crater-forming tumor. Spontaneous healing over a period of two to four months may be observed, but surgical excision remains the treatment of choice.

Leukemia

Leukemia is defined as a malignant disease of the white blood cells, resulting from clonal proliferation of immature hematopoietic stem cells. Chronic and acute, aleukemic and leukemic as well as myeloid and lymphatic leukemias must be differentiated.

Gingival symptoms are often an initial manifestation, especially with acute myeloid and monocytic forms. Gingival swelling, petechiae, ecchymoses and ulcerations are characteristic (Barrett 1984).

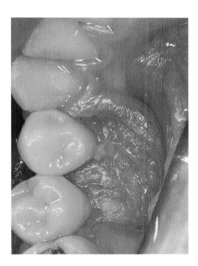
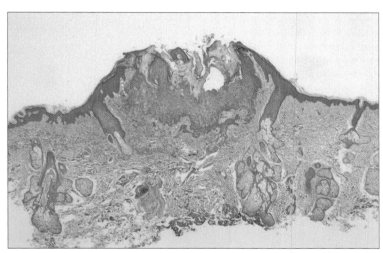

441 Keratoacanthoma
The histologic picture of keratoacanthoma exhibits a deep, keratin-filled central crater surrounded by hyperplastic and partially dysplastic epithelium. This biopsy was taken from the skin (H & E, x 20).

Left: Lingual to the first and second mandibular premolars, note a painless lesion that is partially surrounded by a distinct border. This is consistent with the rare, intraoral keratoacanthoma.

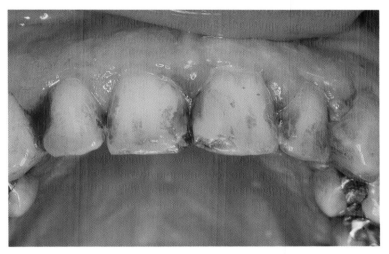

442 Acute myeloid leukemia
This patient exhibits the initial manifestations of an acute leukemia. Several interdental papillae, especially in the left maxillary region, exhibit hyperplasia and initial ulceration of the papilla tips. In addition, note the acute, local hemorrhage between the right lateral incisor and canine, as well as the typical brown pigmentation on the anterior teeth, representing previous hemorrhage.

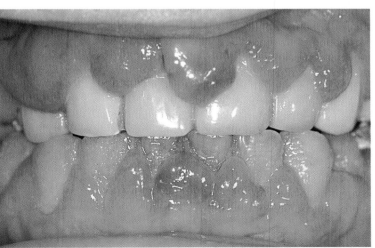

443 Acute myeloid leukemia
In this patient, the initial symptoms were confined to gingival hyperplasia. The hemorrhagic symptoms occurred only later. Tooth mobility resulted from the leukemic infiltration of the periodontal tissues. In such cases, intraoral surgical procedures should always be avoided. The treatment of choice involves oral hygiene measures and the provision of protective stents (Strassburg and Schneider 1993).

The prognosis for children with *acute* lymphoblastic leukemia is good; in adults, however, the prognosis is often unfavorable.

Chronic leukemia begins insidiously and exhibits few clinical signs and symptoms; it occurs most often in adults. Patients with chronic leukemia may exhibit a pale oral mucosa and a prolonged bleeding time.

In cases of acute leukemia, the pathogenic factor is primarily the lack of granulocyte function; even minor trauma can have serious consequences. In addition, the massive production of tumor cells can lead to thrombosis of small blood vessels, with subsequent infarction. The situation may also be complicated by superinfection. Careful cleaning of the necroses with hydrogen peroxide and the insertion of a protective plate or stent can reduce the intraoral symptoms.

444   Acute myeloid leukemia
The gingiva and mucosa are pale and exhibit the typical signs of this disease process. In addition to enlargement of the interdental papillae and generalized swelling, one notes also the initial signs of ulceration on the papilla tips as well as hemorrhage and ecchymosis.

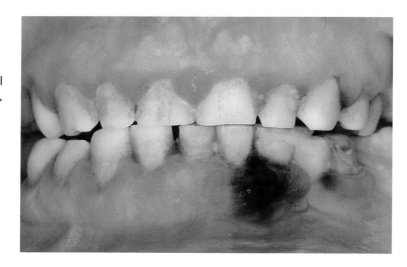

445   Monocytic leukemia
Labial and palatal gingiva and mucosa exhibit an extensive necrosis with multifocal submucosal hemorrhage. (Monocytic leukemia is a form of acute myeloid leukemia.)

Right: Histologic picture of myeloid leukemia. The entire section is evenly infiltrated by tumor cells (H & E, x 80).

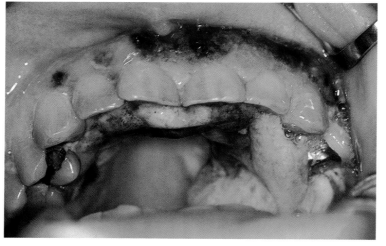
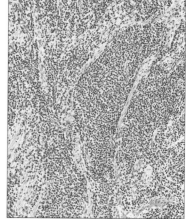

446   Leukemia—histology
Histologic section of a leukemic infiltrate subjacent to the oral epithelium. The myelocytic infiltrate is irregularly distributed. This section does not exhibit any areas of ulceration (H & E, x 120).

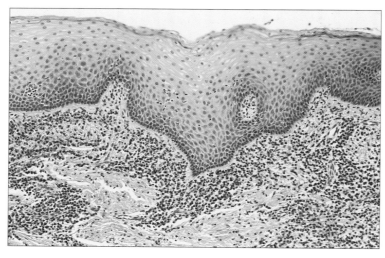

Non-Hodgkin's Lymphoma

Non-Hodgkin's lymphoma can occur as a T-cell or B-cell lymphoma. In the oral cavity, the B-cell lymphoma is more often observed. In most cases, there is regional or generalized lymphadenopathy. In addition, the patient may suffer hepatosplenomegaly, anemia and hemorrhagic diathesis.

In the oral cavity, malignant lymphoma often appears in the form of pillow-like, soft, dark red, frequently ulcerated tumors on the palate, gingiva and floor of the mouth, or in the area of the tonsils. Tooth mobility may be increased.

In AIDS patients, malignant lymphoma is often observed orally and is one of the diseases that define the AIDS syndrome. Even with polychemotherapy, the prognosis is exceptionally poor (Langford et al. 1991, Delecluse et al. 1997). (For additional information on non-Hodgkin's lymphoma, see pp. 144 and 186.)

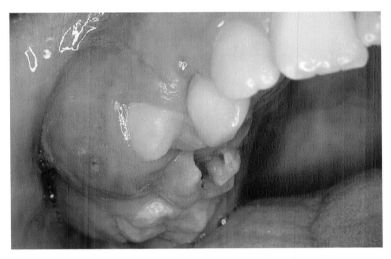

Non-Hodgkin's lymphoma

447 Early clinical findings
This 10-year-old female complained of toothache in the right maxilla. Clinical examination revealed extensive caries in the second deciduous molar.
An odontogenic infection was suspected. However, antibiotic administration did not reduce the swelling. This patient was in poor general health and was hospitalized.

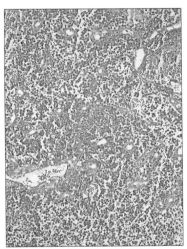

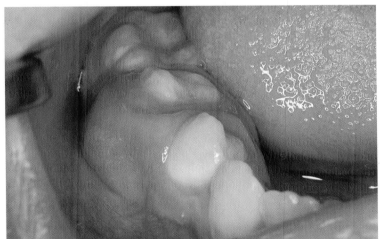

448 Subsequent findings
Several days after the swelling in the right maxilla was discovered (Fig. 447), a similar swelling developed in the right mandible. The submandibular lymph nodes were palpable. A biopsy was taken.

Left: Histologic section of the non-Hodgkin's lymphoma, which has an appearance similar to that of a lymphocytic lymphoma (H & E, x 80).

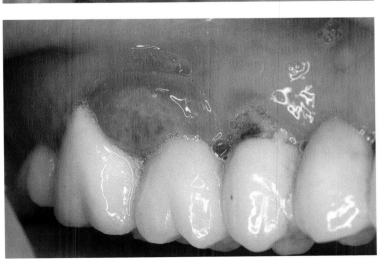

449 AIDS-associated non-Hodgkin's lymphoma
The AIDS-associated non-Hodgkin's lymphoma occurs as large, rapidly growing neoplasias of the oral mucosa, with a clinical appearance similar to that of an epulis with ulcerations. Alveolar bone destruction occurs quickly and extensively.

Gingival Carcinoma

Squamous epithelial carcinoma of the gingiva accounts for up to 20% of all intraoral carcinomas (Cawson et al. 1996). Males are more often affected. Gingival carcinoma occurs three times more frequently in the mandible than in the maxilla. In dentulous patients, the gingival carcinoma is easy to misinterpret, because the clinical signs are similar to those of odontogenic infections and periodontitis. Epulis-like tumor proliferation may also be observed. Osseous destruction can be detected radiographically. Tooth mobility will be increased if the tumor grows along the periodontal ligament. In rare cases, the carcinoma may arise from epithelial rest cells of Malassez, in which case it is referred to as a primary intraosseous squamous cell carcinoma. Regional metastases are frequent, occurring in 30–84% of cases. It is possible that other etiologic and pathogenic factors are involved in gingival carcinoma. in comparison to other oral cavity carcinomas (Barasch et al. 1995). (See also p. 198.)

Gingival carcinoma

450 Clinical appearance
Near the left mandibular premolars and molars one can see an epulis-like lesion with a slightly nodular surface and a fibrin coating. The teeth were slightly mobile. The patient reported only that she noted a mild, dull pain during chewing.

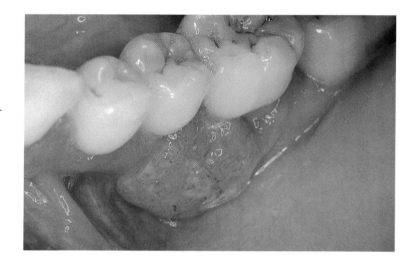

451 Radiograph
The periapical film reveals bone loss between the second premolar and the first molar. Radiographic examination, however, does not provide a differentiation between bone loss due to periodontitis and that caused by gingival carcinoma.

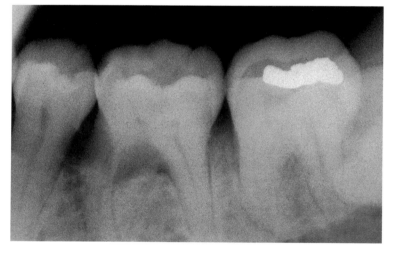

452 Histology
Subjacent to the unremarkable surface epithelium (right) there are several islands of tumor with initial keratinization and some atypical mitoses (H & E, x 140).

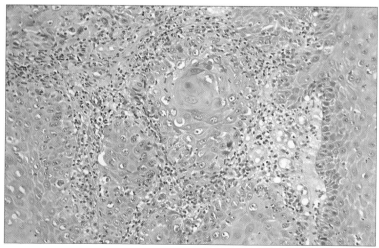

Other Lesions

Wegener's Granulomatosis, Malignant Melanoma

Wegener's granulomatosis is characterized by progressive granulomatous and necrotizing vasculitis of the upper respiratory tract and the kidney. Of diagnostic importance are the elevated titers of antineutrophilic autoantibodies, which react with antigens and cytoplasm of granulocytes and monocytes. Intraoral lesions are found on the gingiva, but also on the tongue, palate, the cheeks and the lips. The clinical appearance is a hemorrhagic, nodule-like hyperplasia of the gingiva with ulceration. The histologic picture reveals necrotizing granuloma with multinucleated giant cells, and a necrotizing vasculitis of small arteries and veins (Eufinger et al. 1992, Lilly et al. 1998).

Malignant melanoma of the gingiva occurs as a primary melanoma or as a metastatic melanoma (Sonner and Reichart 1994) from other mucosal or skin regions. The prognosis for intraoral melanoma is extraordinarily poor.

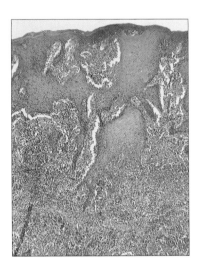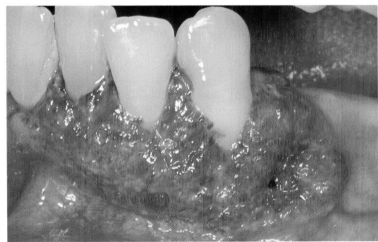

453 Wegener's granulomatosis
The gingiva of the left mandibular region exhibits the typical granular hemorrhagic lesion.

Left: Subjacent to the hyperplastic epithelium, one notes a very heavy inflammatory reaction, including a broad spectrum of immunocompetent cells. Further characteristics include the necrotizing vasculitis of small arteries, and multinucleated giant cells (H & E, x 40).

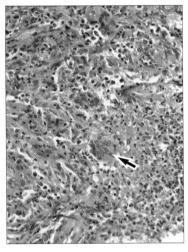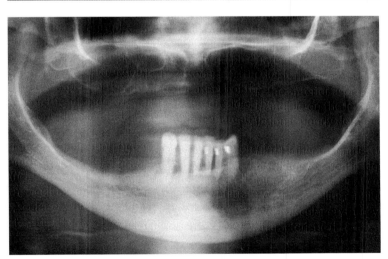

454 Wegener's granulomatosis—panoramic radiograph
This is the same patient shown in Fig. 453. The radiograph clearly reveals the osseous destruction in the anterior aspect of the mandible on the left side. The lesion is poorly demarcated.

Left: Higher magnification of the histologic section in Fig. 453, left. Multinucleated giant cells (arrow) in a dense cellular infiltrate with extravascular erythrocytes are characteristic (H & E, x 150).

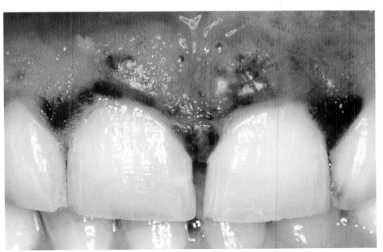

455 Malignant melanoma
The marginal gingiva, particularly the interdental papillae of the maxilla, has been infiltrated by malignant melanoma cells. Secondary melanoma is less common than the primary form. Of primary malignant melanomas, 50% occur on the hard palate, 25% on the gingiva of the maxilla. Thirty percent of oral melanomas develop from areas of hyperpigmentation.

Courtesy I. van der Waal

Juvenile Xanthogranuloma

Xanthoma and xanthogranuloma belong to the family of fibrohistiocytic tumors, or fibrous histiocytoma. These lesions may be benign, malignant or intermediate. The juvenile xanthogranuloma is benign or self-limiting. These tumors usually appear in the region of the skin or the skeletal musculature; they are extremely rare in the oral cavity. The clinical picture is a flat, but slightly raised, yellowish nodule on the gingiva, the tongue or the palate. The histologic picture reveals intertwined strands of spindle cells, xanthomatous or myxoid areas as well as the so-called Touton giant cells.

Gingival Cyst of Adults

In adults, the gingival cyst is rare and is localized in the canine-premolar region of the mandible, similar to the lateral periodontal cyst. The pathogenesis remains unclear, but the cyst may arise from odontogenic epithelial cell rests. The clinical picture reveals a spherical cyst about 1 cm in diameter at the border between the mobile and immobile mucosa (Fardal et al. 1994).

456 Juvenile xanthogranuloma
A symptom-free yellow-whitish spot about 5 mm long and 3 mm wide was noted on the gingiva of an 11-year-old patient in the area of the first and second maxillary premolars. Excision of the lesion and subsequent examination confirmed a juvenile xanthogranuloma.

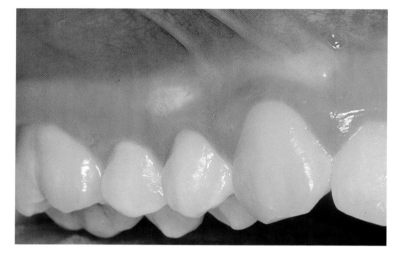

457 Juvenile xanthogranuloma—histology
The low-power view revealed an intact oral epithelium, beneath which the xanthogranuloma is localized. The Touton giant cells are embedded in a dense, cellular inflammatory infiltrate (H & E, x 60).

Right: At higher magnification, one notes multiple multinucleated giant cells in the connective tissue papillae and the lamina propria (H & E, x 240).

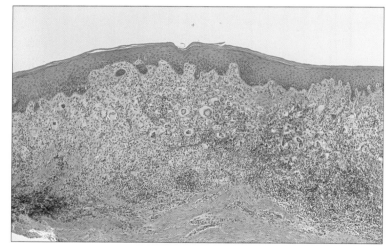
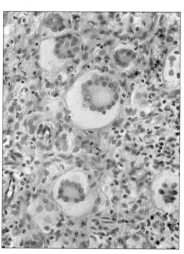

458 Gingival cyst of adults
A protuberance is noted between the lateral incisor and the canine on the right side of the mandible. The adjacent teeth reacted positively to a vitality test. The histologic picture revealed a cyst lined by a non-keratinized stratified squamous epithelium.

Right: The radiograph reveals a radiolucency between the mandibular right canine and the lateral incisor. Smaller cysts often appear as only minor radiolucencies.

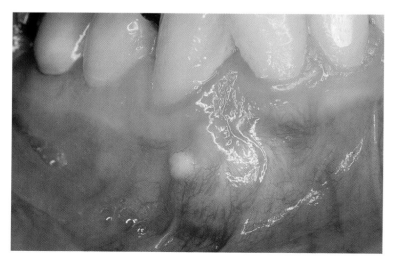
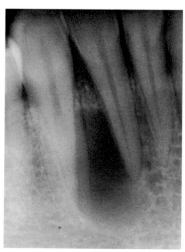

Sarcoidosis

Sarcoidosis is one member of a family of oral granulo-matoses that is characterized histologically by noncaseous, epithelioid granuloma (Ivanyi et al. 1993, Vettin et al. 1988). Sarcoidosis particularly affects the pulmonary lymph nodes, the liver, the skin, the eyes, bones, nerves and salivary glands. Oral manifestations are uncommon, but the gingiva is sometimes involved. The lesions are usually painless swellings.

The diagnosis is made through clinical and laboratory findings, especially through a biopsy, and a positive Kveim skin test. The therapy is based upon corticosteroid administration. (See also pp. 57, 86 and 124.)

Alpha-Mannosidosis

Alpha-mannosidosis is a very rare storage disease related to this special sugar (Ishigami et al. 1995). The oral manifestations include hyperplasia-like tissue accumulation on the gingiva, but also on the palate and the buccal mucosa.

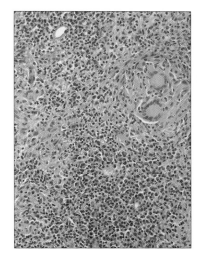
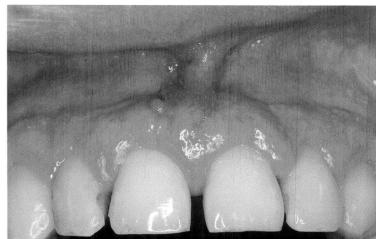
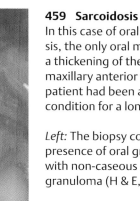

459 Sarcoidosis
In this case of oral granulomatosis, the only oral manifestation is a thickening of the gingiva in the maxillary anterior region. The patient had been aware of this condition for a long time.

Left: The biopsy confirmed the presence of oral granulomatosis with non-caseous epithelioid granuloma (H & E, x 100).

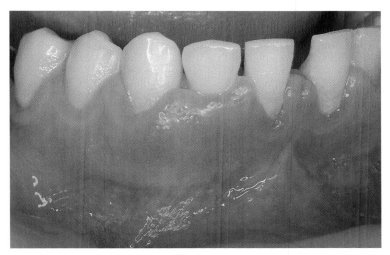
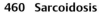

460 Sarcoidosis
This female presented with diffuse hyperplasia in the mandibular anterior region. She also reported symptoms in the lungs, which assisted in substantiating the diagnosis as sarcoidosis.

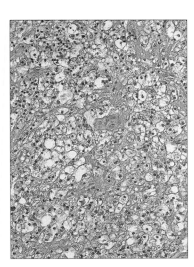
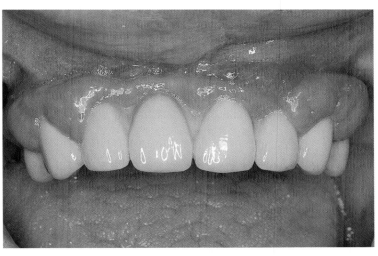

461 Alpha-mannosidosis
The gingiva is hyperplastic, similar in appearance to the gingiva hyperplasia caused by hydantoin therapy (see Figs. 424, left and 425 on p. 161). A straightforward gingivoplasty improved this patient's intraoral condition.

Left: Histologic picture of alpha-mannosidosis, exhibiting characteristic heavily vacuolated histologic cells (storage cells) as well as giant cells (H & E, x 100).

Wiskott–Aldrich's Syndrome

The Wiskott–Aldrich's syndrome is a rare disease whose pathogenesis involves primary immunodeficiency. Children with this disease already exhibit a high level of susceptibility to infections. The clinical course is often fatal. Oral manifestations are seldom observed, except for discrete hemorrhagic gingival lesions.

Chemotherapy-Induced Ulcerations

Stomatitis caused by cytostatic therapy appears as extensive epitheliolysis and very painful ulcerations; these are frequent side effects of antineoplastic therapy, because in addition to the effects of these powerful drugs on highly mitotically active malignant cells, healthy tissues such as the epithelium of the oral mucosa are also affected. The only treatment for the oral lesions is rigorous oral hygiene and the prevention of secondary infections. The oral lesions generally heal quickly and spontaneously when the medication is discontinued.

462 Wiskott–Aldrich's syndrome
The mandibular gingival margins exhibit small areas of erythema, indicating hemorrhage. The differential diagnosis should include disorders involving thrombocytopenia (Porter and Scully 1994).

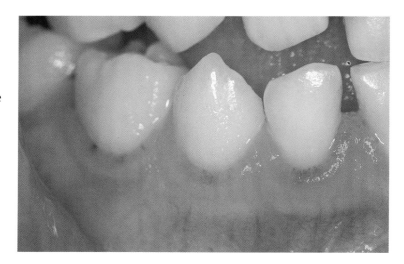

463 Ulcerations caused by cytostatic medications
This HIV patient with non-Hodgkin's lymphoma received a course of cytostatic therapy involving numerous medications. Extensive ulcerations with epitheliolysis and hemorrhage into the tissues could be observed in the region of the gingiva, the cheeks and the lateral borders of the tongue. Rinsing with hydrogen peroxide or iodine-based solutions can help to prevent secondary infections.

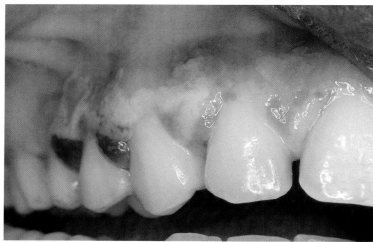

464 Gingival ulceration due to cytostatic treatment
This ulceration at the junction of the attached gingiva and the vestibular mucosa was associated with methotrexate therapy. The lesion was fibrin-covered and already in the initial stages of the healing process.

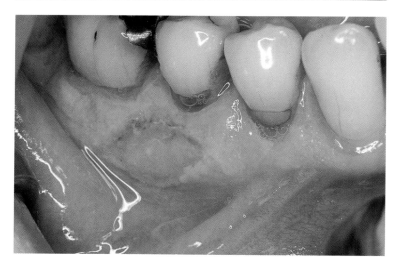

Pigmentation—Exogenous

Exogenous pigmentation of the oral mucosa, such as smoker's melanosis or particularly the amalgam tattoo, is relatively frequently observed; it may be either extensive or localized. The gingiva and the mucosa of the alveolar process are most often involved.

The clinical appearance of an amalgam tattoo is a well-circumscribed, bluish, black or gray discoloration. Such lesions are almost always observed in the superficial mucosa. Amalgam restorations that are damaged during tooth extraction often leave residues of the metal within the extraction wound; after healing, the mucosa will exhibit black discolorations. The differential diagnosis should include other types of pigmentation, such as nevi and above all the malignant melanoma.

The removal of metal particles and the excision of the pigmented areas of the mucosa can be attempted. If there is suspicion of a malignant melanoma, *no* cosmetic surgical manipulations should be performed.

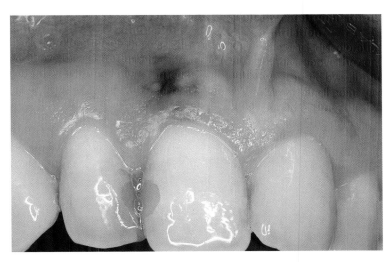

465 Tattooing through self-mutilation
The black discoloration of the gingiva above the central incisor was caused by self-mutilation with a pencil point. Over a long period of time, this female "drilled" the pencil again and again into the same site, causing graphite to be deposited in the mucosal tissues.

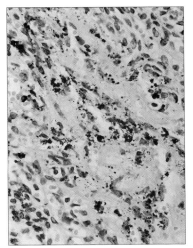

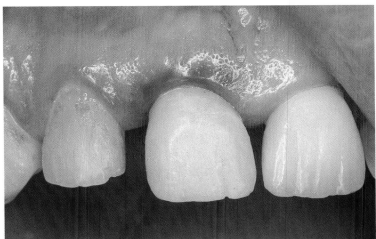

466 Metal tattoo
In this patient, a crown made of porcelain fused to metal elicited a gray discoloration of the marginal gingiva.

Left: Histologic picture of an amalgam tattoo, revealing the distribution of metal particles within fibroblasts and macrophages (H & E, x 120).

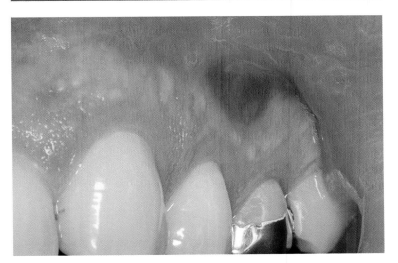

467 Metal tattoo
An endodontic procedure using a silver pin was performed on the maxillary second premolar. The gray and black discolorations near the apex of the second premolar resulted from deposition of silver sulfide in the tissues. This type of discoloration is harmless, but other forms of melanotic lesions must be strictly ruled out of the differential diagnosis.

Edentulous Jaw

The loss of teeth leads to involution and atrophy of the corresponding areas of the alveolar process, and eventually to alveolar collapse. The approximation of the buccal and lingual osseous lamellae of the alveolus leads to narrowing of the jaw and ultimately to a loss of vertical dimension. The loss of force application by the tooth root leads to continuous atrophy and simultaneously to a loss of osseous quality. In elderly individuals, osteoporosis also plays a role.

This chapter will present various types of inflammatory and neoplastic as well as iatrogenic lesions often observed in the edentulous jaw. For the most part, these diseases are not specifically characteristic for the edentulous jaw, but are also observed in the dentulous maxilla and/or mandible. The application of bone replacement materials and membranes, as well as their radiographic and histologic presentations and complications, will also be discussed.

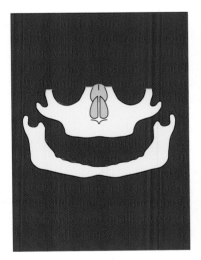

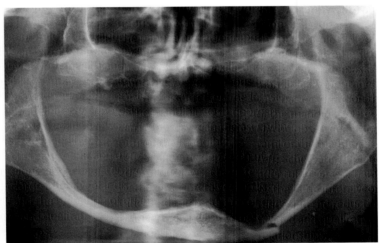

468 Atrophy with spontaneous fracture
The panoramic radiograph reveals an extreme situation with atrophy of both maxilla and mandible. A spontaneous fracture has occurred on the left side of the mandible. Osteoporosis can be observed in the ascending rami of the mandible.
Left: Schematic depiction of edentulous jaws, characterized by the large interalveolar distance and the reduction of quantitative and qualitative osseous relationships.

469 Senile midface and lower face
The body of the mandible and the ascending rami remain intact while the alveolar process is continuously atrophied. This leads to the "caved-in" appearance of the midface and the often pronounced wrinkling of the lower facial soft tissues.

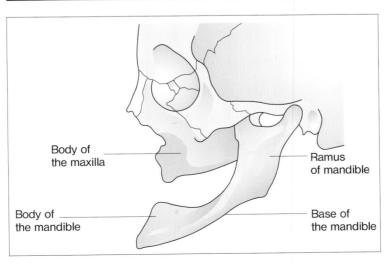

Body of
the maxilla

Ramus
of mandible

Body of
the mandible

Base of
the mandible

Infections—Bacterial and Mycotic

Denture Stomatitis

Denture stomatitis is a chronic inflammatory lesion that is frequently observed in denture wearers (prevalence rate 27–67% of patients). Newton (1962) classified three types:

- Type 1: Pinpoint erythema
- Type 2: Diffuse, extensive erythema
- Type 3: Papillary or nodular hyperplasia

Etiologic factors include old, ill-fitting dentures, the colonization of the dentures by microbial plaque, especially *Candida albicans*, and sometimes the residual monomer in the denture base itself. Since histologic examination has not demonstrated penetration of the mucosa by Candida hyphae, it has been assumed that extracellular proteases from *Candida albicans* support the inflammatory process from their location on the denture base, traversing the distance to the mucosa. (See also p. 131.)

470 Denture stomatitis
The clinical picture of denture stomatitis is characterized by spotty or extensive erythema, particularly in the palatal vault and less often on the alveolar process itself. Treatment consists of topical application of antimycotic agents, which can be painted onto the denture base. In some cases, it is necessary to fabricate a new denture, or recontour or reline the old denture. Failing these measures, recurrence of the stomatitis can be expected.

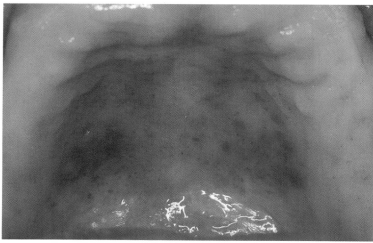

471 Papillary hyperplasia
Papillary hyperplasia is characterized by small, erythematous nodules on the palatal vault. Treatment consists of surgical removal by means of electrosurgery or laser surgery.

Right: Histologic picture of papillary hyperplasia. Some of the papillae are covered with epithelium and exhibit crypts of varying depths. Pronounced epithelial desquamation is obvious. Hyphae are usually not discernable (H & E, x 40).

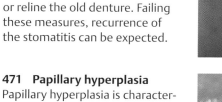

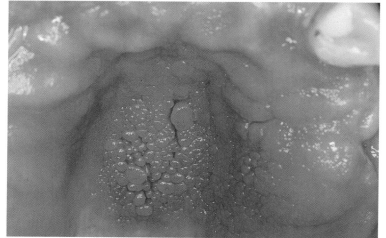

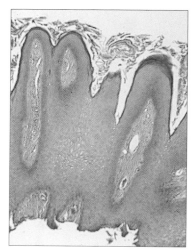

472 Hyperplasia resulting from denture irritation
In the anterior area of the maxillary alveolar process (indicated by the forceps), one observes multiple curtain-like areas of tissue hyperplasia, which resulted from continuous trauma by the denture border. Modification of the denture base will not lead to spontaneous regression of such hyperplasia. Surgical excision is required, with simultaneous or subsequent vestibuloplasty.

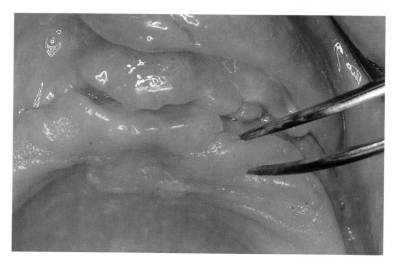

Mechanical and Physical Causes

Denture Irritation Hyperplasia and Denture Ulcer

Denture irritation hyperplasia occurs as a result of continuous traumatization of the denture-covered mucosa. Compared to other hyperplastic connective tissue proliferations, denture irritation hyperplasia is the most common tumor-like swelling of the oral cavity. It occurs because of "low-grade trauma." The clinical picture is one of pink nodules or swelling with occasionally ulcerated surfaces. The histologic picture reveals bundles of collagen fibers subjacent to the squamous epithelium; there is no capsule or pseudocapsule formation. The epithelium is frequently acanthotic. Inflammatory manifestations occur often, especially in cases of ulceration or infection with *Candida albicans*. Because these redundant soft tissue lesions caused by denture-based irritation are usually resected surgically, little is known about their growth potential. Histologic confirmation is required to assure that the swellings are benign. (Further information about *denture-induced ulcers* is summarized in the legends to Figs. 474 and 475.)

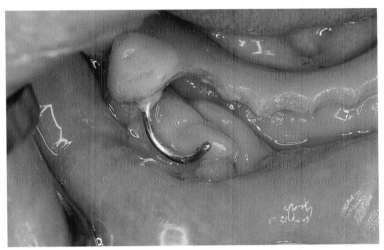

473 Tissue hyperplasia resulting from denture irritation
On the right side of the mandible there is a typical, painless hyperplasia in association with a redundant partial denture clasp that had not been removed. The mucosal irritation emanated from the poor stabilization of the mandibular denture, which was not modified following loss of the remaining anterior teeth.

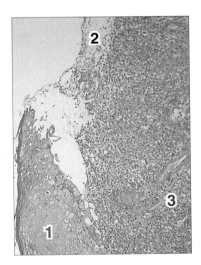

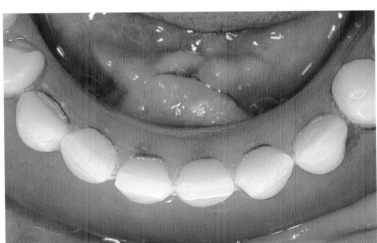

474 Denture-induced ulcer
The denture-induced ulcer is common in people with complete dentures, particularly in the mandible. The ulceration is painful and the adjacent tissues exhibit inflammation.

Left: Histologic examination must rule out squamous epithelial carcinoma (H & E, x 80).

1 Epithelium
2 Fibrin
3 Granulation tissue

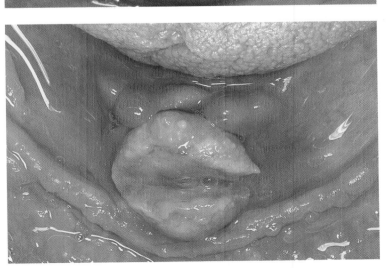

475 Denture-induced ulcer
Following removal of the denture shown in Fig. 474, one observes a large, fibrin-coated ulcer. If the denture-induced ulcer does not heal spontaneously after the patient has not worn the denture for 14 days, suspicion should arise concerning the possibility of a squamous cell carcinoma. Fabricating a new denture or relining the old denture is absolutely necessary.

Infection—Bacterial

Peri-implantitis

Peri-implantitis is an inflammatory alteration of the tissues surrounding the zone where a dental implant penetrates the gingiva; it is in principle similar to the gingivitis and periodontitis experienced by dentulous patients. After decades of using implants, the phenomenon is now considered to be a late complication. In the area where the implant traverses the mucosa, colonization of the sulcus by microorganisms occurs between the implant post and the gingiva. Almost all modern dental implant systems exhibit a highly polished metal surface at the zone of soft tissue contact. However, often there is early involvement of the most coronal threaded portion of the implant, which exhibits a rough surface. Similar to the situation where a tooth is involved periodontally, the soft tissues and surrounding bone become progressively involved (Esposito et al. 1998). Treatment will involve professional prophylaxis, curettage, smoothing the implant surface, and gingivoplasty as well as other methods, such as the use of bone replacement materials or membrane techniques (Lang et al. 1997).

476 Peri-implantitis
Note the obvious inflammatory symptoms, including pronounced soft tissue hyperplasia, around the left and right distal implants.

Right: Histologic view of peri-implantitis. Note the massive infiltration by inflammatory cells, as well as hyperemia and downward growth of the epithelium (H & E, x 20).

1 Oral epithelium
2 Granulation tissue

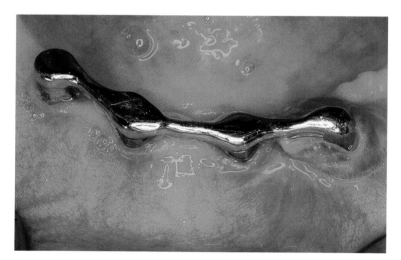
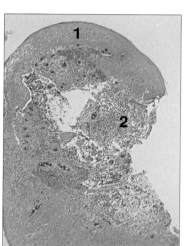

477 Radiograph of peri-implantitis
This section from a panoramic radiograph depicts the implants with peri-implantitis shown in Fig. 476. The level of the bone is about the same around all of the implants. However, a certain reduction of the bone height around the implants has occurred. Formation of true bony pockets around the implants, in the sense of vertical bone loss, is not in evidence.

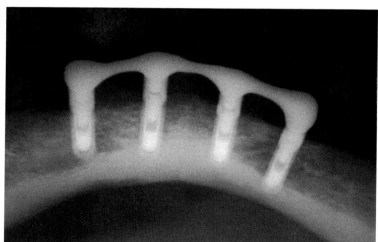

478 Peri-implantitits
In the anterior region of the edentulous mandible, one observes a single-stage dental implant devoid of suprastructure and exhibiting massive plaque accumulation. The soft tissues are severely erythematous and exhibit inflammatory infiltration. The radiograph revealed massive osseous defects.

Right: The implant, which had to be removed, exhibits adherent necrotic tissue along its entire threaded surface.

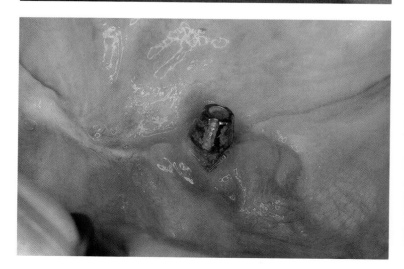
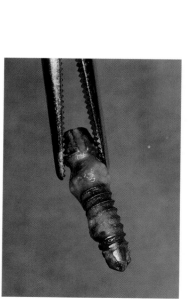

Infections—Mycotic

Aspergillosis

Aspergillus species, particularly *A. fumigatus*, are occasionally the cause of opportunistic infections, particularly following long-term antimicrobial or immunosuppressive therapy.

In recent years there have been many reports of *aspergillosis in the maxillary sinuses* (Beck-Mannagetta et al. 1986 Chambers et al. 1995). In the recorded cases, the situation was caused by root canal filling material being extruded into the maxillary sinus during endodontic treatment. Because many root canal filling materials contain zinc, an aspergilloma is formed around this nutritive substrate (Willinger et al. 1996). Aspergilloma of the maxillary sinus is usually detected by chance on a radiograph and is characterized by a central opacity caused by the root canal filling material. This is an indication for surgical removal of the aspergilloma from the sinus. Aspergilloma may also occur following placement of dental implants, if they encroach upon the sinus.

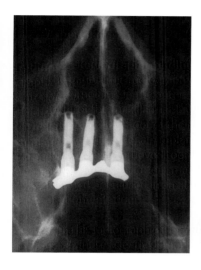
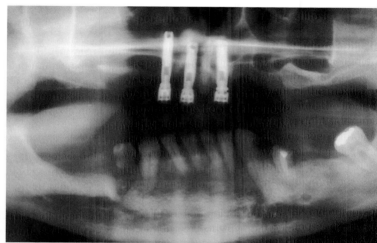

Aspergillosis

479 Radiographic findings
The panoramic radiograph depicts implants in the anterior segment of the maxilla that have perforated the floor of the nose. On the right side, an implant had already been removed together with bone replacement material that had been used in an attempt at augmentation.

Left: This radiograph of the lateral nasal sinuses clearly demonstrates that the implants have perforated.

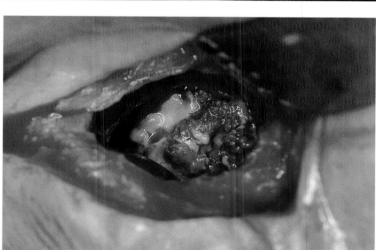

480 Intraoperative view
Surgical entry into the left maxillary sinus revealed the presence of a brown aspergilloma about 3 cm in diameter. The remaining bone replacement material was also removed from the sinus.

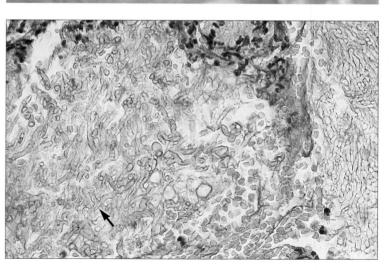

481 Histology
The histologic picture reveals the typical septate and branching hyphae of *Aspergillus fumigatus* (arrow) (H & E, x 100).

Irritations Caused by Foreign Bodies

Hydroxyapatite

The augmentation of the atrophied jaw using hydroxyapatite or other bone replacement material appears to be an ideal alternative to complex surgical procedures such as absolute alveolar bone augmentation by means of free bone transplants or cartilage transplants. The creation of a subperiosteal tunnel along the alveolar process was believed to permit placement of the bone replacement material upon the alveolar bone to provide heightening of the alveolar process, which could be loaded (e.g., by a denture). Quite soon,

however, it was demonstrated that the hydroxyapatite granules were unstable and migrated into the soft tissues (Becker et al. 1988). Soft tissue dehiscences were observed, from which the granules escaped. The major problem was that the implanted material failed to be incorporated and surrounded by new bone. It was observed that the implant material was completely lost over time. Today, hydroxyapatite is rarely used as an augmentation material, but it is sometimes observed as a foreign body in radiographs.

482 Hydroxyapatite
On the right side of the edentulous mandible there is a large soft tissue dehiscence which occurred after attempted ridge augmentation. Several granules can be observed.

Right: Histologic view. The granule on the left exhibits particulation (arrow), as well as splinters (arrowheads). The tight contact and connective tissue encapsulation leads to "grinding" of the granules due to micromovements (Giemsa, x 120).

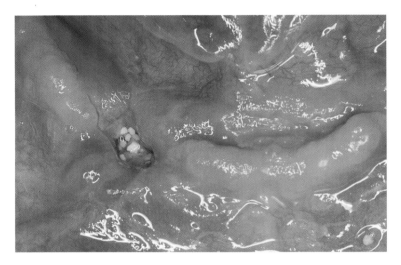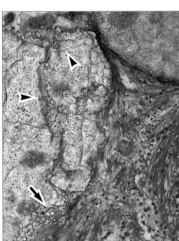

483 Hydroxyapatite augmentation
This section from a panoramic radiograph shows remnants of the hydroxyapatite material (*) on the left mandibular alveolar process; the material has partially penetrated into the bone.

Right: In the cell-rich connective tissue between the granules, one notes a large foreign body giant cell (arrow), which is a sign of a foreign body reaction (Giemsa, x 120).

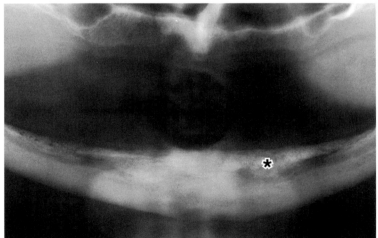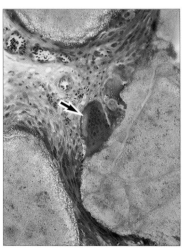

484 Augmentation
This section from a panoramic radiograph reveals the augmentation material that was placed in the right maxilla to treat "flabby ridge."

Right: Alveolar process of the right maxilla. Severe inflammation is noted in the area of augmentation, as well as a fibrin-coated fistula (arrow). Several granules of the augmentation material had escaped via this fistula over time.

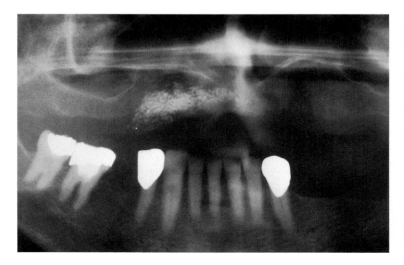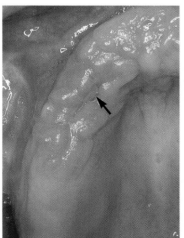

Infection Caused by Foreign Bodies/Oro-antral Fistula

Guided Bone Regeneration, Membrane Techniques

Before or during the placement of dental implants, guided bone regeneration offers the possibility of improving the bony implant bed. This technique targets the selection of specific bone-forming cells using barrier techniques. To achieve this goal, either resorbable or nonresorbable membranes have been used (Schenk 1994). However, numerous authors have described the occurrence of dehiscence, which leads to infection of the entire membrane. This event completely negates any success achieved with the procedure, because the membranes almost always have to be removed.

Oro-antral Fistula

Oro-antral perforation frequently occurs due to atrophy of the maxillary alveolar process. This sometimes leads to the formation of polyps in the antrum, which are not discovered because they may be covered by a denture base.

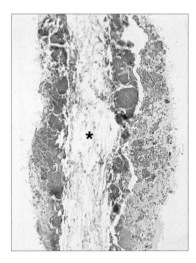 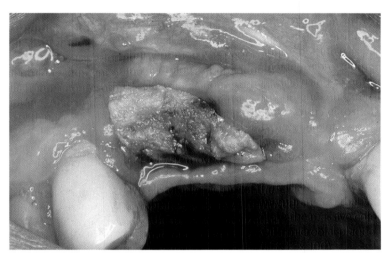

485 Augmentation procedure
A surgical attempt at osseous augmentation was performed in an edentulous segment of the maxilla using a nonresorbable membrane. An extensive dehiscence with necrosis of the soft tissues and infection of the membrane occurred. The membrane had to be removed.

Left: Histologic picture of the membrane (*) that was removed. Note the massive colonization with microbial plaque (H & E, x 100).

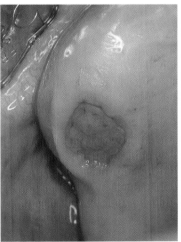 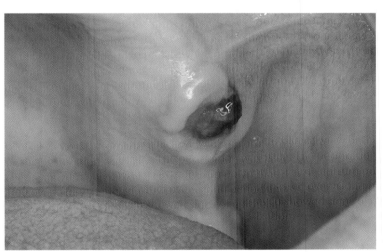

486 Sinus polyp
A soft, brownish mass, which bled readily when prodded, was detected in the alveolus of the left maxillary molars. This antrum polyp had formed within a few days.

Left: Clinical view of the oroantral fistula. The perforation was filled with a large antrum polyp that persisted over a long period and even showed signs of epithelialization.

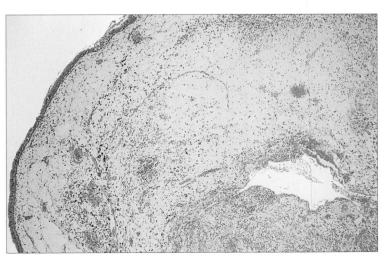

487 Maxillary sinus polyp—histology
Note the loosely organized granulation polyp with hemorrhagic foci and varying degrees of inflammatory cell infiltration. The surface is covered by sinus epithelium (H & E, x 40).

Disturbances of Keratinization

Frictional Keratosis

Frictional keratosis is usually observed on the marginal gingiva and alveolar mucosa in dentulous areas of the jaw; the primary factor is overzealous brushing of the teeth. Sometimes the lesion is also noted beneath a denture, where it is usually limited to the alveolar process and its keratinized mucosa. Other factors, such as tobacco and alcohol, do not play a role beneath the denture. The clinical picture is impossible to differentiate from homogeneous leukoplakia, and thus a biopsy and long-term observation are indicated.

This is particularly the case when other areas of the oral cavity, for example, the floor of the mouth, also exhibit leukoplakia (van der Waal et al. 1997).

Leukoplakia/Carcinoma

Leukoplakia and carcinoma of the palate and the edentulous alveolar process are rare. Idiopathic leukoplakia may affect the entire oral cavity, including the edentulous alveolar process.

488 Frictional keratosis
On the left side of the edentulous maxilla there is an extensive white lesion and a smaller, less distinct lesion on the right alveolar process. The white substance could not be wiped off. The rest of the oral cavity exhibited no evidence of leukoplakia.

Right: Note the white lesion on the mandibular alveolar process. The most important differential diagnosis is leukoplakia. Such lesions seldom recur following laser surgery.

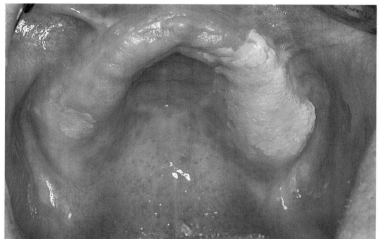
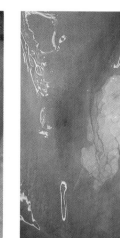

489 Idiopathic leukoplakia
This 70-year-old female had exhibited idiopathic leukoplakia in all areas of the oral cavity for many years. Various therapies had been attempted. On the left alveolar process, and partially on the right, one notes a non-homogeneous leukoplakia with white granular nodules against a red background. Such areas of extensive leukoplakia often provide the basis for the simultaneous or repetitive development of carcinomas, a process called field cancerization.

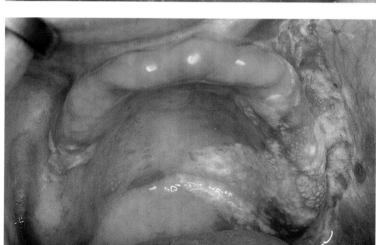

490 Carcinoma
In the anterior mandible vestibulum of this edentulous patient one notes a homogeneous area of leukoplakia (arrow). Distal to this lesion there is an extensive, non-homogeneous, superficially ulcerated and indurated lesion (*). This represents a carcinoma that developed from the leukoplakia.
Right: Biopsy from the border of the suspected carcinoma. The early invasion exhibits the dropping off phenomenon and infiltration into the tissue (H & E, x 80).

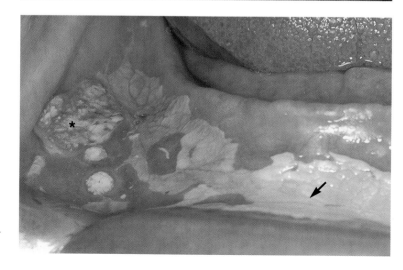
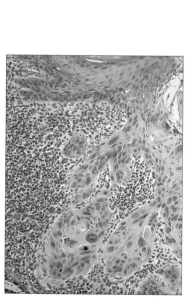

Tumors—Benign and Malignant

Pleomorphic Adenoma

Pleomorphic adenoma of the minor salivary glands of the palate is, in addition to other adenomas, the most common benign tumor in this location. The clinical symptoms are few, often only a mild swelling with a livid bluish color, which is painless upon palpation. The localization corresponds to the distribution of the minor salivary glands in the transition zone between the hard and soft palate. Young individuals may also be affected. In elderly patients who wear dentures, the entire surface of the palate should be carefully inspected and palpated at each appointment, because the differential diagnosis of pleomorphic adenoma also includes adenoidcystic carcinoma.

Mycosis Fungoides

Mycosis fungoides is the most common T-cell lymphoma of the skin. Oral manifestations are only rarely observed, considerably less frequently than with B-cell non-Hodgkin's lymphoma (Hornstein 1996, Hata et al. 1998).

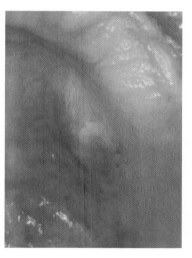 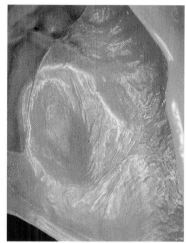

491 Pleomorphic adenoma
Left: In the anterior area of the left palatal vault one observes a flat, bluish swelling that corresponds to a recessed area on the undersurface of the denture.

Right: Inner surface of the maxillary full denture. The relieved portion, which accommodates the tumor (left), can be clearly seen. In this case, the practitioner failed in his responsibility to diagnose the swelling.

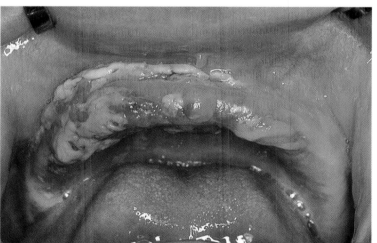

492 Mycosis fungoides
In this female, the edentulous maxillary alveolar process exhibits massive necroses and inflammatory lesions, which indicate the presence of oral mycosis fungoides.

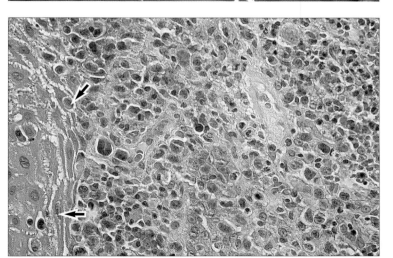

493 Mycosis fungoides—histology
In this histologic picture, the oral mucosal epithelium is located at the left side (arrows), and subjacent to it one notes a primarily large-cell, pleomorphic, anaplastic lymphoma, which is typical for the late stages of mycosis fungoides (H & E, x 150).

Malignant Tumors

Malignant Lymphoma (Non-Hodgkin's Lymphoma)

The oral non-Hodgkin's lymphoma, usually of the B-cell type, is occasionally detected on the palatal vault. B-cell lymphoma may contain lymphoblastic, lymphocytic, plasmocytic or immunoblastic lymphoma, as well as follicular center cell lymphoma (Kiel classification). Malignant lymphoma of the oral mucosa may occur as primary lesions, without any manifestations in other organ systems. There is usually a subsequent systemic dissemination with extramucosal manifestations. The non-Hodgkin's lymphoma may also appear, however, as a secondary lesion in the oral mucosa. Morphologic diagnosis is extraordinarily difficult; required is the identification of monoclonal lymphoid subpopulations.

Carcinoma

Carcinoma of the oral mucosa in an edentulous jaw is observed more frequently in the mandible than in the maxilla. The tumor may often achieve dramatic proportions in elderly patients.

494 Non-Hodgkin's lymphoma
This patient presented with bilateral swellings of the edentulous posterior maxilla that were almost perfectly symmetrical. There were no obvious lesions of the overlying mucosa and no ulceration. In this patient, other extranodal manifestations of the lymphoma had already been diagnosed. Treatment consisted of systemic antineoplastic medication.

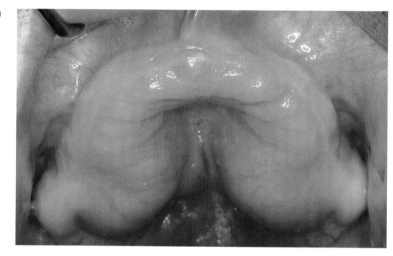

495 Carcinoma
This carcinoma on the left side of the edentulous maxilla is extensive and exhibits the stippling that is typical for carcinoma of the edentulous jaw. Note the sharply demarcated margin adjacent to the vestibulum.

Right: Carcinoma of the mandible in the retromolar region, exhibiting ulceration and obvious tissue proliferation.

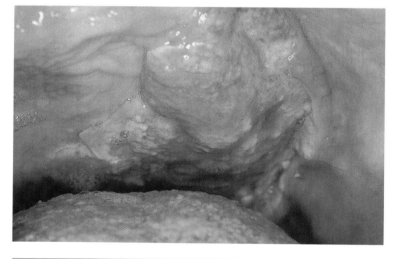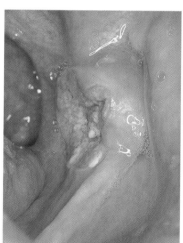

496 Carcinoma
Carcinoma of the left maxilla, with ulceration and infiltration. The patient had worn a maxillary complete denture, which had been fitted with a "suction cup" that created the depression in the palatal mucosa (arrow).
Right: In the lower portion of this picture, the ulcerated, necrotic carcinoma can be seen (**1**). Immediately anterior, one notes the speckled leukoplakia with whitish nodules on an erythematous base (**2**), and anteriorly the homogeneous leukoplakia (**3**).

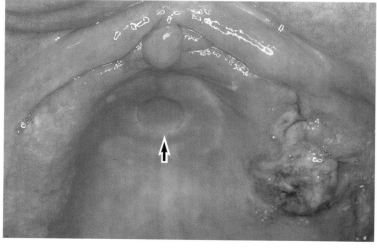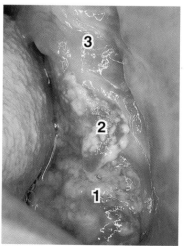

Other Lesions

Free Gingival Grafts and Split Thickness Skin Grafts

Mucosal/gingival and skin grafts are often utilized in the oral cavity in surgical procedures intended to augment the alveolar process (Fröschl and Kerscher 1997) and for covering defects after major soft tissue resections. The most common donor site for tissue transplantation in the oral cavity is the palate. *Skin transplantation* into the oral cavity may be associated with unpleasant sequelae; due to the severe epithelial desquamation, skin transplants into the oral cavity are often infected with *Candida albicans*, which lends a *white color*. Following application of antimycotic medications, however, such skin transplants achieve a pink color that is similar to normal oral mucosa. If hair follicles remain in the skin graft, there may be actual *hair growth* on the skin transplant inside the mouth.

The inexperienced clinician may confuse mucosal/gingival or skin grafts in the oral cavity with leukoplakia.

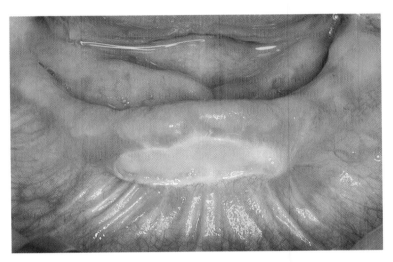

497 Free gingival graft
This free gingival graft in the edentulous anterior mandible is clearly visible; the procedure was performed simultaneously with a vestibuloplasty. A 1-cm wide, fixed zone of attached gingiva was achieved. Histologic examinations have shown that free gingival grafts are well accepted by the adjacent tissues.

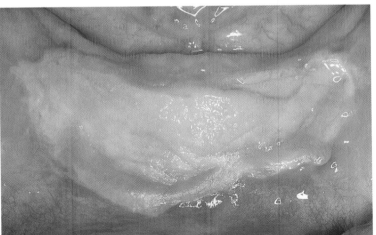

498 Skin transplant
This expansive skin transplant in the mandibular vestibulum exhibits a yellowish-white color, which indicates an infection with *Candida albicans*. Patients sometimes perceive skin transplants as unpleasant, because disturbances of taste and a particular odor may develop.

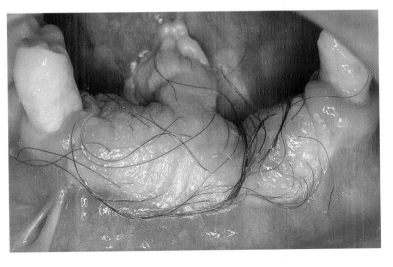

499 Skin transplant
Following a surgical procedure to remove a tumor from the floor of the mouth, the surgical defect was covered with a split thickness skin graft. Unfortunately, the graft was not thinned sufficiently, and it therefore contained hair follicles, which led to the development of hair growth in the oral cavity. The hairs have to be trimmed. In addition, topical antimycotics must be applied to reduce infection by *Candida albicans*.

Jaws

The bones of the jaws and the bones of the facial skeleton may exhibit a large number of pathologic processes, which may take their origins from systemic or local disturbances. In addition to the medical history and the clinical examination, radiographic procedures are absolutely necessary for diagnosis. Proper interpretation of radiographic, computed tomographic or magnetic resonance imaging data demands precise knowledge of the osseous and soft tissue anatomy as portrayed in the various diagnostic systems. In addition, the dentist must possess comprehensive knowledge of the pathologic processes in order to arrive at a final diagnosis. Several specific disease processes will be explored in this chapter, processes that have not been presented in other chapters of this book.

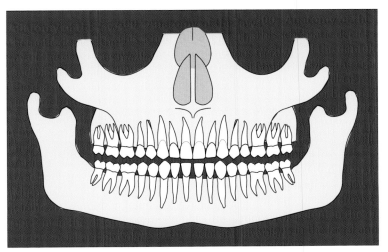

500 Anatomy of the jaws
This schematic depicts the anatomy of the dentulous maxilla and mandible. The cranial boundary of the maxilla is represented by the inferior border of the orbit, while the dorsal border is represented by the zygoma and the zygomatic arch as well as the infraorbital fossa.

The practitioner must possess comprehensive knowledge of the radiographic anatomy, in order to be competent in the diagnosis of lesions in the facial and alveolar skeleton.

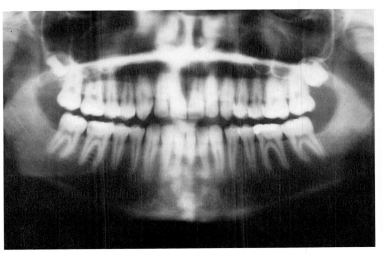

501 Panoramic radiograph—anatomy
This panoramic radiograph of an 18-year-old patient provides an example of the numerous possibilities for "normal" anatomy of the midface and the mandible. The radiograph provides a good overview of the entire facial complex, which is necessary for a comprehensive evaluation of the anatomic situation, including all possible pathologic processes.

Infections—Bacterial

Periapical Granuloma

The periapical granuloma is by far the most commonly diagnosed pathologic radiolucency, accounting for about 50% of all diagnosed radiolucencies. The periapical granuloma can be viewed as the body's successful attempt to neutralize and encapsulate the toxic products from the root canal. The process is a low-grade inflammatory reaction with proliferation of vascular granulation tissue. A periapical granuloma can be viewed as part of the repair process. The radiographic picture is one of a well-circumscribed radiolucency, usually round in shape, encompassing the periapical region. It is impossible to differentiate radiographically between a periapical granuloma and a small radicular cyst (Oehlers 1970).

Submucosal Abscess

An acute odontogenic abscess may develop either intra-orally or extra-orally. The severe and sometimes fatal odontogenic abscesses are quite rare today.

502 Periapical granuloma—intra-oral radiographs
In the periapical region of the mandibular right first molar, one notes a diffuse interradicular radiolucency that appears to expand distally. The root canal fillings are obviously inadequate.

Right: The lateral incisor exhibits a periapical radiolucency after trepanation. The diagnosis of "periapical osteolysis following pulpal necrosis" is likely.

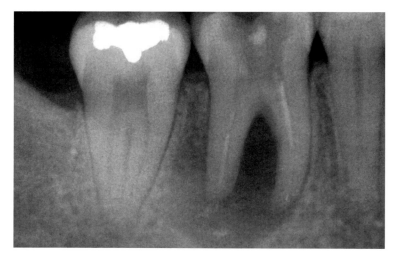
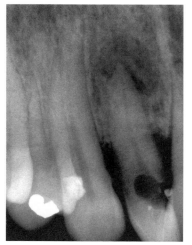

503 Periapical granuloma
The periapical granuloma consists of proliferating epithelial rest cells of Malassez (arrows), capillaries, immature fibroblasts and some collagen. Chronic inflammatory cells (arrowheads), such as lymphocytes, plasma cells and macrophages predominate (H & E, x 80).

Right: Periapical granuloma on the palatal root of a maxillary premolar.

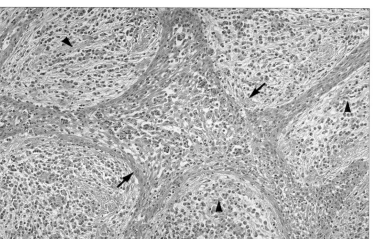
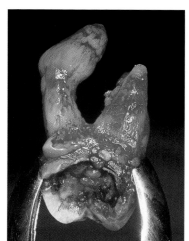

504 Periapical granuloma/odontogenic abscess
Periapical granulomas will often contain nests of odontogenic epithelium (arrows). While the lower epithelial island represents quiescent epithelium, proliferation of the upper island has already begun (H & E, x 80).

Right: Submucosal odontogenic abscess, emanating from the maxillary left lateral incisor. The lesion is fluctuant and should be incised.

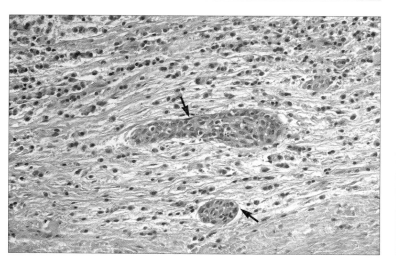
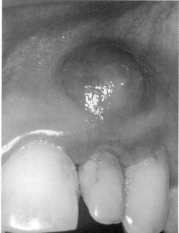

Osteomyelitis

Osteomyelitis of the jaw bone usually derives from an odontogenic source. The term osteomyelitis is used to describe a rather diffuse dissemination of inflammation within the jaw. All portions of the bone, including the periosteum, may be affected, in contrast to ostitis, which exhibits a much more circumscribed and usually periapical inflammation.

Osteomyelitis can occur at any age, but is relatively rare in children. Males and females are approximately equally affected, and the lesions are described as either acute or chronic. The cause of osteomyelitis can usually be traced to nonvital teeth. Other causes include periodontal diseases, jaw fracture, foreign bodies such as wires or osteosynthesis screws, or hematogenic dissemination. Osteomyelitis is more common in the mandible, due to the compact osseous structure and the limited vascular supply.

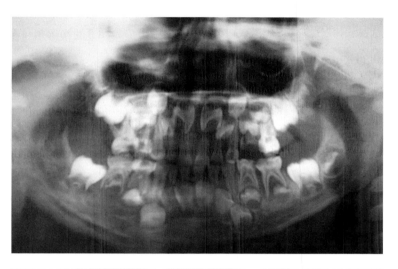

Acute osteomyelitis

505 Panoramic radiograph
A diffuse osteolysis can be ascertained in the right mandible extending into the ascending ramus in this 5-year-old Japanese male. The differential diagnosis should include Ewing's sarcoma.

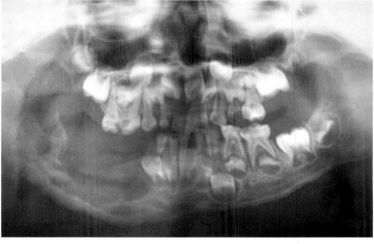

506 Postsurgical appearance
Despite massive antibiotic therapy, it was necessary to perform a resection of the right mandible in order to limit the spread of the inflammation.

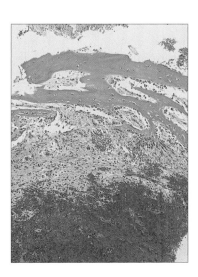
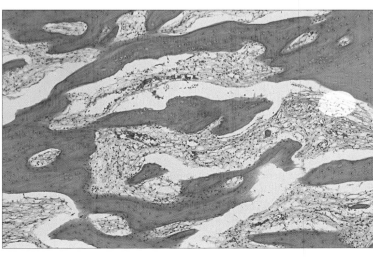

507 Histology
The histologic picture reveals osseous trabeculae with still vital bone as well as a loose connective tissue exhibiting an inflammatory cell infiltration. This histologic section derived from the border of the acute osteomyelitic process (H & E, x 100).

Left: Histologic preparation exhibiting bony trabeculae and massive hemorrhage (H & E, x 80).

Figs. 505–507:
Courtesy K. Sugihara

Chronic Osteomyelitis

Chronic osteomyelitis occurs with or without proliferative periostitis, in the form of a purulent, sclerosing, focal or diffuse lesion. Several special forms of osteomyelitis are acknowledged, for example, chronic periostitis in denture wearers and osteoradionecrosis (see p. 195).

The treatment is usually a combination of surgery and antibiotics; the course of therapy may last for years (Feifel et al. 1997).

Chronic suppurative (purulent) osteomyelitis exhibits simi-lar, although milder, signs of primary acute osteomyelitis. In addition to pain and fever, the teeth in the affected area are highly mobile. The lymph nodes are swollen and painful. In addition, there may be intraoral and extraoral fistulae (van Merkesteyn et al. 1997).

Sclerosing forms of osteomyelitis (see p. 194) must be differentiated from fibrous dysplasia and ossifying/cementifying fibroma (Hell 1986).

The radiographic picture of primary acute osteomyelitis is, for the most part, unremarkable.

Chronic osteomyelitis

508 8-year-old female
An area of chronic osteomyelitis is evident in the right mandible, necessitating the extraction of several deciduous and permanent teeth.
  The primary goal of treatment for osteomyelitis is the elimination of the etiologic factor. In cases of chronic osteomyelitis with sequester formation, the sequestra must be removed.

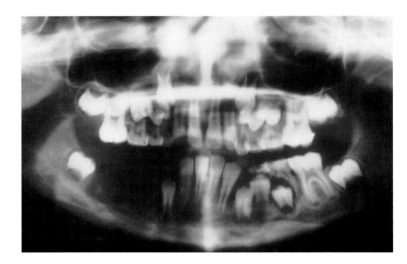

509 Follow-up after 6 years
Despite antibiotic therapy, decortication and application of gentamycin, the osteomyelitis expanded to involve the entire mandible (Figs. 508–510 are from the same patient).

Right: Histologic picture of a sequester with bacterial colonization on devitalized bone and empty osteocytic lacunae (H & E, x 80).

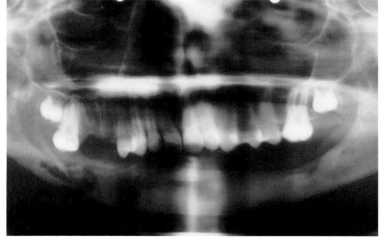
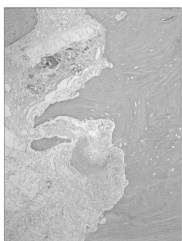

510 Follow-up after 8 years
Radiographic presentation of the same patient, eight years after the chronic mandibular osteomyelitis had begun. The disease had progressed to such an extent that only the basal mandibular bone remained; even the remaining bone exhibits areas of further osteolytic activity.
  In recent years, the treatment for osteomyelitis has included hyperbaric oxygen.
Figs. 508–510:
Courtesy B. Hoffmeister

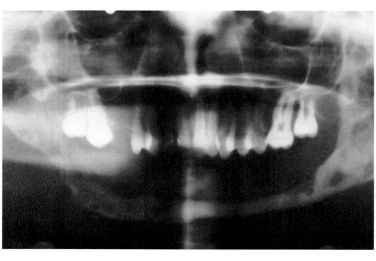

Necrotic bone fragments begin to appear as sequesters only when the lesion enters the chronic stage. A proliferative periostitis may also occur, with actual bony apposition. Szintigraphy using technetium-99m can be employed as an additional diagnostic aid. Using this technique, osteomyelitis appears in the form of "hot spots." False negative findings sometimes occur.

The microbiologic picture of osteomyelitis involves Gram-positive aerobic staphylococci, but also Gram-negative microorganisms, such as *Bacteriodes melaninogenicus*. In the chronic, sclerosing types of osteomyelitis, pathogenic organisms are often difficult to identify.

Periostitis with Sequester Formation

The dental practitioner will occasionally observe periostitis with the formation of peripheral sequetra beneath full dentures.

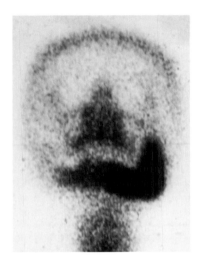
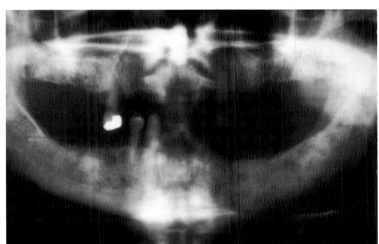

511   Chronic osteomyelitis
The panoramic radiograph reveals a chronic, diffuse osteomyelitis on the left side of the mandible, exhibiting the typical "cloudy" structure and destruction of the cortical bone.

Left: A szintigram depicts the spread of the osteomyelitis better than the panoramic radiograph. The inflammatory process has expanded into the horizontal anterior mandibular ramus.

Courtesy B. Hoffmeister

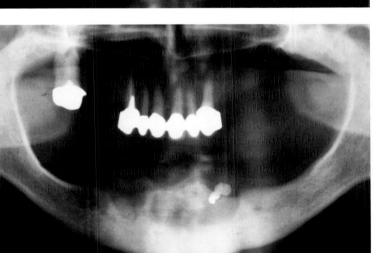

512   Periostitis with sequester formation—panoramic radiograph
The radiograph shows numerous peripheral osseous sequestra in the anterior segment of the mandible. These are a consequence of the periostitis in this region. In this case, the chronic periostitis was probably elicited by a mandibular denture.

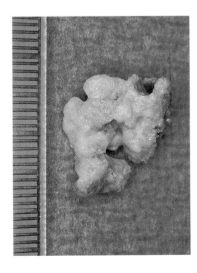
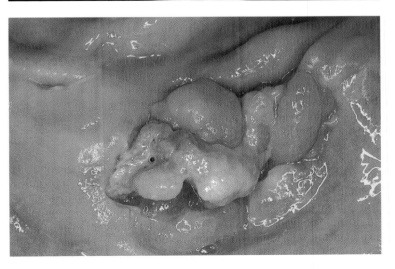

513   Periostitis with sequester formation
The peripheral osseous sequester (shown in Fig. 512) is obvious in the anterior region of the mandible, surrounded by the severely inflamed mucosa of the alveolar ridge and the vestibulum.

Left: The bony sequester consists of nonvital bone with a massive accumulation of microbial plaque. In most cases, the remaining bone of the mandible must be "freshened up" in order to achieve adequate healing.

Sclerosing Osteomyelitis

Diffuse, chronic, sclerosing osteomyelitis is usually observed in elderly patients, commonly those with an edentulous mandible. The clinical course is usually free of symptoms, but exacerbations may occur. The mandible is usually enlarged. The cause of chronic, sclerosing osteomyelitis is not always clear (Groot et al. 1996). This type of osteomyelitis is observed frequently in Black females.

Focal Osteosclerosis

Focal osteosclerosis or focal, chronic, sclerosing osteomyelitis, is characterized by a well-circumscribed radiopaque structure in the area of the root apex. Chronic periapical osteosclerosis may derive from low-grade infections, or it may appear following orthodontic treatment. No treatment is necessary, and bone biopsy is usually not particularly informative because the biopsy normally consists merely of sclerosing bone. The radiographic picture should be used to distinguish this form of sclerosis from hypercementosis or the benign cementoblastoma.

514 Sclerosing osteomyelitis
In this Black female, the panoramic radiograph reveals a chronic sclerosing osteomyelitis of the mandible. Within the entire mandible, varyingly dense radiopacities can be observed.

Courtesy I. Thompson

Right: Sclerosing osteomyelitis exhibits cement-like structures of bone with only few osteocytes (H & E, x 80).

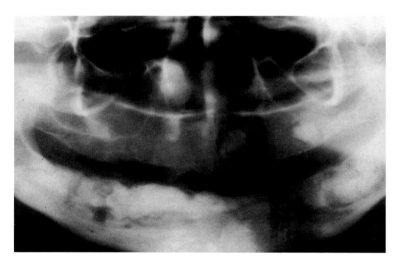 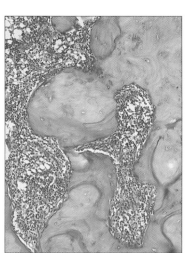

515 Focal osteosclerosis
A diffuse periapical opacity can be observed immediately above the mandibular canal on the distal root tip of the right first mandibular molar. After the tooth was extracted, the sclerosis subsided.

Right: The histologic picture reveals sclerosing bone with abnormal distribution of the bone marrow (Giemsa, x 10).

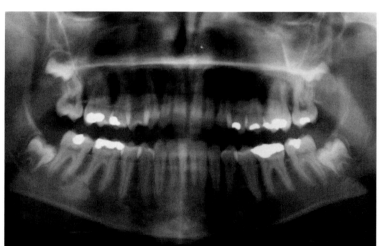 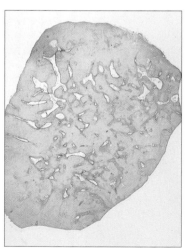

516 Focal osteosclerosis
The panoramic radiograph depicts a typical, dense sclerosis of the mandible in the region of the second premolar and first molar. It is possible that low-grade infections lead to this form of sclerosis.

Right: Histologic picture of focal osteosclerosis without any signs of inflammation or necrosis (H & E, x 60).

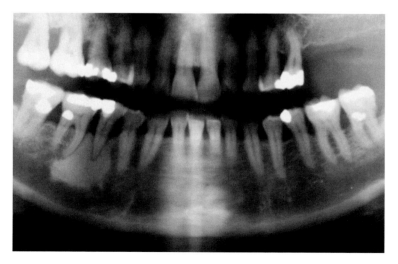 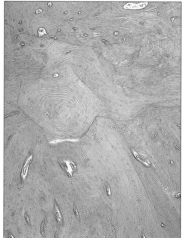

Osteoradionecrosis

Osteoradionecrosis is a much-feared complication following radiation therapy in the orofacial region. The most frequent causes are infections within the jaws due to pulpitis, or tooth extraction immediately preceding the radiation therapy. The degree of radiation damage to the vascular system of the bones of the jaw is an important factor. The mandible is most often affected. Sequester formation is frequent. The treatment corresponds to that for chronic osteomyelitis. Prevention, however, is the primary goal with osteoradionecrosis.

Actinomycosis

Actinomycosis is a disease process that is caused by the bacterium *Actinomyces israelii*. The disease has become less common today and often does not exhibit the classic characteristics of this special infection. The cervicofacial form, in its classic picture, is characterized by indurated infiltrations, multiple fistula formation and a livid bluish discoloration of the skin. The treatment consists of long-term antibiotic administration and surgical intervention (Nagler et al. 1997).

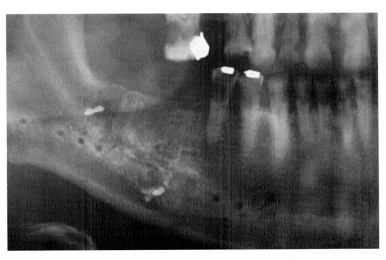

517 Osteoradionecrosis
This section from a panoramic radiograph reveals a diffuse area of osteolysis in the right side of the mandible following the removal of a mandibular osteosynthesis plate. Radiation caries is obvious on numerous teeth. This is a direct result of the irradiation and the associated massive xerostomia. Such severe complications can only be prevented through optimum preparation of the patient for radiation therapy, which should include fluoridation of the teeth.

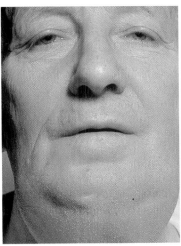 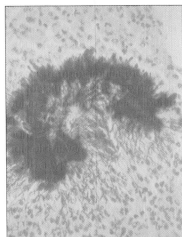

518 Actinomycosis
Left: A massive swelling occurred in the floor of the mouth several weeks after the extraction of a mandibular molar. This temporary delay is typical, because *Actinomyces israelii*, being an anaerobic organism, requires time to mount the infection.
Right: The histologic picture of actinomycosis reveals a typical colonization of *Actinomyces israelii*, which can be recognized as so-called sulfur granules within the pus with the naked eye (H & E, x 120).

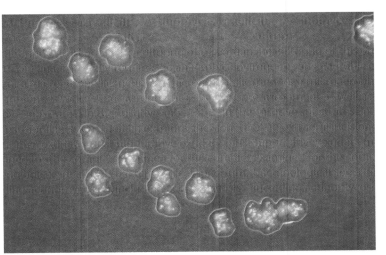

519 Actinomyces israelii in culture
The culturing of this organism requires an anaerobic environment or a microaerophilic environment as well as special nutritive substrates. In the case of an extraoral incision, the suppurative exudate must be examined for the complete bacteriological spectrum, including actinomycosis.

Benign Tumors

Chondroma, Gardner's Syndrome

Chondroma is characterized by the formation of mature cartilage without the histologic characteristics of chondrosarcoma, such as increased cellularity, pleomorphism or mitoses. Chondroma is rare in the jaw region. The tendency for chondroma to recur and to transform into a chondrosarcoma has caused clinicians and pathologists to doubt even the existence of the benign chondroma. The most frequent sites of occurrence are the palate and the anterior maxilla. The radiographic picture is one of a poorly demar-

cated radiolucency. Treatment consists of radical surgical removal.

Gardner's syndrome is characterized by multiple osteomas of the jaw, impacted supernumerary teeth, polyp formation in the colon and rectum, cutaneous and subcutaneous tumors as well as osteomas of the long bones. The disease is inherited as an autosomal dominant trait. Timely diagnosis is important because after age 40 the intestinal polyps can malignantly transform (Antoniades et al. 1987).

520 Chondroma—radiograph
This section from a panoramic radiograph exhibits the ascending ramus of the mandible (white arrow) and the articular process (black arrow), which is enlarged in the cranial direction.

Courtesy B. Hoffmeister

Right: Three-dimensional model of the coronoid and the articular processes. It is clear from this model that tumor formation has occurred ventrally and cranially on the head of the condyle (arrow).

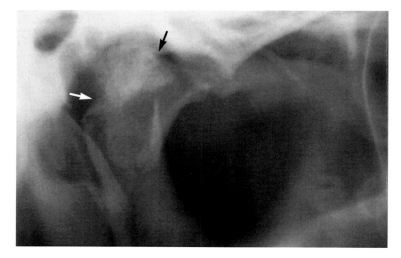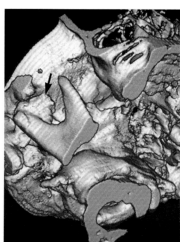

521 Chondroma—histology
The histologic picture of chondroma is characterized primarily by small chondroid cells that contain only one nucleus. Areas of calcification and necrosis may also be observed (H & E, x 100).

Right: A diffuse radiolucency can be noted above the central and lateral incisors. A diagnosis of "chondroma" cannot be based solely upon the radiograph. A bone biopsy is absolutely necessary.

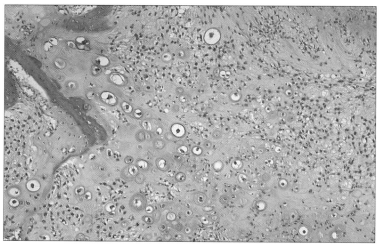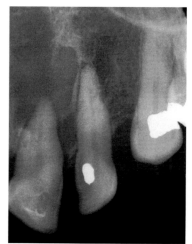

522 Gardner's syndrome
The panoramic radiograph exhibits a large, variably dense radiopacity, especially in the right mandible. This corresponds histologically to an osteoma. The patient was still young, but will be kept under observation throughout his life in order for any malignant polyps in the intestine to be detected at the earliest possible time.

Courtesy B. Hoffmeister

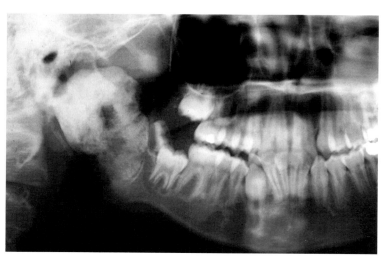

Central Hemangioma

Central hemangioma of the jaw is usually caused by arterio-venous malformations (Mohammadi et al. 1997). The lesions may be congenital or genetic. Females appear to be affected three times more often than males. Central hemangioma of the maxilla is usually of the cavernous type and can be associated with extremely severe hemorrhage (Tooth extraction in the area of a hemangioma can have fatal consequences!). The differential diagnosis should include central giant cell granuloma, aneurysmal bone cyst, kerato-cyst and ameloblastoma. Arteriography is absolutely necessary to establish the diagnosis.

Malignant Tumors

Plasmacytoma

The plasmacytoma is a B-cell lymphoma that develops through proliferation of atypical plasma cells, with formation of numerous osteolytic skeletal defects. The bones of the skull are more often affected than the jaws. As a result of the disturbed hematopoiesis, anemia result with a hemorrhagic tendency and increased susceptibility to infection (Pisano et al. 1997). (See also p. 113.)

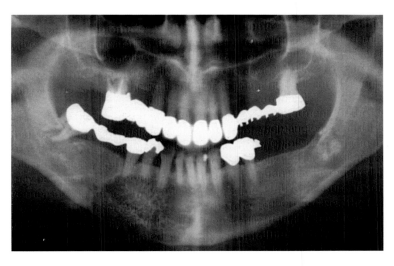

523 Central hemangioma
A relatively well-demarcated radiolucency with a clear, honeycomb-like structure is obvious in the right anterior segment of the mandible.

Treatment for the central hemangioma consists of application of sclerosing agents; in the case of large lesions, embolization may be required as a preoperative measure. In some reported cases, the resected mandible has been sterilized and immediately replaced into the surgical defect.

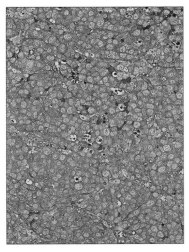
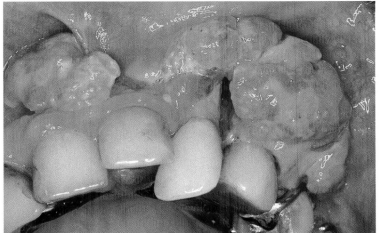

524 Plasmacytoma
The clinical photograph reveals large, partially ulcerated tumor masses in the region of the left maxilla. The left lateral incisor was extremely mobile.

Left: Histologic picture of a uniform plasmacytoma. This type of B-cell lymphoma is referred to as "paraproteinemic B-cell lymphoma." Between 10–15% of plasmacytomas of the light chain type develop amyloidosis (Toluidine Blue, x 150).

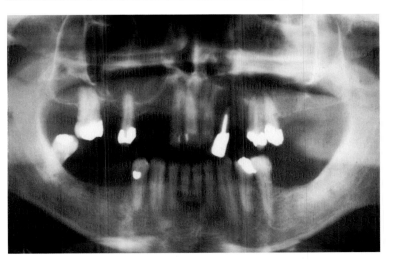

525 Plasmacytoma—radiograph
The panoramic radiograph of the patient depicted in Fig. 524 reveals osseous destruction in the region of the left maxilla, with diffuse disintegration of structures, also toward the maxillary sinus. The plasmacytoma may occur as a solitary lesion, which may later become generalized. The prognosis for plasmacytoma (multiple myeloma, Kahler's disease) is poor.

Carcinoma – Infiltration into Bone

Carcinoma of the oral cavity originates from the mucosa but can also involve the subjacent bone. In contrast, the appearance of a primary intraosseous squamous cell carcinoma developing from odontogenic epithelial cell rests is an extremely rare occurrence. Presence or absence of infiltration into bone is of great importance for the treatment of oral cavity carcinoma.

The radiograph reveals a diffuse, "cloudy" radiolucency, whose borders are poorly demarcated, if at all. Computed tomography (CT) and magnetic resonance imaging (MRI) can be used to advantage to ascertain the precise localization and expanse of the tumor in the bone and in the soft tissue. (See also p. 170.)

Carcinoma of the Maxillary Sinuses

Carcinoma of the sinuses is often detected only quite late, because there are few initial clinical symptoms. Patients often become aware that there is a problem only when the breathing passages become compromised and there is an exudate from the nose or down the posterior wall of the pharynx.

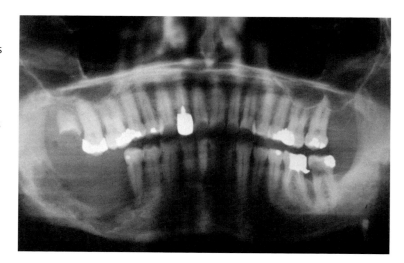
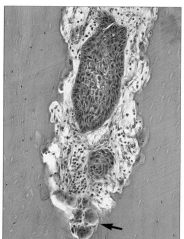

526   Carcinoma – infiltration
This panoramic radiograph reveals a diffuse area of osteolysis extending almost to the basal compact bone in the right mandible. Primary osteoplasty following resection of such extensive infiltrating carcinoma is usually not possible.

Right: Invasion of carcinoma into bone. Note osteoclastic activity as evidenced by the presence of lacunae (arrow) (H & E, x 100).

Courtesy U. Gross

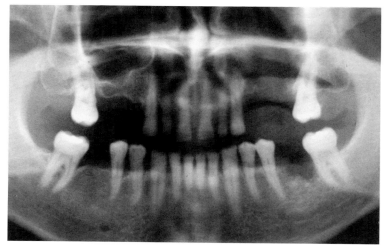
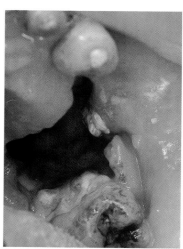

527   Carcinoma of the maxillary sinus
The panoramic radiograph reveals a poorly demarcated lesion near the left maxillary sinus, which appears to be radiopaque in comparison to the right side.

Right: There is a large communication, extending from the alveolar process into the sinus cavity, which is filled with malignant tissue. The patient presented with this condition at the initial appointment.

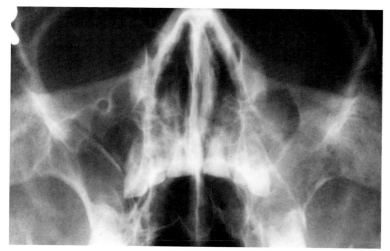
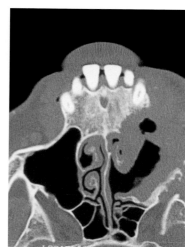

528   Carcinoma of the maxillary sinus
This radiograph of the nasal sinuses of the patient depicted in Fig. 527 reveals the poorly demarcated maxillary sinus on the left side. Anatomic structures, such as the infraorbital foramen, cannot be discerned.

Right: Computed tomography scan of the nasal and maxillary sinuses. The destruction of the maxilla, the zygomatic process, and the osseous tissue surrounding the sinus is obvious.

Metastases to the Jaws

Metastases to the region of the jaw are not common, occurring in about 3% of the malignant tumors of the oral cavity and the jaw (Hirshberg et al. 1994). Most important is the detection of the primary tumor, but this is not possible in all cases. The histologic pictures of the primary and the metastatic tumor must be identical (Rubens 1998, Meyer and Hart 1998, Hiraga et al. 1998). Malignant tumors of the breast, lung, prostate, kidney, colon and rectum are those which most commonly metastasize.

The radiographic picture of metastasis to the jaw presents as a diffuse, poorly demarcated radiolucency. However, in the case of metastasis from a mammary or prostate carcinoma, radiopacity may also be observed. The mandible is more often affected than the maxilla. Anesthesia or paresthesia of the lower lip is a typical symptom. Treatment depends mainly upon the situation with metastases in other organs and the therapeutic control of the primary tumor.

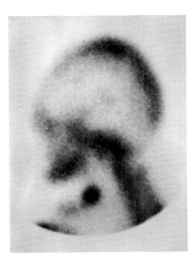
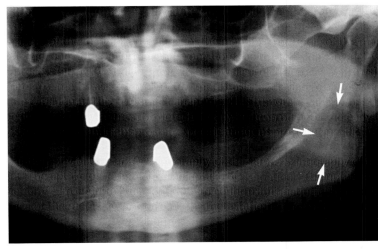

529 Prostate carcinoma—metastasis
At the angle of the mandible on the left side, one notes an osteolytic process (arrows) corresponding to a metastasis from a prostate carcinoma. This tumor can be detected early be means of prostate-specific antigens.

Left: Szintigraphy of the same patient. The uptake of technetium-99m confirms the presence of the metastatic carcinoma.

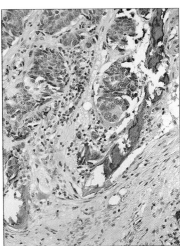
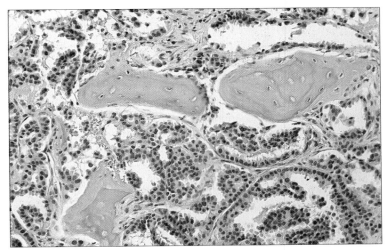

530 Osseous metastasis—histology
The bone has been infiltrated by metastases from a carcinoma of the prostate. Islands of still viable bone are surrounded by the characteristic gland-like structures of the prostate carcinoma (H & E, x 120).
Left: Mammary carcinoma within bone. The bone has been almost completely replaced by tumor tissue. The morphology is identical to that of the primary tumor (H & E, x 100).
Courtesy U. Gross

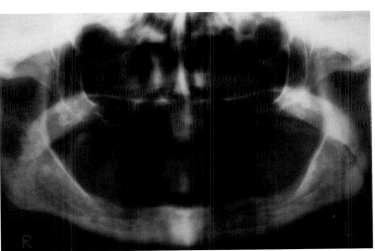

531 Mammary carcinoma—metastasis
The panoramic radiograph reveals a spotty, expansive area of osteolysis within the entire mandible, especially at the left and right angles of the mandible and the ascending rami.

Courtesy B. Hoffmeister

Malignant Tumors

Osteogenic Sarcoma

Osteosarcoma is found primarily in patients between the ages of 10 and 25 years. Males appear to be more frequently affected. Six percent of all osteosarcomas are localized in the jaw region. The osteosarcoma is usually located centrally within the jaw. The clinical symptoms include swelling, mobile teeth, anesthesia or paresthesia, dental pain, or nasal congestion. The radiographic appearance must be used to differentiate between the osteoblastic and osteolytic types: In the case of *osteoblastic* sarcoma, one observes the formation of trabeculae that extend toward the surface of the jaw, from which the term "sunburst effect" originates. For the *osteolytic* type, a symmetrically widened periodontal ligament space is a characteristic sign. Widening of the mandibular canal is often observed.

Treatment consists of radical resection of the tumor, also encompassing healthy tissues. Chemotherapy is also recommended. The prognosis for osteosarcoma of the jaw is more favorable than that of other skeletal localizations (van Es et al. 1997, August et al. 1997).

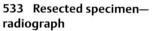

Osteogenic sarcoma

532 Radiographic diagnosis
From the first mandibular premolar into the region of the extracted third molar, one notes an extensive radiopaque area.

Right: The szintigram reveals an accumulation of technetium-99m in the left mandible, which corresponds to the panoramic radiograph. The szintigram alone is not sufficient to indicate a tumor.
Courtesy B. Hoffmeister

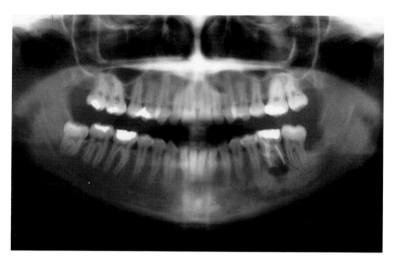
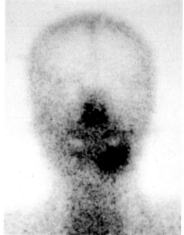

533 Resected specimen—radiograph
This radiograph of the surgical specimen reveals obvious areas of osteoblastic activity extending from the second premolar to the retromolar region.

The prognosis for osteosarcoma of the mandible is better than for the maxilla. Chondroblastic osteosarcoma has a more favorable prognosis. Hematogenic metastases are common. Death occurs due to the uncontrollable nature of the process.
Courtesy B. Hoffmeister

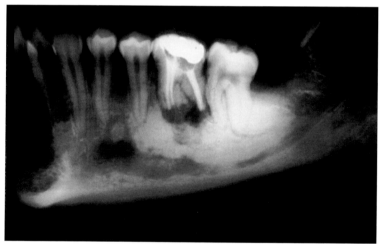

534 Histology
The histologic picture exhibits the small cell osteosarcoma with formation of osteoid material (arrow), which is characteristic particularly for the osteoblastic type (H & E, x 80).

Courtesy U. Gross

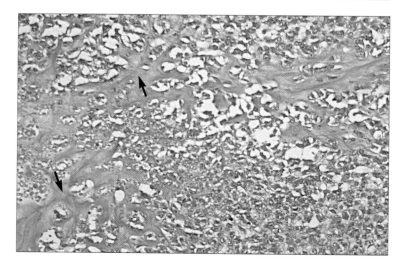

Langerhans Cell Granulomatosis

Eosinophilic Granuloma, Hand–Schüller–Christian Syndrome

Langerhans cell granulomatosis, also known as histiocytosis X, includes the eosinophilic granuloma, Hand–Schüller–Christian disease and Abt–Letterer–Siwe disease. The etiology and pathogenesis of these histiocytoses are unknown. The disease is characterized by proliferation of tissue macrophages and histiocytes, or specialized bone marrow cells known as Langerhans cells.

The *eosinophilic granuloma* occurs in adolescence, and may be unifocal or multifocal. The male:female ratio is 2:1. The skull, mandible, ribs and spinal column as well as the flat bones are most often affected. Radiographically, the lesions appear as poorly circumscribed radiolucencies (Dagenais et al. 1992).

The *Hand–Schüller–Christian disease* occurs in children, primarily in boys. The entire skeleton is affected; the clinical course is usually chronic.

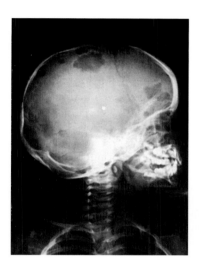 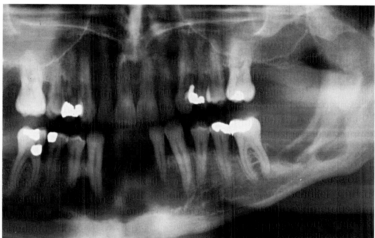

535 Eosinophilic granuloma/ Hand–Schüller–Christian syndrome
There are diffuse areas of osteolysis that may also involve the roots of the teeth. Szintigraphic examination of the skeleton frequently reveals no additional foci of eosinophilic granuloma.

Left: Radiographic overview of the skull in a case of Hand–Schüller–Christian syndrome. Numerous large "punched out" defects are apparent, especially in the skull.

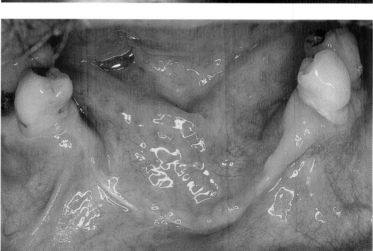

536 Eosinophilic granuloma— clinical finding
Note the atrophied, collapsed alveolar process in the anterior segment of the mandible. Even though the eosinophilic granuloma was not treated, spontaneous re-epithelialization of the defect occurred following spontaneous tooth loss.

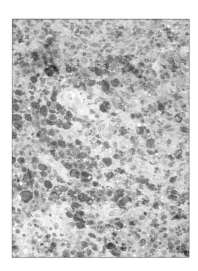 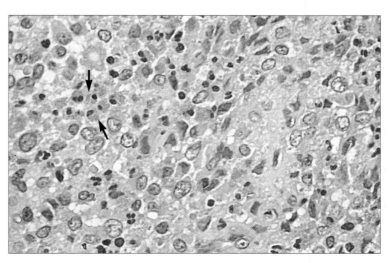

537 Eosinophilic granuloma— histology
The histologic picture reveals histiocytes. However, in the early stage the lesion is frequently predominated by eosinophilic granulocytes (arrows) (H & E, x 400).

Left: The identification of S-100 protein in Langerhans cells is a positive sign for the diagnosis of Langerhans cell granulomatosis (APAAP, x 250).

Courtesy A. Eckardt

Diseases of the Skeletal System

Paget's Disease, Osteogenesis Imperfecta

Paget's disease, also known as osteitis deformans, is a disease of unknown origin with simultaneous destruction and repair of osseous tissues. Paget's disease of bone may occur as monostotic or polystotic lesions. The disease usually occurs after the age of 40, and is more common in males. The clinical course is chronic. Typical symptoms include osseous pain, headache, dizziness, vision loss, deafness and confusion. The skull may continuously enlarge. The maxilla is more often affected than the mandible. Following tooth extraction, disturbances of wound healing often occur. The radiographic picture reveals a "cotton wool–like" structure of the bone. Hypercementosis of the roots of the teeth is common (van der Waal 1991).

Osteogenesis imperfecta is a syndrome consisting of extremely fragile bones, blue sclera, deafness, weakness of the joint ligaments, and dentinogenesis imperfecta. The various types of osteogenesis display specific hereditary patterns.

538 Paget's disease of bone
The histologic picture reveals the typical, almost pathognomonic, mosaic formation of the bone in Paget's disease. The osseous tissue is partially resorbed and then reformed. This repetitive process results in numerous reversal lines. The stroma is fibrous (H & E, x 120).

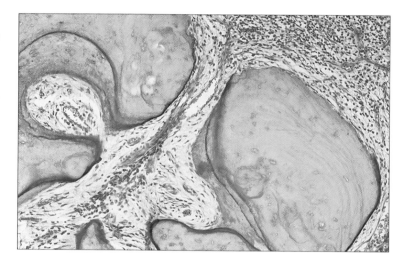

539 Paget's disease of bone/osteogenesis imperfecta
Left: This 60-year-old female patient was deaf. Over many years, she had experienced a distinct enlarging of the skull, which is typical for Paget's disease of bone.
Middle: Radiograph of the sinuses of the same patient. Note the diffuse opacities in the region the maxillary sinuses and the orbits.
Right: Lateral skull film of a patient with osteogenesis imperfecta, with massive enlargement of both mandible and maxilla.

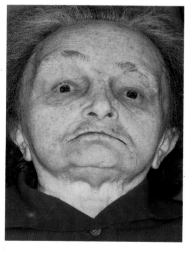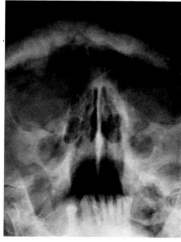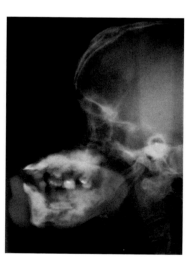

540 Osteogenesis imperfecta
This panoramic radiograph of the female patient depicted in Fig. 539 reveals a diffuse radiopacity that affects both maxilla and mandible, as a consequence of the excessive osteogenesis.

Right: The histologic picture exhibits islands of newly-formed irregular bone surrounded and interwoven by reversal lines. Fiber-rich connective tissue surrounds the osseous trabeculae (Alcian blue, x 100).

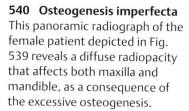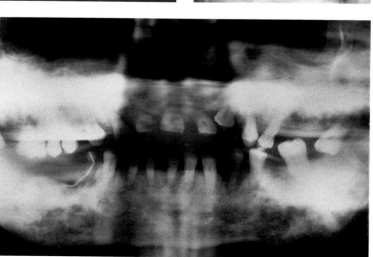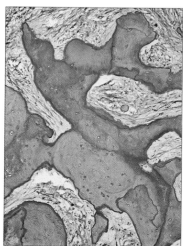

Lesions Induced by Implants

Hydroxyapatite Implants

The filling of large cysts with bone replacement materials (e.g., hydroxyapatite) was recommended in the early 1980s and widely employed. The goal of the procedure was to fill large cystic defects in order to accelerate osseous regeneration of the large lumen. Particles of hydroxyapatite of various sizes and densities were used. Although the material at first appeared to be ideal, it quickly became evident that osseous rebuilding of larger defects, especially in the mandible, did not always occur; in many cases there was only a connective tissue–like encapsulation and penetration of the hydroxyapatite filling material, and the affected region of the mandible remained particularly susceptible to fracture. In a radiograph, the hydroxyapatite ceramic filling material appeared as a grainy radiopacity.

In an attempt to prevent alveolar collapse, dense, root-shaped hydroxyapatite ceramic implants were placed into extraction sockets.

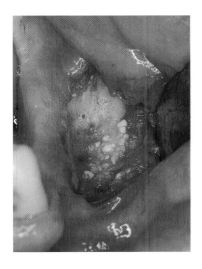
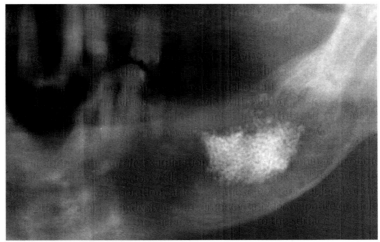

Hydroxyapatite ceramic implants

541 Filling a cystic cavity
This area of a panoramic radiograph reveals the situation after filling a cystic cavity with hydroxyapatite. The granules appear to have been well accepted.

Left: Examination of the surgical site reveals broad osseous incorporation, at least of those hydroxyapatite granules adjacent to the surface.

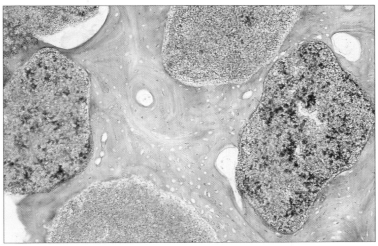

542 Histology
A biopsy of the hydroxyapatite depicted in Fig. 541 demonstrates the osseous incorporation of individual hydroxyapatite granules. One notes only a few lacunae on the ceramic surface.
In contrast to ridge augmentation, in the case of filling a cystic cavity, osseous regeneration is more likely to occur due to the stable position of the granules, but the osseous defects must not be excessively large (Giemsa, x 40).

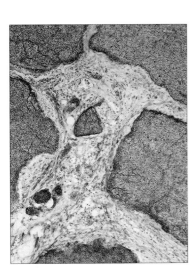
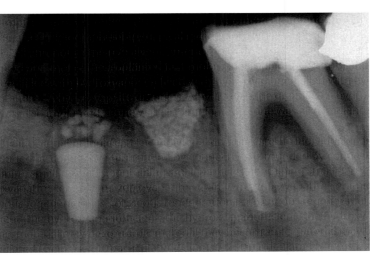

543 Implant into alveolus
This periapical radiograph depicts two alveoli anterior to the re-implanted first molar; the alveoli had been filled with hydroxyapatite granules. A hydroxyapatite cone was also implanted.

Left: The individual granules are surrounded by connective tissue containing small particles of hydroxyapatite ceramic material. If osseous regeneration is not sufficient, the hydroxyapatite ceramic material may become particulated (Giemsa, x 10).

Epithelial Cysts of the Jaws

A cyst (Greek: kystis = bladder) is a pathologic cavity containing liquids, semisolids or gas, but which did not arise due to the accumulation of pus. Cysts often contain cholesterol in the form of rhomboid crystals and may expand to achieve remarkable size through a process not yet fully understood. Cysts may displace neighboring structures, such as roots and teeth; they may also elicit resorption, but this is less common. Cysts are usually lined by epithelium and are common in the head and neck region, occurring in the jaws as well as in the soft tissues.

Odontogenic cysts derive from odontogenic epithelium. They are developmental in origin or the result of an inflammatory process. In addition to the odontogenic cysts, *non-odontogenic cysts* can occur in the jaws and facial tissues; these derive from epithelial cell remnants, which are often entrapped embryologically during organogenesis.

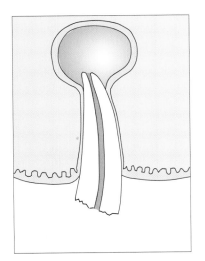

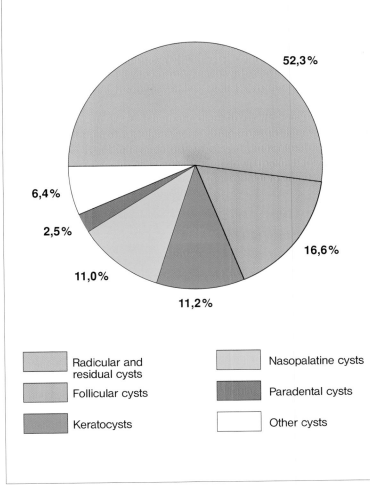

52,3%

6,4%

2,5%

11,0%

11,2%

16,6%

Radicular and residual cysts	Nasopalatine cysts
Follicular cysts	Paradental cysts
Keratocysts	Other cysts

544 Epithelial cysts of the jaws
Frequency distribution of cysts of the jaw according to diagnoses (adapted from Shear 1992). The category "other cysts" contains eleven entities, each with a frequency of less than 1%.

Left: Schematic diagram of a radicular cyst resulting from an inflammatory process at the root tip of a badly broken down maxillary canine with a necrotic pulp.

Classification

There have been various attempts in recent decades to develop a "logical" classification of cysts of the jaws. Most of these classifications are quite satisfactory from the point of view of diagnosis as well as today's state of knowledge. The classification presented in this book is based upon the World Health Organization's publication *Histological Typing of Odontogenic Tumors and Cysts* (Kramer et al. 1992). This classification of cysts that originate from various odontogenic and non-odontogenic epithelial remnants reflects the contemporary understanding of the lesions. Use of this classification is highly recommended, primarily from the point of view of international cooperation and the adoption of a uniform terminology. This will facilitate and improve the communication among students, teachers and scientists.

545   Classification of epithelial jaw cysts according to WHO, 1992

* See text below.

Cysts of Developmental Origin

- Odontogenic Cysts
  - "Gingival cysts" of the newborn (Epstein's pearls) (*)
  - Odontogenic keratocyst (primordial cyst)
  - Follicular cyst
  - Eruption cyst
  - Lateral periodontal cyst
  - Gingival cyst of adults
  - Glandular odontogenic cysts; sialo-odontogenic cyst (*)

- Non-odontogenic Cysts
  - Nasopalatine duct (incisive canal) cyst
  - Nasolabial (nasoalveolar) cyst

Cysts of Inflammatory Origin

- Radicular Cyst
  - Apical and lateral radicular cysts
  - Residual radicular cysts
  - Paradental cysts
  - collateral mandibular infected buccal cysts (*)

The WHO classification of odontogenic and non-odontogenic cysts (Fig. 545) contains three types of cysts (all marked with an asterisk) that have not been included in the following descriptions of the various types of cysts because they are rare or because they have been described only very recently. For example, for several of the cysts (e.g., glandular odontogenic cysts and mandibular infected buccal cyst), we have only a preliminary picture of the clinical and histopathologic characteristics.

The description of the individual types of cysts will follow a pattern whereby the definition according to the WHO classification will be given first, followed by the clinical characteristics including the frequency and the age and gender distribution, the radiological characteristics, the pathogenesis and the histopathology. Therapy will also be briefly discussed, especially surgical measures, such as the classic types of cystectomy and cystostomy.

Odontogenic Keratocyst

These cysts occur in the dentulous segments of the jaws or posterior to the mandibular third molars. They are characterized by a thin connective tissue capsule, lined with keratinized squamous epithelium that is usually five to eight cell layers in thickness and frequently devoid of rete pegs.

Philipsen (1956) introduced the term odontogenic keratocyst (OKC); it represents about 10% of odontogenic cysts (1.5–21.8%). It probably derives from remnants of the dental lamina. The development from basal cells of the oral epithelium has also been hypothesized. Aggressively growing OKCs have also been considered to be cystic tumors.

The age distribution is bimodal, with a peak in the second and third decades of life, followed by another peak in the fifth decade of life and later. Males are more often affected than females (M:F = 1.5:1). One-fourth of all patients with OKCs complain of pain. The clinical appearance includes swelling and intraoral fistula.

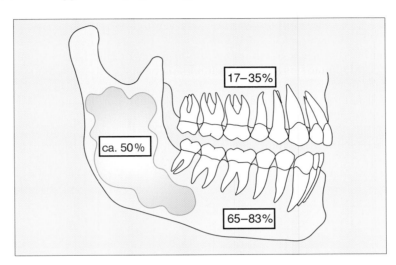

Keratocysts

546 Locations within the maxilla and mandible
Most OKCs develop in the mandible. About half are observed at the angle of the mandible and in the ascending ramus. These data derive from various studies.

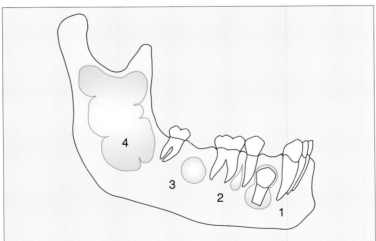

547 Types of Odontogenic Keratocyst
(from Voorsmit 1984)

1 Envelopmental
2 Collateral
3 Replacement ("replacing a tooth bud")
4 Extraneous

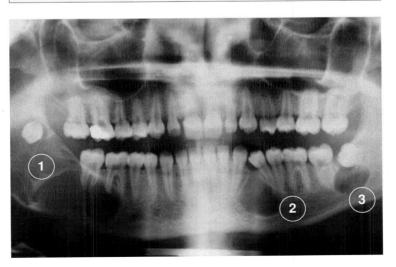

548 Panoramic radiograph
This radiograph of a 26-year-old female exhibits various forms of OKCs. Although there was a suspicion that this patient manifested Gorlin–Goltz syndrome, the clinical and radiographic findings provided no evidence for this syndrome.

1, 3 Follicular type
2 Collateral type

Radiographically, odontogenic keratocysts may appear as follicular, lateral periodontal, primordial or residual cysts. They appear on the radiograph as round or oval radiolucencies, which may be unilocular or multilocular.

Multilocular keratocysts are most often detected in the mandible. The most characteristic feature is cortical expansion. The differential diagnosis should include ameloblastoma, in addition to odontogenic myxoma and follicular cyst. Root resorption may also occur, although rarely. The odontogenic keratocyst is particularly important because of its high rate of recurrence, which varies between 3 and 62%.

In earlier times, *radical therapy* was recommended, including even the resection of affected portions of the jaw. However, the approach today is rather more conservative. Carnoy's solution may be used to swab the cystic cavity in order to devitalize the cystic lining; this, in combination with excision of the mucosa of the overlying alveolar ridge, will lead to reduction of the rate of recurrence. Follow-up over many years is recommended (Voorsmit 1984).

Keratocysts

549 Radiographic diagnosis
Left: Section from a panoramic radiograph. Note the multilocular translucency in the right body of the mandible and the ascending ramus. This represents a recurrence of a cyst 40 years later.

Right: Computed tomography of a 14-year-old patient with recurrent keratocysts. At the base of the left maxillary sinus (arrow), one notes a cystic lesion, which corresponds to a recurrent OKC.

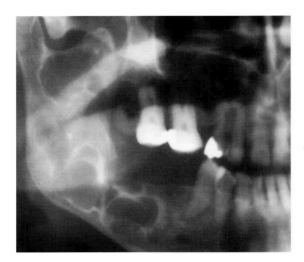
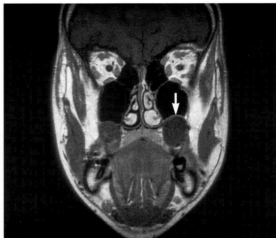

550 Clinical and radiographic picture
Left: The cyst has led to tipping of the left canine and lateral incisor.

Right: The radiolucency is well circumscribed, and the tipping of the adjacent teeth is pronounced. There is no indication of root resorption. This type of odontogenic keratocyst has also been termed a collateral cyst.

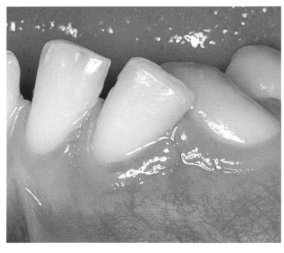
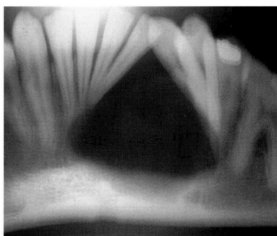

551 Histology
Left: The cyst epithelium exhibits parakeratosis. The basal cells demonstrate pallisading and absence of rete pegs. The arrowheads indicate the view perpendicular to the lining surface shown in Fig. 551 (right). The arrow indicates a mitotic figure. (H & E, x 180)

Right: Scanning electron photomicrograph of the surface of a keratocyst. Epithelial borders are clearly visible as well as microplicae (*) and nuclei (arrows). (SEM, x 11 000)

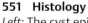
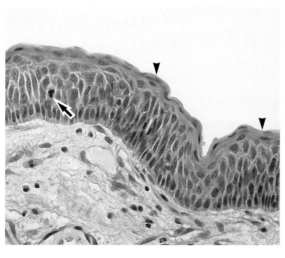
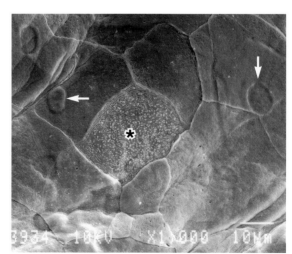

In 1960, *Gorlin* and *Goltz* described a syndrome that carries their names and which consists of odontogenic keratocysts, bifid ribs as well as nevoid basal cell carcinoma. In this syndrome, keratocysts are detected in 65–90% of cases (Gorlin 1995).

Of importance is the possible occurrence of "daughter" or satellite cysts within the cyst wall. These may be responsible for recurrence.

The histologic characteristics of the keratocyst include:

- Absence of rete pegs
- Epithelium consisting of six to eight cell layers
- Pallisading of the basal cells
- Flattening of the epithelial cells toward the lumen
- Undulating appearance of the epithelial surface of the lumen
- Parakeratosis, or occasionally orthokeratosis of the cyst epithelium
- Irregularly folded cyst lumen filled with keratin
- Absence of inflammation in the cystic wall

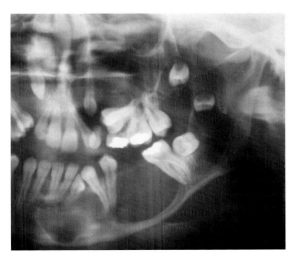
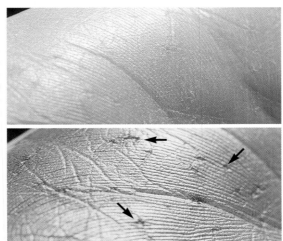
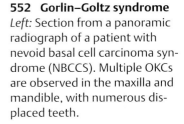

552 Gorlin–Goltz syndrome
Left: Section from a panoramic radiograph of a patient with nevoid basal cell carcinoma syndrome (NBCCS). Multiple OKCs are observed in the maxilla and mandible, with numerous displaced teeth.

Right: Palmar "pits" on the left hand of the same patient. Between 65–90% of affected individuals exhibit NBCCS. Painting the skin with toluidine blue enhances the pits (arrows).

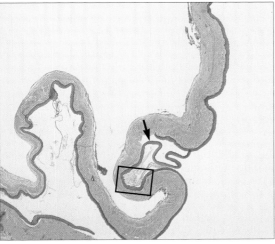
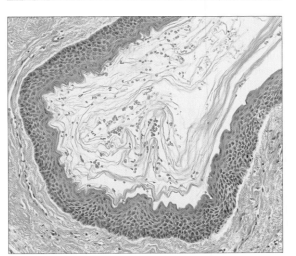

553 Keratocyst—histology
Left: The cyst epithelium is morphologically very uniform and lacks rete pegs. The junction between the epithelium and connective tissues is weak, and in many areas separation occurs (arrow). (H & E, x 8)

Right: Higher magnification of the area framed on the figure on the left. The parakeratotic layers appear wavy. The cyst lumen is filled with desquamated keratin and some erythrocytes. (H & E, x 150)

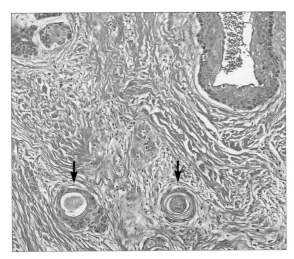
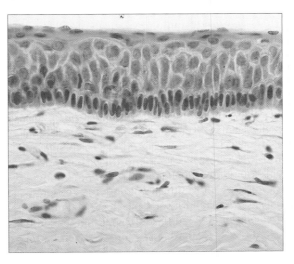

554 Keratocyst—histology
Left: Cyst wall with numerous satellite microcysts (arrows) within the connective tissue capsule. (H & E, x 80)

Right: The distinct basal cell layer consists of pallisading, cylindrical or cuboidal cells. The cell nuclei are located away from the basement membrane. This is an important criterium for distinguishing between OKCs and other keratinizing cysts of the jaw. (H & E, x 280)

Follicular (Dentigerous) Cyst

This type of cyst surrounds the crown of the tooth and is attached to the neck of unerupted teeth. It develops through accumulation of fluid between the reduced enamel epithelium and the crown, or between the layers of the reduced enamel epithelium.

Follicular cysts account for approximately 17% of all odontogenic cysts (Shear 1992). They occur primarily in the second to fourth decades of life and are more common in males (male:female = 1.6:1). The most common localization of the follicular cyst is the mandible, in connection with third molars, followed by the permanent maxillary canines.

The radiographic appearance is one of a unilocular radiolucency around the crown of an unerupted tooth; the reason for its failure to erupt is not always evident. The follicular cyst is always attached at the cementoenamel junction; various subtypes may be observed radiographically (see Fig. 556).

Follicular cyst

555   Anatomic localization
Two-thirds of all follicular cysts are associated with unerupted mandibular teeth, primarily the third molars (adapted from Shear 1992).

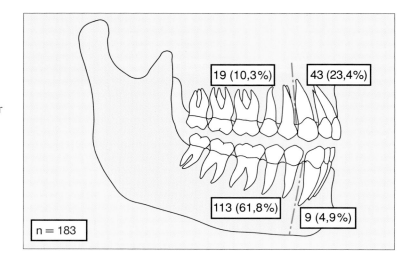

556   Development
This diagram reveals how the dental follicle can develop into the various types of radiographically evident subtypes (adapted from Shear 1992).

1 Central
2 Lateral
3 Circumferential

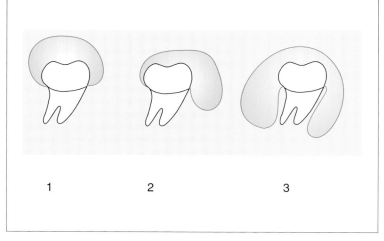

557   Panoramic radiograph
Note the large follicular cysts emanating from the right mandibular first premolar and canine. The differential diagnosis should include radicular cyst of the deciduous tooth. Surrounding the crown of the left second premolar, one notes a small translucency which is a possible indication of a developing follicular cyst.

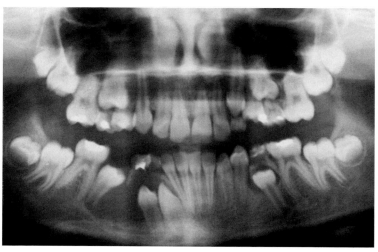

Histologically, the wall of the cyst is made up of a thin connective tissue layer with an epithelium that is two to three cell layers thick and which is reminiscent of the reduced enamel epithelium. The epithelium is not keratinized. Mucous-producing or cilia-bearing cells may be observed.

The follicular cyst and the unicystic ameloblastoma (see p. 226) cannot be differentiated radiographically. Nevertheless, these two pathological processes are fundamentally different entities.

In earlier times, the surgical *therapy* for a follicular cyst often included removal of the retained tooth; today, the goal is to maintain teeth and to employ orthodontic means to align them in the arch. Depending upon the size of the cyst, cystostomy (marsupialization) or cystectomy may be attempted. In children and adolescents, filling the cyst cavity with foreign materials or host bone should only be performed in exceptional cases. Recurrence of follicular cysts following removal is the exception.

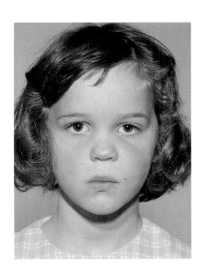
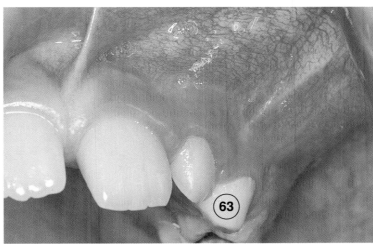
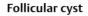

Follicular cyst

558 Clinical findings
An indurated swelling is noted in the region of the left maxillary vestibulum. The left central incisor is tipped and the deciduous maxillary canine (63) is retained.

Left: The extraoral photograph shows swelling of the left cheek, which extends to the nose. The overlying skin in this 8-year-old girl appears normal.

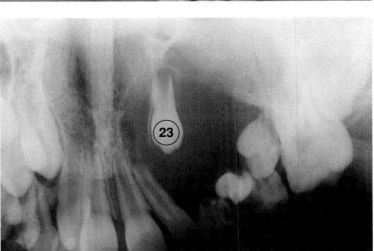
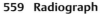

559 Radiograph
The radiograph of the girl shown in Fig. 558 clearly reveals the unerupted maxillary canine (23). In this case the attachment of the cystic wall to the crown of 23 cannot be determined radiographically. The differential diagnosis in adolescent patients should include adenomatoid odontogenic tumor.

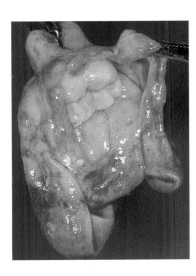
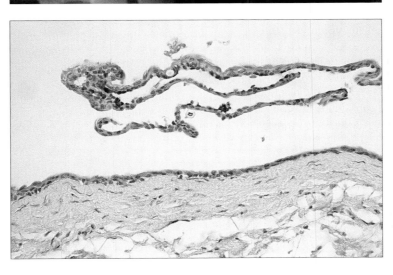

560 Histology/surgical specimen
The epithelium and also the connective tissue capsule are thin and exhibit no signs of inflammation. A portion of the epithelium has detached and lies freely within the cystic lumen (H & E, x 120).

Left: The surgical specimen includes the mandibular third molar. The cyst is attached at the cementoenamel junction. The thin wall of the cyst has been opened to reveal the occlusal surface of the tooth.

Eruption Cyst

Eruption cysts are located over the crown of an erupting tooth. They represent a variant of the follicular cyst in the soft tissues outside of the alveolar bone.

Eruption cysts present clinically as a bluish swelling in the region where tooth eruption is immediately imminent. This type of cyst represents less than 1% of all odontogenic cysts (Shear 1992).

Gingival Cyst of Adults

The gingival cyst of adults develops from odontogenic epithelial remnants. It accounts for less than 0.5% of odontogenic cysts and appears in the fifth and sixth decades of life. It is most commonly localized to the gingiva of the canine-premolar or the canine-incisor regions of the mandible. Controversy continues regarding its origin (Nxumalo and Shear 1992). The wall of the cyst exhibits one to two layers of a thin squamous epithelium. Similar to the lateral periodontal cyst, one may observe circumscribed epithelial plaques of fusiform or clear-cell types.

561   Eruption cyst in an infant
Eruption cyst in the region of the erupting maxillary deciduous central incisor. The bluish-black color is characteristic.

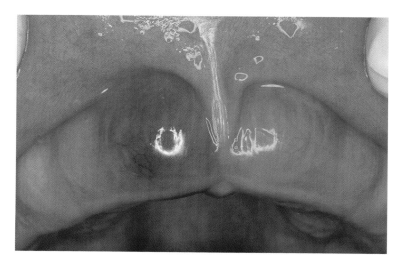

562   Eruption cyst
Note the bluish swelling in the region of the maxillary left canine, which was impacted. Treatment consists of simply removing the cystic wall.

Right: Excision biopsy
(H & E, x 30).

1 Cystic epithelium with an adjacent inflammatory reaction
2 Connective tissue of the oral mucosa
3 Gingival epithelium

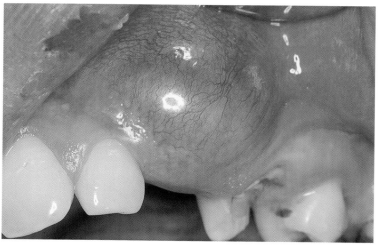

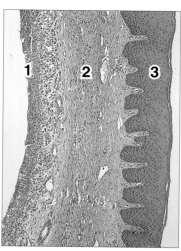

563   Gingival cyst of adults
Left: Typical localization between the mandibular right lateral incisor and canine.
Middle: Schematic diagram of the possible origin of a gingival cyst (*) of an adult, from the junctional epithelium after eruption of the tooth (Shear 1992).
Right: Histologic specimen
(H & E, x 15)

1 Cyst epithelium
2 Connective tissue of the oral mucosa
3 Gingival epithelium

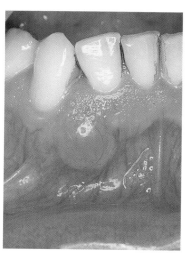

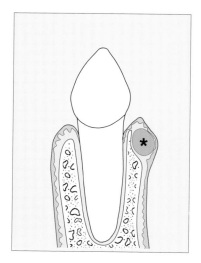

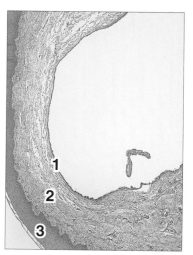

Lateral Periodontal Cyst

The lateral periodontal cyst occurs lateral to or between the roots of vital teeth. This cyst develops from cellular remnants of the dental lamina, and never as a result of inflammatory stimuli. In the differential diagnosis, the lateral periodontal cyst must be differentiated from the collateral odontogenic keratocyst, the gingival cyst of adults as well as an inflammatory cyst that can develop laterally to the tooth root. The lateral periodontal cyst accounts for less than 1% of all odontogenic cysts. Males are more often affected; the age peak is in the sixth decade of life.

Lateral periodontal cysts do not elicit clinical symptoms; they are usually discovered during routine radiographic examination of the teeth. Adjacent teeth remain vital. Routine probing of the gingival sulcus will not reveal any communication with the cyst. Treatment consists of enucleation. Recurrence is rare (Carter et al. 1996, Altini and Shear 1992).

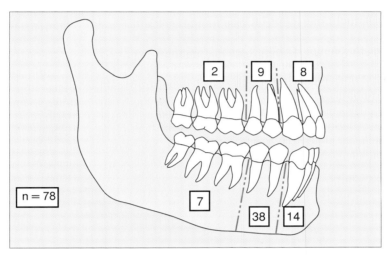

Lateral periodontal cyst

564 Frequency of anatomic localization
The diagram depicts the anatomic localization of 78 cases (Philipsen and Reichart, unpublished). Seventy-five percent of all cases occur in the mandible, of which 50% occur in the premolar region.

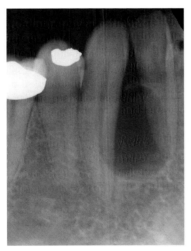
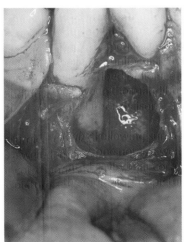

565 Radiography and findings during surgery
Left: The periapical radiograph reveals a unilocular, oval, well-circumscribed radiolucency between the mandibular canine and lateral incisor.

Right: Following surgical cystectomy, one notes a well-demarcated cavity that corresponds to the radiographic picture.

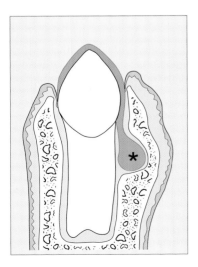
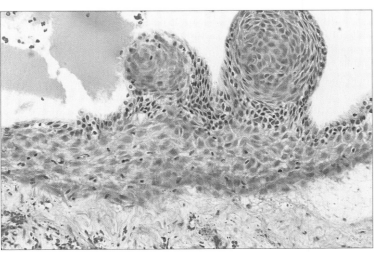

566 Histology
Histologic picture of a section of the cyst wall. The non-keratinized squamous epithelium exhibits individual round "plaques" with fusiform cells
(H & E, x 280).

Left: Schematic diagram illustrating the possible histogenesis of the lateral periodontal cyst (*). The cyst develops by dilation of the reduced enamel epithelium of the follicle before tooth eruption (adapted from Shear 1992).

Nasopalatine Duct Cyst

The nasopalatine duct (incisive canal) cyst is thought to be derived from embryonic epithelial remnants of the nasopalatine duct in the incisive canal. It is the most common non-odontogenic cyst, comprising approximately 10% of all cysts of the jaw. Males are more often affected (M:F = 2:1). The cyst appears most frequently between the fourth and sixth decades of life. Radiographs reveal that the cyst is localized to the middle of the palate, above or between the roots of the central incisors, which react positively to vitality tests.

Nasolabial Cyst

The nasolabial (naso-alveolar) cyst is localized outside the bone in the nasolabial folds below the alae nasi on the alveolar process at the side of the nose. This soft tissue cyst is rare, comprising about 0.5% of all cysts. Females are more often affected (F:M = 3.7:1); it occurs most frequently in the fourth and fifth decades of life. The most obvious clinical sign is swelling of the nasolabial grooves. Although the nasolabial cyst cannot be depicted radiographically unless contrast medium is used, it may sometimes exhibit impressions in the bone of the maxilla (Shear 1992).

567 Nasopalatine duct cyst
Well-circumscribed palatal swelling (arrows) distal to the maxillary central incisors. The vitality test of the teeth was positive, thus ruling out an inflammatory cyst.

Right: The occlusal radiograph reveals an oval radiolucency (arrows) above the root tips of the central incisors. It may be difficult to decide whether the radiolucency is a nasopalatine duct cyst or a large incisive fossa.

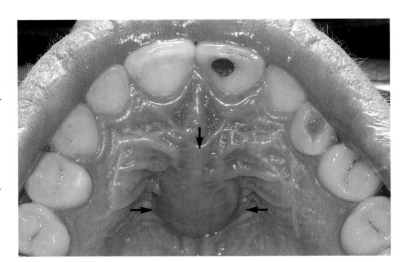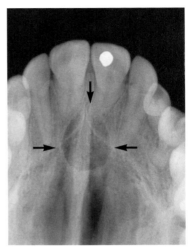

568 Nasopalatine duct cyst—histology
Histologic picture of the wall of the cyst. The histologic appearance of the epithelial lining is extremely variable. In this case, one notes a pseudostratified, prismatic epithelium. The most common appearance is that of squamous epithelium.
(* Fresh hemorrhage in the connective tissue of the cystic walls)
(H & E, x 180)

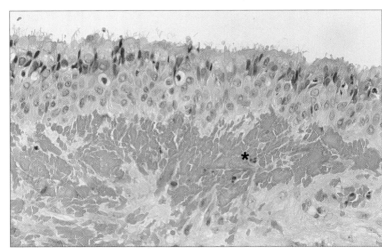

569 Nasopalatine duct cyst/nasolabial cyst
This scanning electron microscopic view of a nasopalatine duct cyst exhibits the ciliated epithelium (arrow: cilia-bearing cells; arrowheads: intracellular craters resulting from empty mucous cells) (SEM, x 11 000).

Right: The nasolabial cyst elevates ala nasi on the left side. Patients do not report any pain.

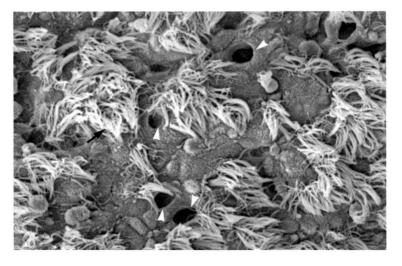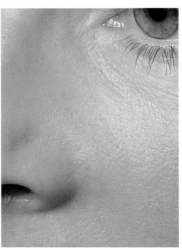

Radicular Cyst

The radicular cyst derives from the epithelial rest cells of Malassez in the periodontium and develops as a direct result of inflammation, which is usually caused by pulpal necrosis. Radicular cysts usually appear at the root apex, but may also develop on the lateral aspect of the root. The radicular cyst is by far the most common cyst in the jaw, comprising more than 50% of all odontogenic cysts. The most frequent site is the anterior segment of the maxilla. Radicular cysts are most common in the third to fifth decades of life. Males are more frequently affected than females (M : F = 1 : 4.1).

Many radicular cysts are symptom-free and are frequently detected only serendipitously on periapical radiographs of nonvital teeth. It is not always possible radiographically to differentiate between a radicular cyst and a chronic apical granuloma. However, radicular cysts are usually larger and exhibit a sharply demarcated border, which represents a delicate zone of osteosclerosis.

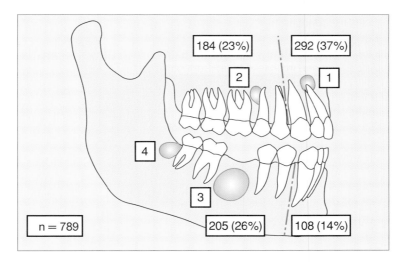

Radicular cyst

570 Anatomic localization
Sixty percent of all radicular cysts occur in the maxilla and a third of all cysts in the anterior segment of the maxilla (adapted from Shear 1992).

1 Periapical type
2 Lateral type
3 Residual cyst
4 Paradental cyst

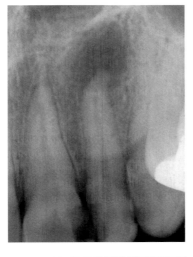
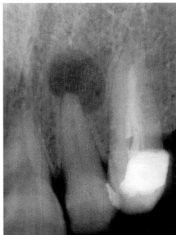

571 Radiographic findings
Left: The area of periapical osteolysis exhibits a poorly demarcated border. It is difficult to differentiate between a periapical "granuloma" and a periapical radicular cyst.

Right: This may be called a "typical radiographic appearance" of a periapical radicular cyst. The radiolucency is round or oval, with a sharply demarcated border.

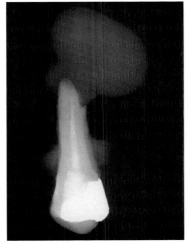
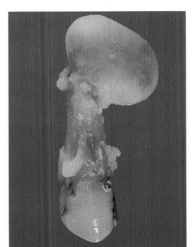

572 Periapical radiograph and extracted tooth
Left: Radiograph of the maxillary second premolar shown on the right, exhibiting a root canal filling that does not extend to the apex. Note also the incipient resorption, which is less commonly observed with radicular cysts.

Right: Macroscopic picture of the extracted tooth. It is uncommon to see a radicular cyst of this size maintaining its attachment to the tooth following extraction.

Incipient radicular cysts often persist within the jaw following extraction of the tooth; such cysts are referred to as *residual cysts*.

Pathogenesis

The most widely held theory of the pathogenesis of radicular cysts involves three phases:

- In the *initiation phase*, there is an inflammation-induced proliferation of epithelial cell remnants of Malassez, but the mechanisms are not completely understood.

- During the phase of *cyst formation*, an epithelially-lined cyst forms within a proliferating epithelial mass as a result of centrally located cell degeneration and cell death.

- During the phase of *cyst enlargement*, it is likely that osmotic pressure differences play a role. The hydrostatic pressure within a cyst is approximately 70 mm (H_2O) and is therefore higher than the capillary blood pressure. In addition, bone resorption occurs due to the action of prostaglandins; collagenases probably also play a role. Focal fibrinolysis may play an adjunctive role.

Radicular cyst

573 Pathogenesis/periapical radiograph
a Initiation
b Cyst formation
c Cyst enlargement

Right: Typical radiograph of a periapical radicular cyst arising from a small, retained root fragment. The circumscribed appearance is particularly evident with the narrow radiopaque border. Cysts of this size are treated by cystectomy.

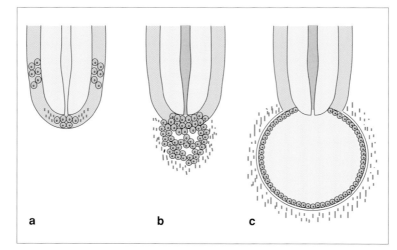
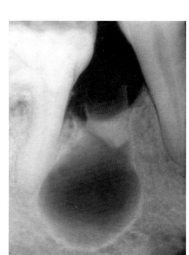

574 Radiographic findings
The panoramic radiograph reveals a large radicular cyst arising from the left second mandibular molar and extending to the mandibular canal. Periapical osteolysis can also be observed in the region of the root tips of the first molar.

Right: The periapical radiograph reveals a periapical radicular cyst with a thick, diffuse, radiopaque border. This is a sign that the lesion is of long standing.

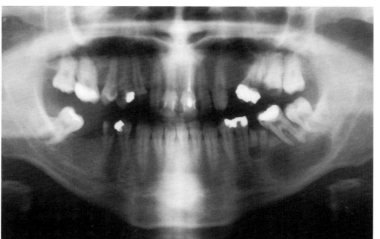
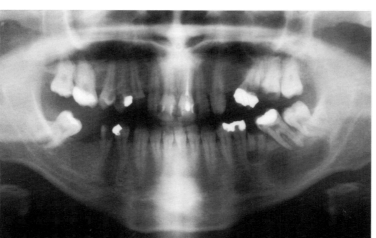

575 Residual cyst
A large residual cyst can be observed in the premolar region on the right side of the mandible. The treatment of choice for periapical radicular cyst is classic cystectomy; in selected cases, cystostomy (marsupialization) may be performed (Reichart 1999).

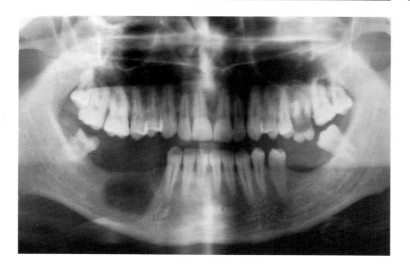

Histology

Low magnification reveals a round or oval cyst, but it is usually irregular or collapsed, or consists of interrupted segments. The cyst wall may be 5–7 mm thick. Yellowish nodules, which consist of cholesterol, may accumulate on the wall of the cyst and project into the lumen. Almost all radicular cysts are completely or partially lined with *squamous epithelium*. The epithelial lining may be up to 50 cell layers in thickness, but most cysts exhibit 6 to 20 cell layers. The epithelium may be clearly hyperplastic with an intensive inflammatory reaction, whereby polymorphonuclear granulocytes predominate. Orthokeratinization or parakeratinization of the epithelial lining is rare, and if present is a consequence of metaplasia. If it occurs, it must be differentiated morphologically from that of an odontogenic keratocyst.

Occasionally one observes *mucous-producing cells* in the epithelium of a radicular cyst. In addition, one may observe ciliated cells, possibly as a result of metaplasia in the epithelium.

In about 10% of all radicular cysts, *hyalin bodies* are observed in the epithelium. They are linear, straight, or curved, or of a hairpin shape and sometimes they are concentrically lami-

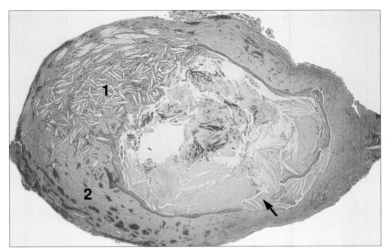

Radicular cyst—histology

576 Thick-walled cyst
This low-power histologic picture shows a thick-walled, periapical radicular cyst. The epithelial lining is discontinuous (arrow), and there is an accumulation of cholesterol-containing granulation tissue (**1**). Numerous cholesterol slits are observed within the cyst cavity. The wall of the cyst contains numerous dilated vessels (**2**). (H & E, x 6)

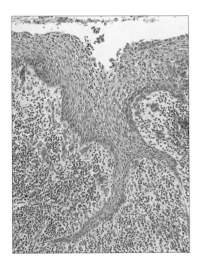

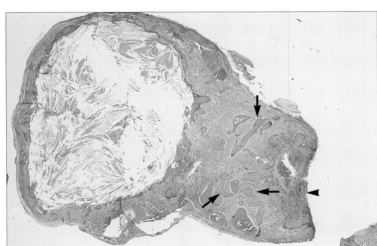

577 Thin-walled cysts/epithelial hyperplasia
The wall of this cyst is thinner than that in Fig. 576. The arrowhead points to the region of the cyst wall that had previously been connected to the tip of the root. The arrows point to various areas where proliferation of epithelial rests of Malassez is occurring (H & E, x 6).
Left: Epithelial hyperplasia of the wall of the cyst revealing a dense inflammatory infiltrate consisting of lymphocytes, plasma cells and PMNs (H & E, x 120).

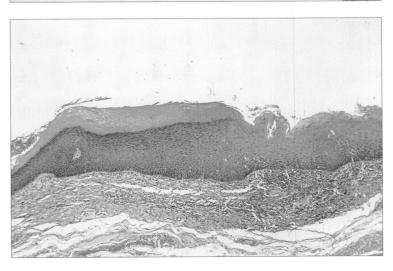

578 Focal orthokeratinization of cystic epithelium
This histologic picture of an inflammation-induced keratinizing cyst must not be confused with an odontogenic keratocyst. The epithelium is usually much thicker and the typical keratocyst signs, such as pallisading cylindrical basal cells, are lacking (H & E, x 80).

nated. The bodies measure up to about 0.1 mm. In spite of intensive research, very little is known about the origin and composition of hyaline bodies.

Cholesterol deposits are found in the fibrous capsule of 30–40% of radicular cysts, where they elicit a foreign body reaction. Cholesterol crystals give the cystic fluid its characteristic yellow, shimmering appearance. An estimation of the soluble protein level in aspirated cyst fluid may be a valuable aid in the preoperative diagnosis of cysts.

The *fibrous capsule* of the radicular cyst consists peripherally of condensed collagen; adjacent to the epithelial lining it consists of loose connective tissue. The intensity of the acute or chronic inflammatory infiltration varies. Plasma cells predominate; they express antibodies against microbial toxins from the root canal. During the phase of enlargement, some cysts are richly vascularized, and hemorrhage is not uncommon. Calcifications of various forms may also occur.

Radicular cyst—histology

579   Section through the wall of a cyst
The lining exhibits a regular squamous epithelium (**1**). The connective tissue capsule contains numerous cholesterol slits (**2**) and phages that harbor hemosiderin (**3**). (H & E, x 140)

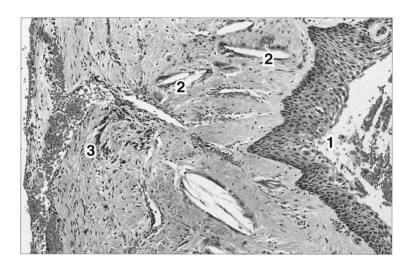

580   Cholesterol deposits
Large deposits of cholesterol are apparent in the connective tissue of this cystic wall. The cholesterol slits are cigar-shaped. In the center of the section one can observe an accumulation of phagocytized hemosiderin (arrows). (H & E, x 15)

Right: Higher magnification of the cholesterol slits in the cystic wall. The arrows indicate aggregations of multinucleated giant cells adjacent to the cholesterol deposits (van Gieson, x 140).

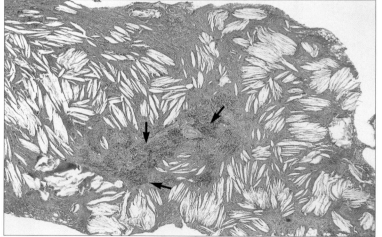
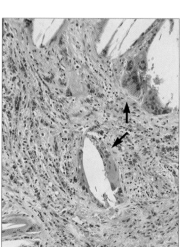

581   Lipophages in the cystic wall
At higher magnification the cystic wall exhibits numerous lipophages. This phenomenon is not uncommon and is usually observed in the region adjacent to cholesterol deposits (H & E, x 180).

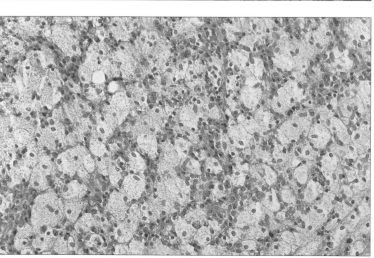

Paradental Cyst (Craig cyst)

The paradental cyst occurs on the lateral aspect of the root of a partially erupted mandibular third molar; the medical/dental history often reveals a preexisting pericoronitis. The cyst is usually localized on the buccal aspect of the root.

The histologic picture of the paradental cyst reveals a hyperplastic, nonkeratinized squamous epithelium that is indistinguishable from that of the radicular cyst. Rests of Malassez and reduced enamel epithelium are considered the most likely sources of the cystic epithelium. The treatment of choice involves cystectomy with simultaneous extraction of the third molar (Ackermann et al. 1987).

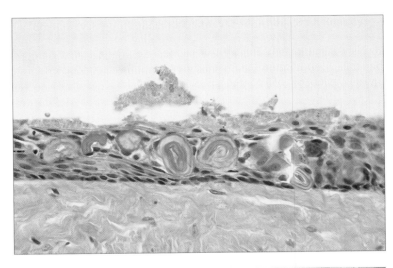

582 Radicular cyst—epithelial wall
The epithelial wall exhibits numerous hyaline bodies of the layered, polycyclic type (H & E, x 240).

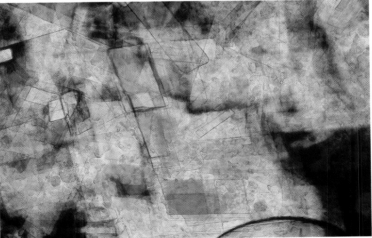

583 Radicular cyst—cholesterol crystals
The cholesterol crystals depicted here are free-floating in the fluid aspirated from a radicular cyst. The crystals form rhomboid tablets of varying dimension. (Polarized light, x 30)

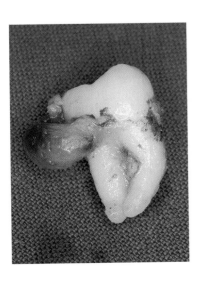
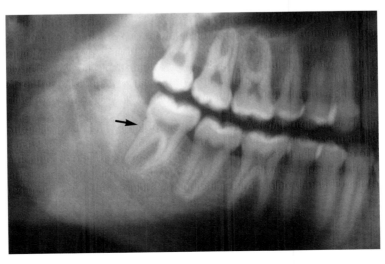

584 Paradental Cyst
This section from a panoramic radiograph reveals an area of osteolysis (arrow) on the distal surface of the third molar, corresponding to a paradental cyst.

Left: Surgical specimen. A small cyst can be seen at the cementoenamel junction of the distobuccal aspect of the partially erupted mandibular third molar.

Odontogenic Tumors

The origin of odontogenic tumors is to be found in the organogenetic, histogenetic, and embryologic bases of normal tooth development. Neoplastic proliferation emanates from stem cells, which originate from normal tissues. During tooth development, it is possible to differentiate histogenetically between cells of ectodermal origin (ameloblasts, epithelium of the dental lamina, squamous epithelium of the oral mucosa), ectomesenchymal cells (odontoblasts, cementoblasts), mesenchymal cells of the normal supportive and connective tissues, as well as neuroectodermal cells (Reichart and Ries 1983, Heikinheimo 1993). The permutations of these quite different cells lead to the multifaceted picture of the odontogenic tumors. Thus, in this sense, it is the deviation from normal odontogenesis that serves as the basis for odontogenic tumors and defective development.

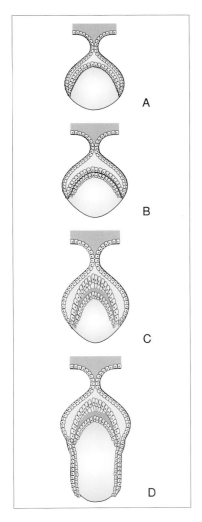

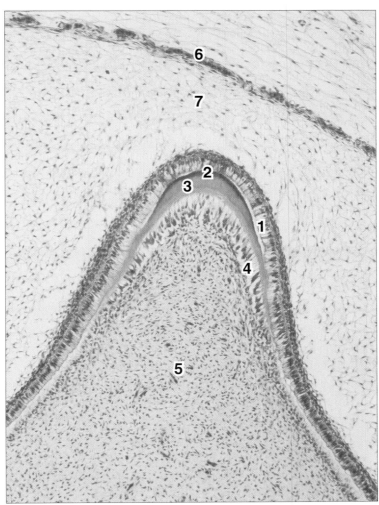

585 Odontogenesis
This low-power histologic picture reveals the late bell stage of normal tooth development, with the ameloblast layer (**1**), the already deposited enamel matrix (**2**) as well as the subjacent predentin (**3**) and the neighboring odontoblast layer (**4**). The primitive pulp (**5**) is adjacent. The upper portion of this picture shows the external enamel epithelium (**6**). The stellate reticulum (**7**) is visible between the ameloblast layer and the outer enamel epithelium (H & E, x 150).

Left: Stages of odontogenesis (Eversole et al. 1971)

A Bell stage with induction of neighboring ectomesenchyme
B Odontoblast differentiation
C Formation of predentin
D Formation of root sheath

Classification

The classifications that have been proposed in the last 20 years are based upon the principles of histogenesis and induction. The latter is the most basic principle for odontogenesis—the interplay among ectodermal, ectomesenchymal and mesenchymal components in a perfect harmony, resulting in tooth formation. Disturbances of the induction phenomenon lead to malformations or neoplasias, which can be attributed to the histogenesis of the primordial tissues of the tooth germ. Reichart and Ries (1983) introduced the principle of ectomesenchyme into the classification of

odontogenic tumors; four cell types represent the possible stem cells of odontogenic tumors:
- Epithelial cells (squamous epithelium of the oral mucosa, epithelium of the dental lamina, ameloblasts)
- Ectomesenchymal cells (odontoblasts and cementoblasts)
- Mesenchyme (fibrocytes, fibroblasts, adipose tissue, hemangioendothelium, osteocytes, osteoblasts, chondrocytes)
- Neuroectodermal cells (neuroblasts, Schwann cells, melanocytes).

586 Classification
The classification proposed by the World Health Organization in 1992 represents the classification of odontogenic tumors that is recognized today.

Benign Tumors
- *Odontogenic epithelium without odontogenic ectomesenchyme*
  - Ameloblastoma
  - Squamous epithelial odontogenic tumor
  - Calcifying epithelial odontogenic tumor
  - Clear-cell odontogenic tumor
- *Odontogenic epithelium with odontogenic ectomesenchyme, with or without dental hard tissue formation*
  - Ameloblastic fibroma
  - Ameloblastic fibrodentinoma and ameloblastic fibro-odontoma
  - Odontoameloblastoma
  - Adenomatoid odontogenic tumor
  - Calcifying odontogenic cyst
  - Complex odontoma
  - Compound odontoma
- *Odontogenic ectomesenchyme with or without included odontogenic epithelium*
  - Odontogenic fibroma
  - Odontogenic myxoma
  - Benign cementoblastoma

Malignant Tumors
- *Odontogenic carcinomas*
  - Malignant ameloblastoma
  - Primary intraosseous carcinoma
  - Malignant variants of other odontogenic epithelial tumors
  - Malignant changes in odontogenic cysts
- *Odontogenic sarcomas*
  - Ameloblastic fibrosarcoma (ameloblastic sarcoma)
  - Ameloblastic fibrodentinosarcoma and ameloblastic fibro-odontosarcoma
  - Odontogenic carcinosarcoma

This classification was accepted in 1992 by the World Health Organization (Kramer et al. 1992).

Tumors are classified as benign or malignant depending upon their biological behavior. Some benign tumor entities are non-neoplastic; these are classified as hamartomas or developmental anomalies in a broad sense. They are lesions whose growth rate appears to be regulated—for example, the odontoma, which does not exhibit any further tendency to grow following completion of tooth development.

The group of *benign tumors* consists of:
- Tumors with odontogenic epithelium but without odontogenic ectomesenchyme
- Tumors with odontogenic epithelium and odontogenic ectomesenchyme with or without formation of dental hard tissue
- Tumors with odontogenic ectomesenchyme with or without included odontogenic epithelial remnants.

Malignant odontogenic tumors are rare and may appear as malignant odontogenic carcinoma (malignant ameloblastoma, primary intraosseous carcinoma, etc.) or as odontogenic sarcoma (ameloblastic fibrosarcoma, odontogenic carcinosarcoma, etc.).

Ameloblastoma

In earlier times, the ameloblastoma was called "adamantinoma"; however, it produces no dental hard substances, so this terminology was not justified. The tumor is locally destructive and exhibits invasive growth, but without formation of metastases. According to its definition, the ameloblastoma is considered to be benign; from the therapeutic point of view, however, it must be viewed as a malignant process, demanding radical surgical excision.

In 1995, the biological profile of ameloblastoma was analyzed by evaluating 3,677 cases that had been published in the world literature (Reichart et al. 1995). The average age of patients with ameloblastoma was 39.9 years. The average age for Blacks with ameloblastoma was 28.7 years, and 41.2 years for Asians. Males and females are equally affected.

Primary symptoms such as painless swelling and slow growth are uncharacteristic. The prevalence of all types of ameloblastoma in the mandible versus the maxilla is 5.5:1.

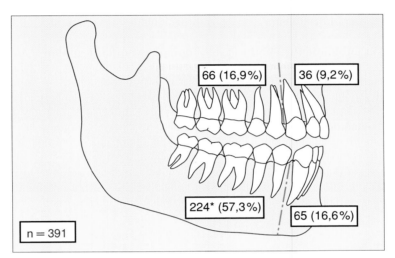

Ameloblastoma

587 Anatomic localization
Sonner (1993) evaluated 391 reported cases of ameloblastoma. The frequency of solid intraosseous ameloblastoma of the maxilla compared to that of the mandible in the molar and premolar regions was 1:3.4 and in the anterior area 1:1.8 (* including the angle of the mandible and the ascending ramus).

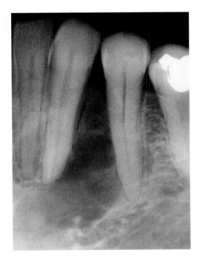
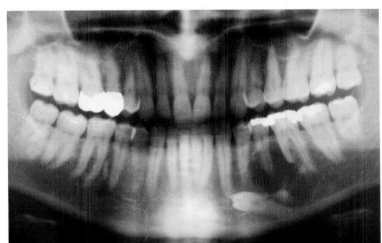

588 Radiographic findings
This panoramic radiograph depicts a homogeneous, well-demarcated radiolucency above a supernumerary premolar. The lesion also involves the second premolar and the partially resorbed mesial root of the first molar.

Left: Small, multilocular ameloblastoma between the mandibular canine and the first premolar.

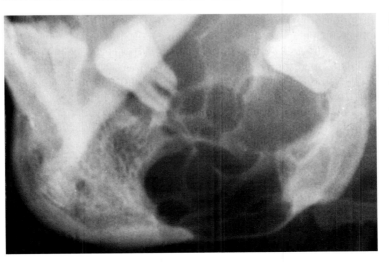

589 Radiographic finding
This is an oblique-lateral projection of the mandible, revealing a large, cystic, multilocular ameloblastoma of the horizontal ramus, partially extending into the ascending ramus as well. The basal cortical bone remains intact.

In 50% of cases, the ameloblastoma appears radiographically as a *multilocular* lesion (multicystic/polycystic) with clear demarcation. It is important to bear in mind that the unilocular variant occurs in patients with an average age of 29, while the multilocular variant occurs in patients with an average age of 40.8 years (Reichart et al. 1995).

Histologically, one third of the lesions appear as the *plexiform*, and one third as the *follicular* type; other variants such as the *acanthomatous* ameloblastoma occur in elderly patients. Of interest is the difference in frequency of recurrence of the various histologic types: for example, in cases of plexiform ameloblastoma, recurrence in noted in 16.7% of cases, while in the case of follicular ameloblastoma the recurrence rate is 29.5%.

The ameloblastoma must be treated radically; chemotherapy and irradiation are contraindicated. Fifty percent of all recurrences are noted only five years postoperatively, necessitating a life-long follow-up of these patients (Gardner 1996).

Ameloblastoma

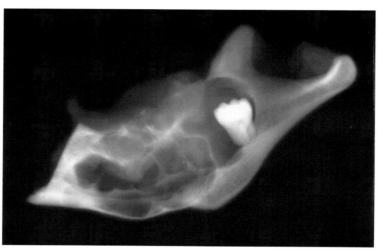
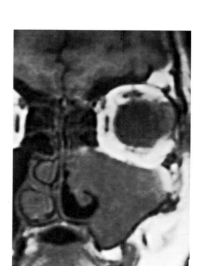

590 Radiographic findings
Surgical specimen revealing a large, multilocular ameloblastoma associated with a displaced, impacted third molar.
Right: Magnetic resonance imaging of the midface. The maxillary sinus exhibits diffuse shadowing. Destruction of the lateral nasal wall can be observed. Maxillary ameloblastomas are especially dangerous due to the danger of expansion cranially and orbitally.
Courtesy B. Hoffmeister

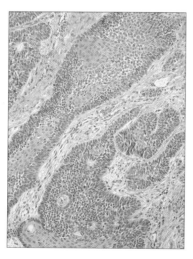
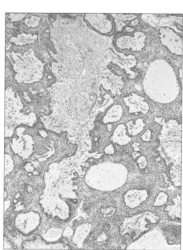

591 Histology
Left: The follicular ameloblastoma is characterized by isolated follicles, or islands, within a loose connective tissue matrix (H & E, x 80).

Right: Plexiform ameloblastoma with the tumor epithelium arranged in a network pattern. Cyst formation occurs mainly due to stromal degeneration (H & E, x 40).

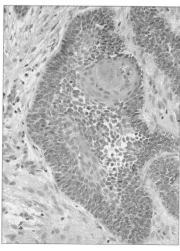
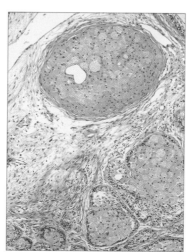

592 Histology
Left: This acanthomatous ameloblastoma is characterized by focal keratinization of the stellate reticulum within the ameloblastoma islands and strands (H & E, x 80).

Right: Ameloblastoma of the granular cell type, characterized by large round cells with acidophilic granules (H & E, x 60).

Peripheral Ameloblastoma (PA)

The peripheral ameloblastoma accounts for 2% of all ameloblastomas (Reichart et al. 1995). It develops from the epithelium of the oral mucosa or from remnants of the dental lamina. Average age of patients at the time of diagnosis is 51 years; this is 15 years beyond the mean age of patients with intraosseous, central ameloblastoma. The mandible is more frequently affected than the maxilla (mand.: max. = 2.5 : 1). The lesions occur in the mandibular anterior and premolar regions twice as often as in the molar regions or the ascending ramus. The PA is a firm, exophytic growth often diagnosed as "fibrous epulis". The primary radio-graphic finding is the so-called "cupping" with superficial erosion of the bone, or there is no evidence of bony involvement at all.

The PA is most commonly of the acanthomatous subtype. Histologic evaluation of excised tissue may be fraught with diagnostic difficulties in those cases where an intraosseous ameloblastoma infiltrates through the bone and eventually makes contact with the basal cell layer of the oral epithelium. This may give the impression of a PA, which, in fact, is not the case. Simple excision of the lesion is sufficient; the recurrence rate is low. Because of the benign behavior of the PA, it has been questioned whether the PA is a true counterpart of the central, infiltrative ameloblastoma.

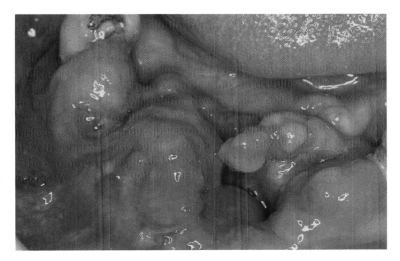

Ameloblastoma

593 Clinical appearance
This clinical picture gives the impression of a squamous cell carcinoma. However, it actually proved to be a large central ameloblastoma from which individual teeth spontaneously exfoliated. The extent of the lesion is unusual for PA.

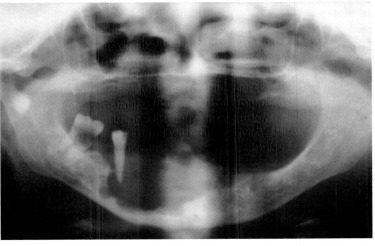

594 Radiographic findings
The panoramic radiograph reveals unusual and extraordinarily, expansive bony destruction in both anterior and posterior segments of the mandible, probably representing a central ameloblastoma. Histology shows fusion of the tumor with the overlying mucosa.

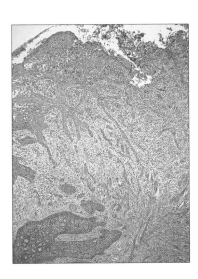
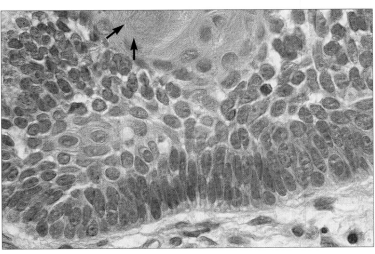

595 Histology
At this high magnification, the typical cylindrical ameloblastoma cells are obvious at the periphery of the tumor. In addition, one notes the keratinization (arrows), confirming that this ameloblastoma is of the acanthomatous type (H & E, x 300).

Left: Low-power view of the tumor. Strands of the ameloblastoma tissue penetrate from the oral epithelium (upper left) into the depths of the lamina propria (H & E, x 60).

Unicystic Ameloblastoma (UA)

The unicystic ameloblastoma is a variant of the intraosseous, infiltrative ameloblastoma (Philipsen and Reichart 1998). The latter is characterized by islands, strands and irregular configurations of odontogenic tumor epithelium, consisting of centrally located, stellate reticulum–like cells which are surrounded by pre-ameloblast-like cells.

In contrast, the unicystic ameloblastoma—as the name implies—is in essence a cystic lesion lined by ameloblast-like cells. One may note one or several nodules extending from the cystic wall and projecting into the lumen (intralumenal or plexiform variants). Some UAs exhibit infiltration of the connective tissue wall of the cyst (intramural variant). These consist of invasive islands or strands of the classic intraosseous solid or multicystic ameloblastoma.

The median age at diagnosis of the follicular cyst type (with an impacted tooth) is 16.5 years, and for the nonfollicular type, 35.2 years (without an impacted tooth). The ratio of males to females is 1.5:1 for the follicular type and 1:1.8 for the nonfollicular type. The mandible is most often affected (maxilla: mandible = 3:1 to 13:1).

Unicystic ameloblastoma

596 Anatomic localization
Similar to the conventional, or classic, ameloblastoma, the UA is localized primarily at the posterior segment of the mandible (Philipsen and Reichart 1998). This schematic diagram depicts the distribution of 24 cases of the follicular type. The third molars are most often affected.

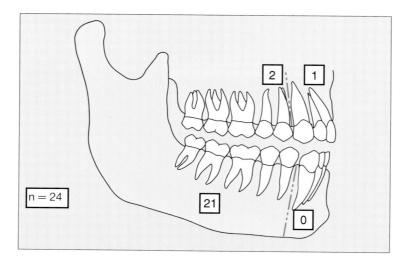

597 Histologic types
Philipsen and Reichart (1998) differentiate four groups of UA:
1   Simple type with ameloblastic cyst epithelium
1,2 Simple type with intralumenal growth
1,2,3 Simple type with intramural growth
  • arising from cyst epithelium, or
  • arising from cyst epithelium with islands of tumor cells
1,3 Simple type with intramural growth

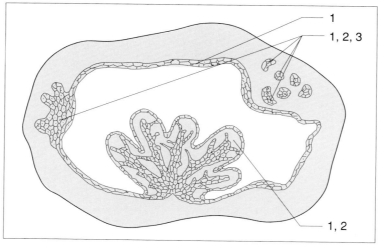

598 Radiographic appearance
Note the unilocular radiolucency around an impacted mandibular second molar. The primordium of the third molar can be observed in the ascending ramus (arrow). This case presents the typical findings of a follicular UA with an impacted and retained molar. The differential diagnosis should also include follicular (dentigerous) cyst.

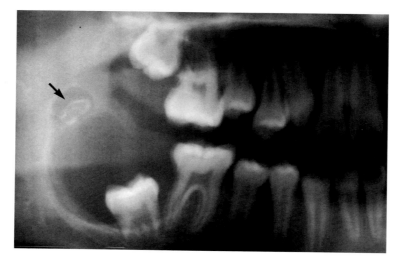

From a pathologic point of view, the UA is unicystic even though its radiographic appearance is not always unilocular, but often multilocular. The lesion can be categorized histologically into four subtypes (Philipsen and Reichart 1998):

- Group 1: simple type with ameloblastic cyst epithelium
- Group 1, 2: simple type with intralumenal growth
- Group 1, 2, 3: simple type with intralumenal and intramural growth
- Group 1, 3: simple type with intramural growth

The minimum criterium for a histologic diagnosis of UA is the identification of a cyst with a lining of odontogenic epithelium of an ameloblastomatous character.

Groups 1 and 1,2 can be treated conservatively (enucleation), while Groups 1, 2, 3 and 1, 3 must be resected in the same way as classic ameloblastomas.

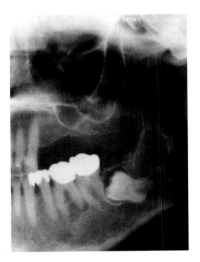
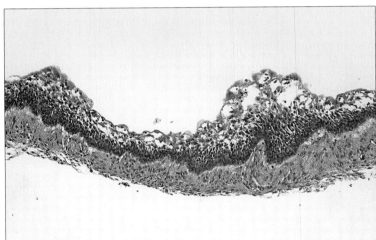

Unicystic ameloblastoma

599 Example of Group 1
The Group 1 UA exhibits a cyst wall with ameloblastic epithelium, but without infiltrative growth (H & E, x 80).

Left: This section from a panoramic radiograph reveals a multilocular radiolucency involving the impacted third molar.

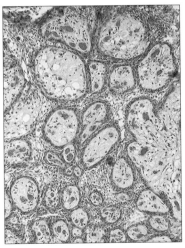
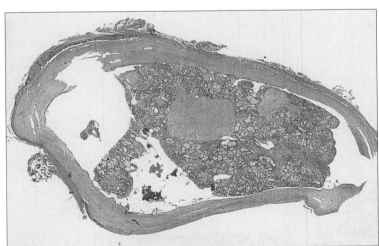

600 Example of Group 1, 2—histology
Low-power view of a unicystic plexiform ameloblastoma of Group 1, 2. There is epithelial proliferation in the intralumenal region, which mimics an ameloblastoma of the plexiform type (H & E, x 5).

Left: At higher magnification, the plexiform structure of the ameloblastic intralumenal proliferation can be observed, with cyst formation in the connective tissue (H & E, x 80).

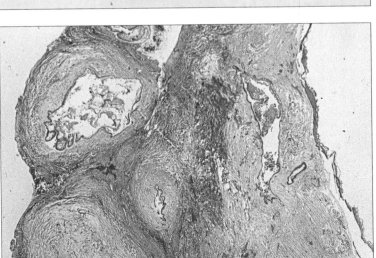

601 Example of Group 1, 3—histology
Histologic view of a UA of Group 1, 3, revealing infiltration of ameloblastic epithelium into the cyst wall. The tumor islands within the cyst wall may be follicular or plexiform type (H & E, x 80).

Desmoplastic Ameloblastoma (DA)

The "classic" ameloblastoma appears in a variety of cyto-morphologic subtypes, such as the acanthomatous and clear-cell variants, and the keratoameloblastoma. Several years ago, an additional variant was described, which was characterized by desmoplasia and pronounced collagenization of the stroma: the desmoplastic ameloblastoma. Desmo- and osteoplastic variants have also been described (Philipsen et al. 1992). The literature contains about 75 published cases. The average age is 51.3 years, with a range of 51–59. This is more than a decade later than the classic ameloblastoma; the gender distribution is similar.

The characteristic localization of this subtype is the anterior segments of the jaws. The radiographic picture is of a diffuse, poorly demarcated unilocular or multilocular radiolucency with multiple flocculent radiopacities. The initial diagnosis is often a fibro-osseous lesion. Radical therapy is indicated because the incidence of recurrence is at least as high as with the classic ameloblastoma.

Desmoplastic ameloblastoma

602   Anatomic localization
The frequent localization in the maxilla is remarkable; the DA can involve large areas of the maxilla. This should be interpreted as especially aggressive behavior.

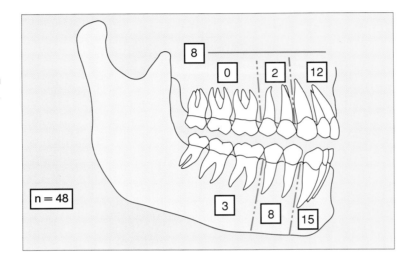

603   Histology/CT
This histologic picture reveals the existing bone into which a plexi-form ameloblastoma in a dense, collagen-rich connective tissue matrix is invading (H & E, x 80).

Right: Computed tomography of a DA of the maxillary sinus and the anterior maxilla. Radiolucencies and radiopacities occur simultaneously (from Philipsen et al. 1992).

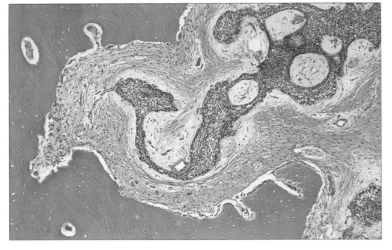
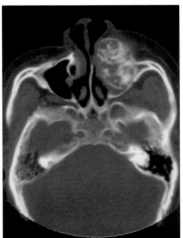

604   Histology/radiograph
The trichrome stain reveals the growth of new, immature bone (*), surrounded by an osteoid border (green) with active osteoblasts (Trichrome, x 150).

Right: The intraoral radiograph reveals resorption and obliteration of the pulp. It also reveals a mixed radiopaque and radiolucent structure, which is reminiscent of a fibro-osseous lesion (from Philipsen et al. 1992).

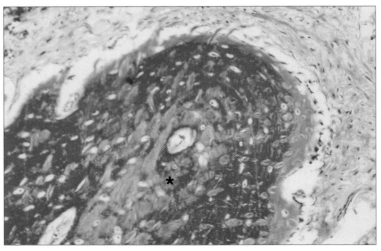
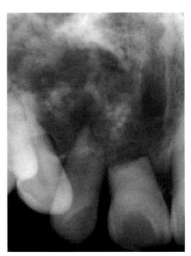

Squamous Odontogenic Tumor and Calcifying Epithelial Odontogenic (Pindborg) Tumor

The *squamous odontogenic tumor* was first described in 1975, and 36 cases were reviewed in 1996 (Philipsen and Reichart). The average age was 38.2 years (range 8–74 years). Males were more often affected than females (1.8:1). The more common, central variant exhibits unilocular radiolucency. The treatment of choice is a conservative surgical approach.

The *calcifying epithelial odontogenic tumor* (Pindborg 1955) occurs most frequently between 30 and 50 years of age,

with no gender differences. The radiograph may reveal unilocular or multilocular radiolucencies with occasional calcified structures of varying size and density. Extraosseous calcifying odontogenic tumors have also been described (Houston and Fowler 1997). While the treatment for the extraosseous variant consists of simple excision, the central form demands a more radical approach. Long-term follow-up is recommended.

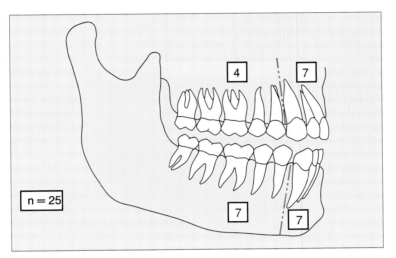

605 Squamous odontogenic tumor—anatomic localization
The 25 tumor cases were distributed relatively equally in the maxillary and mandibular quadrants. Tumors have also been described that occupied an entire quadrant or multiple areas of the jaw.

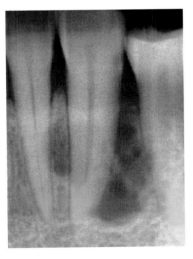
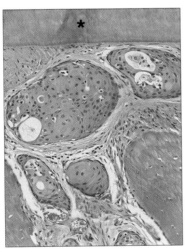
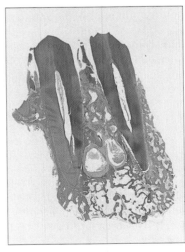

606 Squamous odontogenic tumor
Left: Note a small, multicystic radiolucency between the mandibular canine and first premolar.
Middle: Epithelial islands close to the tooth root (*). These are derived from cell rests of Malassez. The epithelial islands often demonstrate microcystic degeneration (H & E, x 80).
Right: Between the roots of the canine and the premolar, one observes an SOT (H & E, x 1.5).

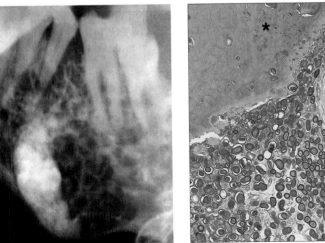
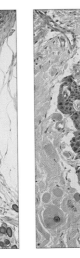

607 Calcifying epithelial odontogenic tumor
Left: The radiograph reveals a mixture of radiolucent and radiopaque areas at the angle of the mandible and in the ascending ramus. *Courtesy J. J. Pindborg*

Middle: Typical calcification, appearing as concentric, lamellar structures (* = tooth root). (H & E, x 80)

Right: Epithelial cell structures with eosinophilic cytoplasm. Note the polymorphism of cells and nuclei (H & E, x 80).

Adenomatoid Odontogenic Tumor

The adenomatoid odontogenic tumor (AOT) was previously called the adenoameloblastoma, a term that led many surgeons to institute unnecessarily aggressive therapy. Philipsen and Birn (1969) were the first to recognize the significance of this tumor and gave it the appropriate name. Philipsen et al. (1991) published a literature review of 500 cases. The number of published cases today approximates 1,000.

From a topographic view, the AOT occurs in both peripheral and central variants, whereby the latter can be divided into a follicular type (with an impacted tooth), and an extrafollicular type (without an impacted tooth). The AOT grows slowly with few symptoms. The slow tumor growth leads to displacement of teeth, and less often to root resorption. The failure of a permanent tooth to erupt, frequently the maxillary canine, may lead to discovery of the tumor.

The *follicular* AOT type resembles a follicular cyst and is difficult to differentiate radiographically from this type of cyst. Forty percent of all impacted teeth are maxillary canines; 59% of all AOT-associated teeth are maxillary or

Adenomatoid odontogenic tumor (AOT)

608 Age distribution
The age distribution of 397 cases reveals that the AOT is a tumor of the teenage years. The mean age of the follicular variant is 17 years. The limited and high age peak is unusual for odontogenic tumors. (Based on Philipsen et al. 1991)

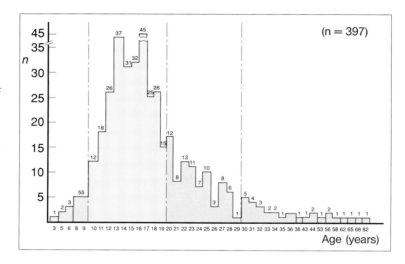

609 Gender and localization
This bar graph depicts the gender distribution and localization of AOT. Females are more often affected. The ratio is about 2:1. (Based on Philipsen et al. 1991)

Right: Anatomic localization of the follicular variant (associated with an impacted tooth). The canines of the maxilla are by far the most often affected. (Based on Philipsen and Reichart 1999)

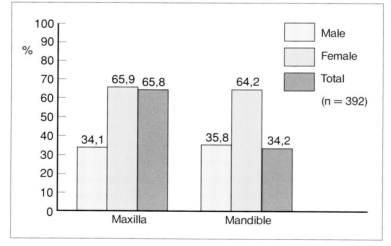

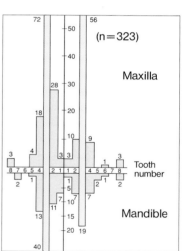

610 Clinical and radiograph findings
Left: Circumscribed radiolucency around the crown of the maxillary canine. Note the diffuse distribution of minute radiopacities.
Middle: Surgical specimen from the maxillary canine with an AOT. In contrast to a follicular cyst, the AOT is not attached at the cementoenamel junction.
Right: CT of an AOT. The left maxillary sinus is filled by the tumor. In addition to the impacted tooth, note the numerous minute radiopacities around 28 (*).

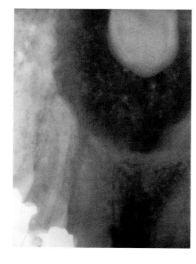

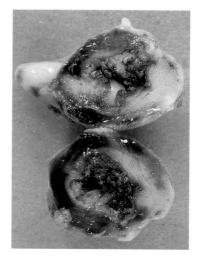

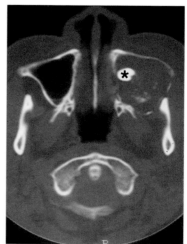

mandibular canines. The *extrafollicular* type of AOT is radiographically similar to a residual cyst or a "globulomaxillary cyst," while the peripheral type corresponds to a gingival fibroma (fibrous epulis). In comparison to the central variant (97%), the various other types are rare (Philipsen and Reichart 1999). Extrafollicular types exhibit a higher mean age at the time of diagnosis (24 years).

It is most important to remember that the AOT should be *treated conservatively*. This is valid for all of its variants; in the case of the follicular type, it is reasonable to attempt to preserve the impacted canine, with a view toward subsequent orthodontic therapy. Recurrence has not been reported and there is no similarity to the ameloblastoma.

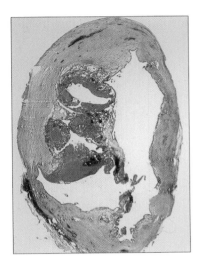
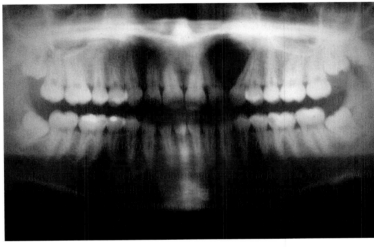
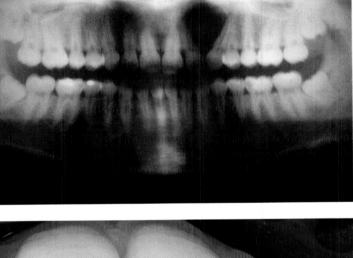
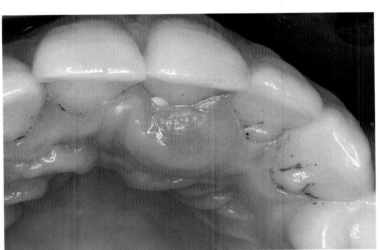

Adenomatoid odontogenic tumor (AOT)

611 Extrafollicular variant
The panoramic radiograph reveals an inverted, pear-shaped radiolucency between teeth 22 and 23. The differential diagnosis must include "globulomaxillary cyst" (from Kuntz and Reichart 1986).

Left: Histologic view of a thick-walled cyst with intralumenal tumor formation and areas of cystic degeneration. (H & E, x 2.5).

612 Peripheral variant
Palatal to the upper left central incisor, one observes an epulis-like swelling. All of the anterior teeth were vital.

Left: The periapical radiograph reveals a radiolucency between the left central and lateral incisor. Histologic examination reveals the diagnosis of adenomatoid odontogenic tumor. (From Philipsen et al. 1992)

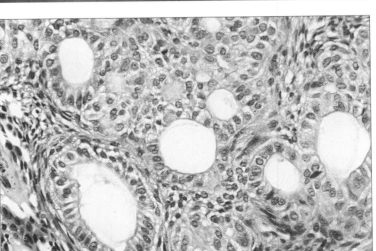

613 Histology
Tubular, or duct-like, structures ("adenomatoid") are typically observed in the region of cellular tumor structures. These duct-like structures are lined by cuboidal or flat-cylindrical epithelial cells; the ovoid nuclei are situated away from the lumen (H & E, x 150).

Adenomatoid odontogenic tumor (AOT)

614   Histology
This section reveals the typical tumor cell configuration, with occasional "duct" formation. The lumena are for the most part empty, but may also contain eosinophilic material or cellular debris. Duct-like structures are not observed in all tumors (H & E, x 180).

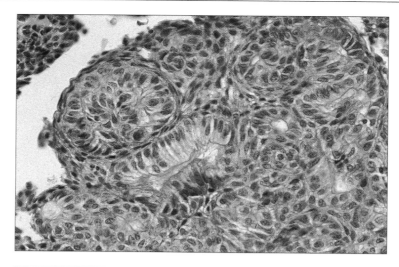

615   Histology
Areas of calcified material may be present in some tumors. One often notes irregularly calcified regions, which are believed to be dystrophic calcification. Such areas of calcification often exhibit concentric structuring (H & E, x 150).

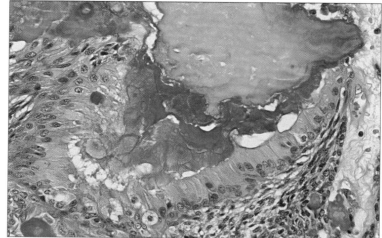

616   Histology
In addition to calcified material, there are often small, non-calcifying, amorphous "droplets" or bodies, which appear in the H & E section as eosinophilic bodies (arrows; H & E, x 100).

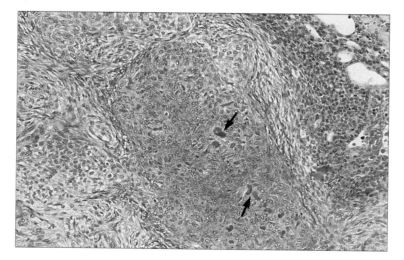

617   Ultrastructure
The electron photomicrograph clearly depicts the extracellular position of the tumor bodies. These are usually of varying, frequently bizarre configuration. At higher magnification, one also notes tubular elements, which can be interpreted as secretion products of epithelial cells (TEM, x 8000). (From Philipsen and Reichart 1996)

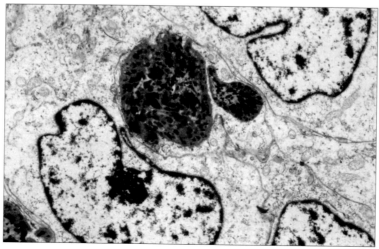

Ameloblastic Fibroma

The ameloblastic fibroma is a rare, benign neoplasia in which odontogenic epithelium and the ectomesenchymal components are neoplastic (Kramer et al. 1992). Seventy-eight percent of cases are diagnosed before age 20 (Philipsen et al. 1997). If cases occurring beyond the age of 30 are eliminated from the statistical evaluation of ameloblastic fibroma, the mean age is 12.4 years. Males are more frequently affected than females (1.4:1). Most ameloblastic fibromas are typically detected in the posterior region of the mandible. Failed eruption of teeth may present a diagnostic clue. Impacted teeth are observed in 75% of cases. Radiographically, the tumor appears as a well-circumscribed, unilocular or multilocular radiolucency. Histologic examination may reveal tiny ameloblastic fibromas within the opercula of nonerupted first or second molars (Philipsen et al. 1992).

In very rare cases, an ameloblastic fibroma may transform into an ameloblastic fibrosarcoma (Reichart and Zobl 1978).

The ectomesenchymal component is thereby transformed, but not the odontogenic epithelium.

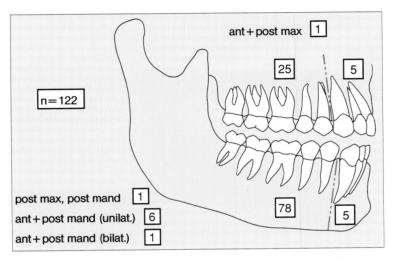

Ameloblastic fibroma

618 Anatomic localization
The posterior segments of the mandible are most frequently affected, followed by the posterior segments of the maxilla. Some cases may affect both anterior and posterior regions of the maxilla or mandible.

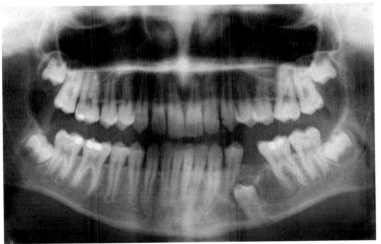

619 Radiographic finding
A multilocular radiolucency is apparent in the region of the left mandible near the impacted second premolar. The mesial root of the first molar is contained within the radiolucency. The differential diagnosis should include follicular cyst. A pre-operative biopsy is absolutely essential in such cases.

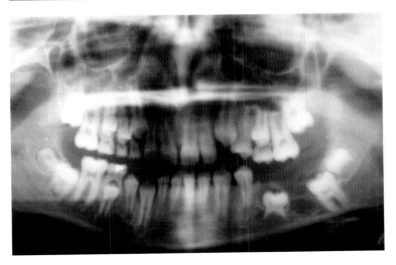

620 Radiographic finding
On the left side of the left mandible, a multilocular radiolucency is present in the region of the congenitally absent second premolar. The first and second molars have been displaced dorsally. The second deciduous molar is retained and impacted. The final diagnosis of ameloblastic fibroma can only be established histologically.

The therapy for ameloblastic fibroma should be conservative, although a cumulative recurrence rate of 18% has been reported (Philipsen et al. 1997). Careful surgical enucleation with clinical and radiographic follow-up is sufficient as the initial therapy.

Of particular interest is the relationship of the ameloblastic fibroma to the ameloblastic fibro-odontoma, and to the complex and compound odontomas. This tumor group is characterized by induction phenomena that are typical for normal odontogenesis. Philipsen et al. (1997) have described in some detail the degree to which the individual

tumors and hamartomas (odontomas) are related to each other or whether they represent individual pathologic processes.

Ameloblastic fibroma

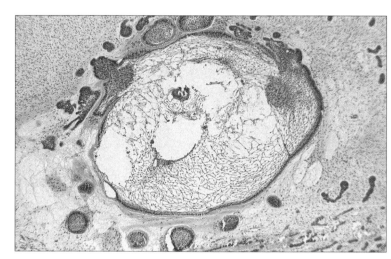

621 Histology
The epithelial tumor component is characterized by proliferating islands and strands of odontogenic epithelium. The strands are reminiscent of the dental lamina. The large island in the center reveals loosely structured stellate reticulum. The ectomesenchymal component appears as cell-rich mesenchyme, which corresponds to the dental papilla or primitive pulpal tissue (H & E, x 60).

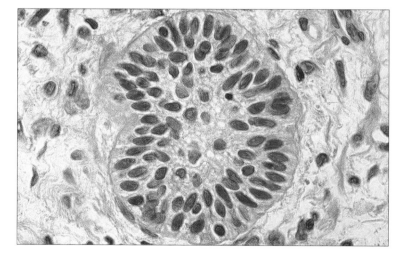

622 Histology
Higher magnification of an epithelial island in an ameloblastic fibroma. At the periphery one notes highly cuboidal or prismatic ameloblast-like cells. The tumor island is separated from the ectomesenchymal tissue by a basement membrane (H & E, x 200).

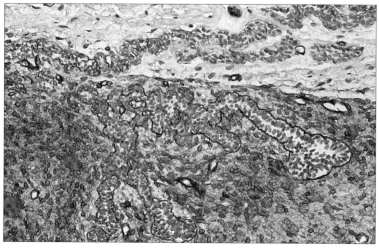

623 Immunohistochemistry
Tumor strands of the ameloblastic epithelium are obvious at the boundary between the ectomesenchyme and the mesenchyme. Collagen type VI is clearly visible in the entire tumor stroma, but not in the adjacent mesenchyme. The epithelial tumor islands are surrounded by a band of type VI collagen (APAAP, x 200). (Becker et al. 1992)

Ameloblastic Fibrodentinoma

The WHO classification (Kramer et al. 1992) defines this lesion as a neoplasm with inductive phenomena that lead to dentin formation. The ameloblastic fibrodentinoma is rare; up until 1997 only 25 cases had been published (Philipsen et al. 1997). Two additional cases were recently reported (Akal et al. 1997). Eighty percent of cases are diagnosed before the age of 20. The mean age is 13.6 (range: 4–30 years). Males are more often affected than females (2.4:1). Seventy-five percent of cases are localized in the posterior area of the mandible. The ameloblastic fibrodentinoma grows slowly and exhibits few symptoms. Because this lesion is associ-

ated with the formation of dentin or dentinoid substance, the radiographic picture of the tumor is a mixture of radiopacities and radiolucencies.

From the pathogenic point of view, the ameloblastic fibrodentinoma may be regarded as a stage between ameloblastic fibroma and ameloblastic fibro-odontoma. The so-called "immature dentinoma" (Takeda 1994) is considered to be a special form of this lesion.

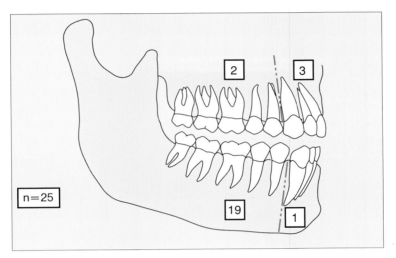

Ameloblastic fibrodentinoma

624 Anatomic localization
Because only very few cases have been published, it is not possible to provide a definitive appraisal of the localization of this tumor. It appears, however, that the posterior segment of the mandible is more frequently affected.

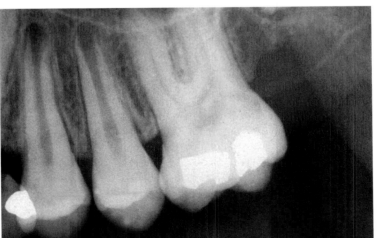

625 Radiographic finding
Distal to the first molar, one observes a radiolucent/radiopaque lesion, which corresponds to the appearance of a small ameloblastic fibrodentinoma. The treatment for ameloblastic fibrodentinoma consists of conservative excision of the tumor. Recurrence has not been reported.

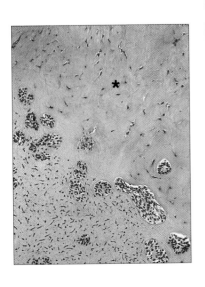
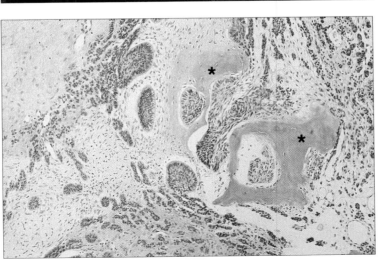

626 Histology
As with the ameloblastic fibroma, one observes strands and islands of odontogenic epithelium within a cell-rich, primitive ectomesenchyme. A particular characteristic is the abortive dentin (*) (dentinoid, osteodentin) formed in this tumor (H & E, x 60).

Left: Depicted is the border between the ectomesenchyme with its typical epithelial islands and the osteodentin structures (*) (H & E, x 60).

Ameloblastic Fibro-odontoma

Similar to the ameloblastic fibrodentinoma, the ameloblastic fibro-odontoma produces dentin, but also enamel. In 1997, Philipsen et al. published a literature review of 86 cases. Ninety-nine percent of all cases occur before age 20. The average age is 9 years (range: 1–22 years). Males are more frequently affected than females (1.4:1). Most ameloblastic fibro-odontomas occur in the posterior region of the mandible (54%). The ameloblastic fibro-odontoma is an expanding tumor that grows painlessly; it is often noticed initially due to the development of facial asymmetry. Eighty-three percent of these tumors are associated with impacted teeth. The radiographic appearance of the ameloblastic fibro-odontoma is unilocular or multilocular with a central opacity that corresponds to the often large tumor mass.

The treatment of choice is conservative removal of the tumor. Impacted teeth may be left *in situ* for subsequent orthodontic realignment. Recurrence following removal has not been reported.

Ameloblastic fibro-odontoma

627   Anatomic localization
The ameloblastic fibro-odontoma is localized most frequently in the posterior segments of the mandible, but it may occur in all areas of the posterior and anterior segments of both jaws.

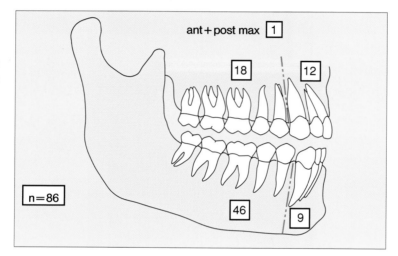

628   Radiographic finding
The left mandibular first molar is impacted. A rather homogeneous radiopacity is obvious directly above the impacted tooth. A small homogeneous opacity can also be observed above the crown of the developing third molar, within the follicle.
   This ameloblastic fibro-odontoma was surgically removed, but the first molar was left *in situ*. The first molar erupted subsequently, despite the root dilaceration.

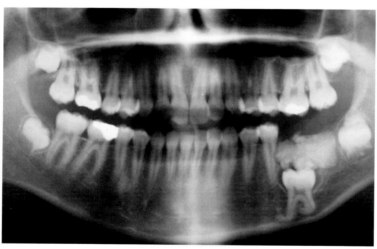

629   Radiographic finding
A large, sharply demarcated cystic lesion is obvious in the angle of the mandible on the right side. Within the lesion, one notes a large, dense radiopacity. Impacted tooth 47 can be seen caudal to the lesion. (from Reich et al. 1984)
   If this tumor is left untreated, it will evolve into a complex odontoma (see p. 238).

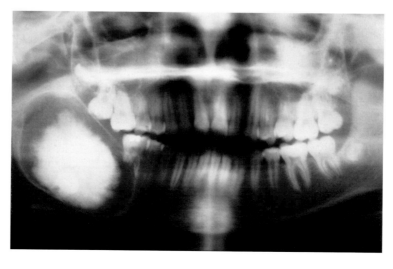

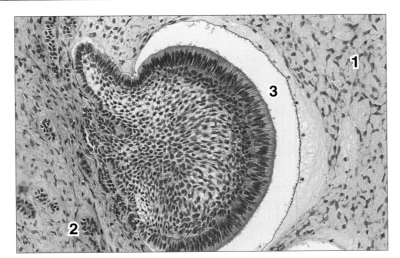

Ameloblastic fibro-odontoma

630 Histology
The structure is similar to a dental follicle, with ectomesenchymal connective tissue (**1**) and dense connective tissue stroma (**2**) which contain small islands of odontogenic epithelium. Ameloblasts can be seen along the periphery of the tumor island. The cell-free zone corresponds to the enamel matrix layer (**3**), which was lost during the process of decalcification of the surgical specimen (H & E, x 100).

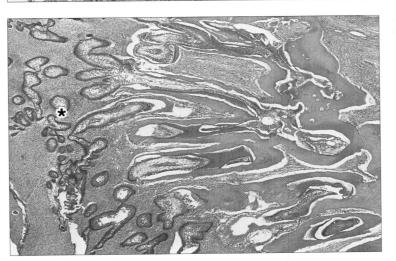

631 Histology (low power)
Histology of the ameloblastic fibro-odontoma depicted in Fig. 629. This lesion exhibits a capsule. Within the capsule is an ameloblastic fibro-odontoma consisting of enamel, dentin and areas of cementum. In the lower right corner of the picture, the impacted, deformed second molar is visible (*) (H & E, x 1.5).

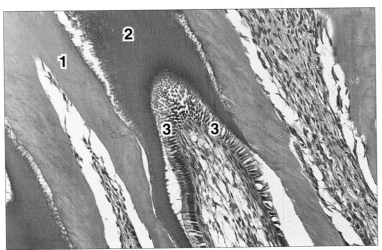

632 Histology (detail)
This magnification depicts the periphery of the ameloblastic fibro-odontoma shown in Fig. 631. Islands of ameloblastic epithelium (*) are observed in a dense connective tissue matrix. Elongated structures of dentin, enamel and cementum are adjacent (H & E, x 40).

633 Histology (magnified section)
This higher magnification of the periphery of the tumor depicts dentin structures (**1**), enamel matrix (**2**), and connective tissue. Also visible are the rows of ameloblasts (**3**). The similarities between these structures and a complex odontoma are obvious (H & E, x 120).

Complex Odontoma

The complex odontoma contains all of the dental hard tissues. Some of the structures are well formed but irregular (Kramer et al. 1992). The average age at diagnosis is 19.9 years (range: 2–74 years). Eighty-four percent of these tumors occur before age 30. Males are more commonly affected than females (1.5:1) (Philipsen et al. 1997). Most complex odontomas are localized in the posterior region of the mandible. Growth is painless, slow and expansive. The size of the tumors may vary considerably.

Radiographically, the complex odontoma appears as an amorphous, solitary mass of calcified material. Tooth-like structures do not appear. Impacted teeth are observed in 10–45% of cases (Philipsen et al. 1997). The complex odontoma is considered to be a self-limiting, developmentally-induced malformation (hamartoma). Conservative enucleation is sufficient therapy, and recurrence has not been reported.

Complex odontoma

634 Anatomic localization
Percentage localizations for the complex odontoma, derived from various publications (**1** to **4**). The posterior segment of the mandible is the most common site (based on Philipsen et al. 1997). *Right:* The periapical radiograph reveals a complex odontoma in the canine region of the mandible. The lesion is sharply demarcated and exhibits a radiopaque central structure of varying intensity.

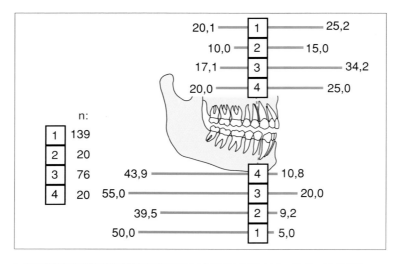
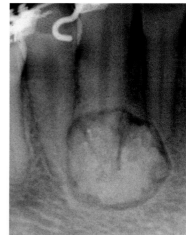

635 Radiographic findings
The panoramic radiograph depicts a complex odontoma in the region of the left maxilla. The second premolar is deeply impacted. In its place, one notes a mixed radiopaque structure.

Right: Computed tomography is often a valuable additional diagnostic technique. In this case, it reveals the complex odontoma with its irregular radiopaque structures in the maxillary sinus.

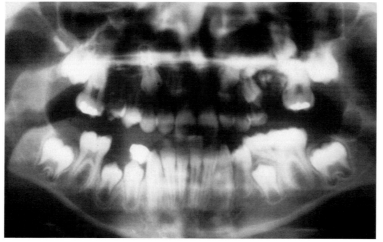
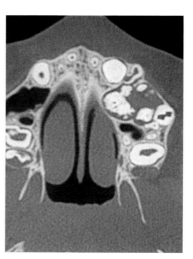

636 Histology
Histologic view of the complex odontoma in Fig. 635. It consists of a mixture of hard substances, epithelial structures, and empty spaces formerly occupied by enamel matrix. The complex odontoma always exhibits a capsule (H & E, x 20).

Right: Enamel matrix (*), dentinoid or cementoid structures as well as connective tissue with remnants of odontogenic epithelium (arrows) are visible (H & E, x 20).

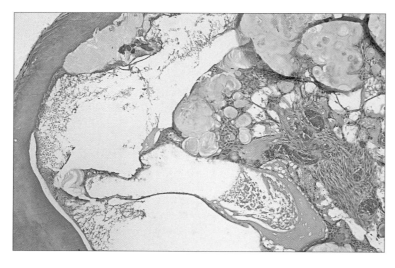
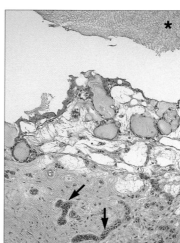

Compound Odontoma

Unlike the complex odontoma, the compound odontoma is a malformation (hamartoma) in which the calcified dental tissues are better organized, resulting in tooth-like structures (Kramer et al. 1992). The relative frequency of the compound odontoma represents 9–37% of all odontogenic tumors, making it the most common odontogenic tumor. The average age at diagnosis is 17.2 years (range: 0.5–73 years) (Philipsen et al. 1997). Seventy-five percent of all cases are diagnosed at around age 20. Males are slightly more commonly affected than females (1.2:1). The anterior maxilla is the site of most compound odontomas.

The diagnosis is frequently made on the basis of the failure of a permanent tooth to erupt. The radiograph reveals several or often many "microteeth" or tooth-like formations; in 40–50% of cases, an impacted permanent tooth is associated with the compound odontoma. The therapy consists of conservative surgical removal, when possible without extraction of the permanent tooth, which can usually be treated orthodontically.

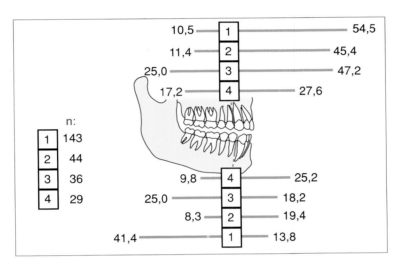

Compound odontoma

637 Anatomic localization
These percentage data derive from four publications (**1** to **4**) (Philipsen et al. 1997). The anterior segment of the maxilla is most often affected. This is quite different from the complex odontoma (see Fig. 634), whose most frequent localization is the posterior segment of the mandible.

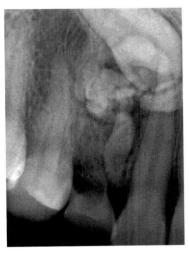

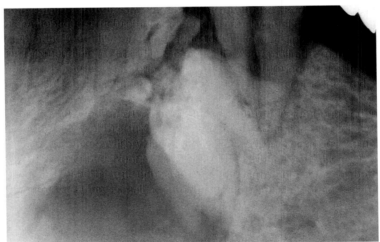

638 Radiographic findings
Multiple radiopaque structures, some appearing tooth-like, are noted in the mandible. As a result of periodontitis, these structures had become infected.

Left: A compound odontoma is evident in the region of the maxillary deciduous canine, whose root is partially resorbed. Note the appearance of both large and small odontoid structures.

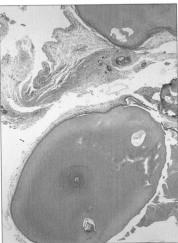

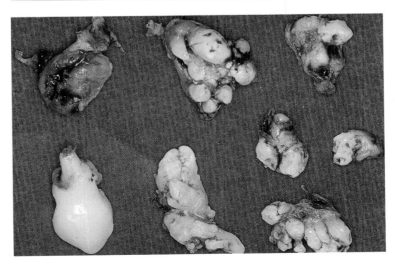

639 Surgical specimen/histology
The compound odontoma consists of variously sized tooth-like structures, the number of which may reach 300. A postoperative radiographic check is necessary to ensure complete removal of all fragments of the odontoma.

Left: Transverse section through a tooth-like structure from a compound odontoma. The growth of the compound odontoma ceases when tooth eruption is complete (H & E, x 10).

Calcifying Odontogenic Cyst

The calcifying odontogenic cyst (COC) is considered to be an odontogenic cyst, but also a cyst with a neoplastic tendency. Toida (1998) reviewed the rather complex terminology and classification. The WHO classification defines this lesion as a non-neoplastic cyst with an epithelial lining of "ghost epithelial cells"; these cells may calcify, and the formation of dysplastic dentin is possible. The COC may also occur in the soft tissue of the tooth-bearing areas. Occasionally, it may be associated with an odontoma. The COC occurs equally in males and females, primarily before the second decade of life (Buchner et al. 1990). Maxilla and mandible are affected

equally. The radiographic picture is of a well-circumscribed radiolucency with enclosed radiopaque structures. Histologic examination may reveal ameloblastoma-like areas; this is an indication of a neoplastic tendency ("dentinogenic ghost cell tumor"). The treatment is conservative, except for those cases exhibiting a neoplastic component.

Calcifying odontogenic cyst

640   Anatomic localization
This diagram depicts the localization of intra-osseous variants of the COC.

1 Cystic variant
2 Odontoma-associated variant

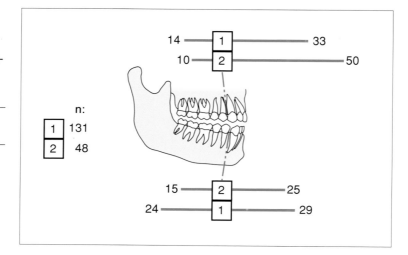

	n:
1	131
2	48

641   Radiographic findings
This panoramic radiograph reveals a cystic lesion on the right side of the maxilla. Note the opaque, cloudy structure above the canine-premolar region. The roots of these teeth have been displaced.

Right: The periapical radiograph clearly shows the displacement of the teeth, especially the canine and the premolar. The radiopacity of various density exhibits an irregular border.

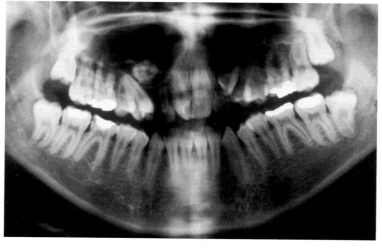
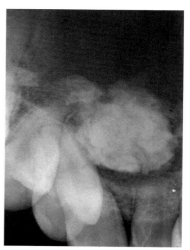

642   Histology
This low-power view depicts sections of the cystic epithelium (arrows) as well as large conglomerates of "ghost cells" (*), and dentinoid (arrowheads), which have a weakly eosinophilic appearance (H & E, x 60).

Right: Higher magnification of the cystic epithelium (arrow) and the ghost cells (*), whose cell nuclei have been lost (H & E, x 80).

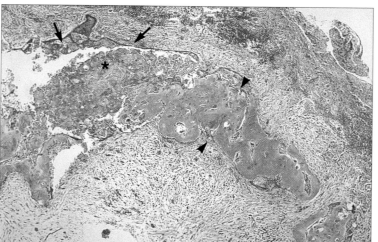
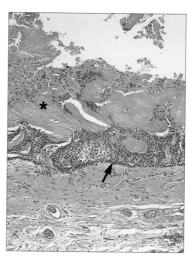

Odontogenic Fibroma

The odontogenic fibroma is defined as a fibroblastic neoplasia containing varying amounts of apparently active odontogenic epithelium (Kramer et al. 1992). This fibroma is relatively rare. The odontogenic fibroma continues to elicit controversial discussion with regard to its entire concept and definition (Gardner 1996). There is general agreement about classifying this lesion as the so-called "simple" type and the WHO type of odontogenic fibroma. The connective tissue of the simple fibroma resembles the dental follicle morphologically, while that of the WHO type consists of a more cellular connective tissue with islands and strands of odontogenic epithelium. Histologically, the odontogenic fibroma must be differentiated from a hyperplastic tooth follicle, from a desmoplastic ameloblastoma and from the central granular cell fibroma. Calcified areas of dysplastic cementum and bone may occasionally be found. A central variant of the odontogenic fibroma is differentiated from an extraosseous type. The therapy consists of conservative surgery.

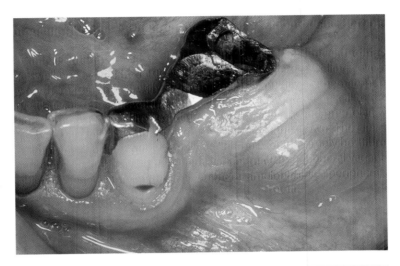

Odontogenic fibroma

643 Clinical findings
A large swelling covered by a mildly erythematous mucosa is observed buccal to the mandibular second premolar, which bears a full crown. The clinical diagnosis would simply be "fibrous epulis." This peripheral variant may resemble a peripheral ameloblastoma.

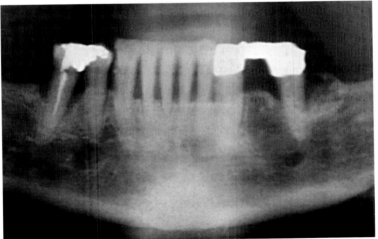

644 Radiographic findings
This section from a panoramic radiograph reveals osseous destruction resembling vertical periodontal pocket formation around the left mandibular premolar. The bone distal to the tooth has a slightly eroded and irregular appearance.

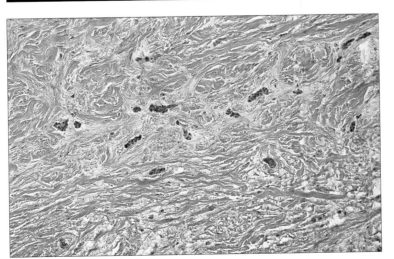

645 Histology
The histologic picture includes dense, collagen fiber-rich connective tissue with scattered small islands of dormant odontogenic epithelium. This is consistent with the diagnosis of odontogenic fibroma, WHO-type. The odontogenic fibroma will occasionally contain numerous epithelial islands and strands (H & E, x 40).

Odontogenic Myxoma

The odontogenic myxoma is defined as a locally invasive neoplasm which consists of round and stellate-shaped cells within a mucoid stroma (Kramer et al. 1992). The odontogenic myxoma is relatively rare and its growth is primarily intraosseous. It is observed most often between the second and third decades of life; males and females are affected with equal frequency. This tumor is more common in the mandible than in the maxilla. The growth of this tumor is relatively rapid, caused by accumulation of mucoid ground substance.

In the radiograph, an odontogenic myxoma appears as a unilocular or multilocular radiolucency. The so-called "soap-bubble" appearance is frequently observed. Impacted teeth are often associated with odontogenic myxoma. This tumor derives from the ectomesenchyme. The differential diagnosis must include ameloblastoma. The treatment consists of broad resection. Recurrence can be expected in about 35% of cases.

Odontogenic myxoma

646 Radiographic and clinical findings
A multilocular, soap bubble-like radiolucency is obvious extending from the angle of the mandible to the first molar. This is typical for odontogenic myxoma.

Right: In the region of the second and third molars, which had been extracted previously, one notes an expansive soft tissue tumor.

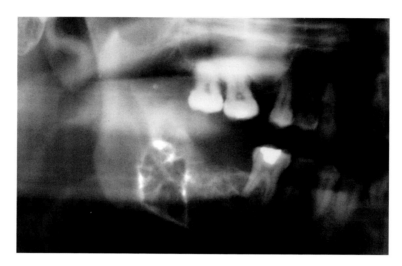
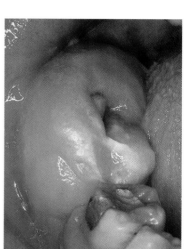

647 Histology
Spindle-like and stellate cells within a collagen-poor connective tissue containing copious myxoid ground substance. If dense bands of collagen are present, the lesion may be described as a myxofibroma. Odontogenic myxoma grows without a capsule (H & E, x 150).

Right: Odontogenic myxoma in the region of the right angle of the mandible with a soap bubble appearance and poorly demarcated borders.

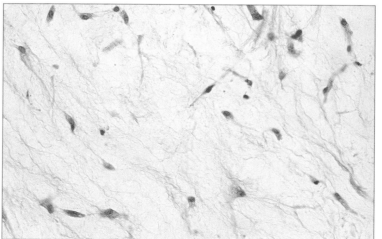
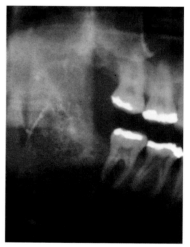

648 Histology
Immunohistochemical depiction of collagen type I. The fibroblasts within the stroma of the tumor exhibit an intracytoplasmic reaction. The surrounding mesenchyme is of non-ectomesenchymal origin and does not exhibit this reaction (PAP, x 80). (From Schmidt-Westhausen et al. 1994)

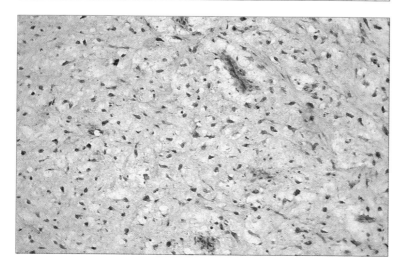

Benign Cementoblastoma

The benign cementoblastoma is defined as a neoplasia characterized by the formation of sheets of cementum-like tissue with numerous reversal lines. No mineralization is noted at the periphery or in the more active growth area (Kramer et al. 1992). The benign cementoblastoma occurs most frequently in the premolar or molar regions, particularly in the mandible. Males are more often affected. Most cases are diagnosed between the second and third decades of life. This tumor is almost always observed in close relationship with one or more tooth roots.

The benign cementoblastoma appears radiographically as a sharply circumscribed lesion. The radiopaque portion of the tumor is surrounded by a narrow radiolucent zone whose width is constant. The histologic picture of the benign cementoblastoma in close association with the root of a tooth exhibits cementum formation and a zone of non-mineralized, active growth. The treatment includes extraction of the tooth, and the tumor usually remains attached. Simple surgical removal of the benign cementoblastoma is adequate (Ulmansky et al. 1994).

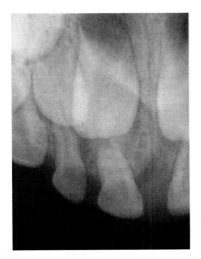
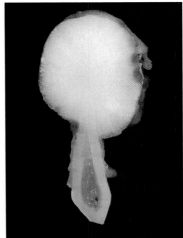
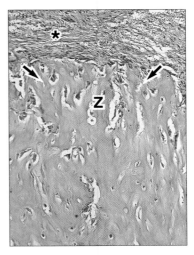

Benign cementoblastoma

649 Diagnostic Findings
Left: The periapical radiograph reveals a benign cementoblastoma attached to the left deciduous central incisor.
Middle: Surgical specimen of a cementoblastoma whose connection to the root of the tumor is obvious.
Right: At the periphery of the tumor, toward the connective tissue (*), one notes a non-mineralized zone (arrows) of the cementum (**Z**). (H & E, x 60)

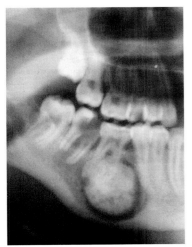
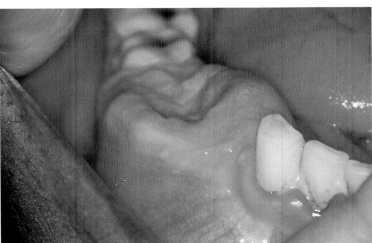

650 Clinical appearance
The clinical picture reveals a large, epulis-like swelling, which was hard upon palpation, between the right mandibular canine and second molar.

Left: Typical radiographic picture of a benign cementoblastoma, emanating from the mandibular first molar. The characteristic peritumor radiolucency is clearly visible.

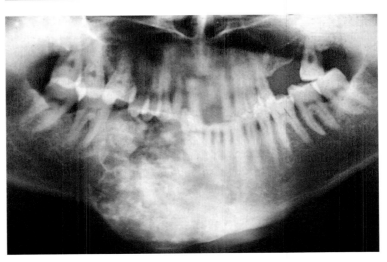

651 Radiographic finding
This panoramic radiograph is of the patient depicted in Fig. 650 (right). One observes a large, mixed radiolucent/radiopaque lesion on the right side of the mandible, which is reminiscent of a gigantiform cementoblastoma. This large lesion is less clearly demarcated than the classic benign cementoblastoma.

Ameloblastic Fibrosarcoma, Odontogenic Carcinoma

Among the rare malignant variants of the odontogenic tumors are odontogenic sarcoma and carcinoma. Odontogenic sarcomas include the ameloblastic fibrosarcoma, ameloblastic fibrodentinosarcoma and fibro-odontosarcoma.

The *ameloblastic fibrosarcoma* resembles the ameloblastic fibroma, wherein the ectomesenchymal components exhibit sarcomatous transformation. These tumors are extremely rare; a recent literature review presented a total of 51 cases (Muller et al. 1995). The ameloblastic fibrosarcoma occurs at an average age of 27.5 years; thus, more than 20 years later than the ameloblastic fibroma.

The *odontogenic carcinoma* may develop through malignant transformation of an existing ameloblastoma or directly from remnants of odontogenic epithelium, or from a cystic follicle (Lau et al. 1998).

652 Ameloblastic fibrosarcoma—radiographic finding
The panoramic radiograph of a young Black male reveals a large area of osteolysis in the left mandible, including the ascending ramus. Following histologic examination, the diagnosis of ameloblastic fibrosarcoma was established.

Courtesy I. Thompson

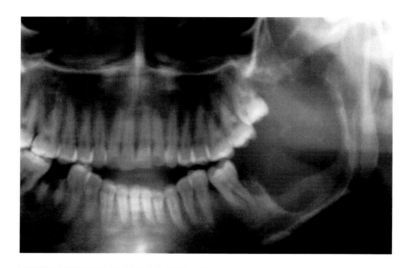

653 Ameloblastic fibrosarcoma—histology
Histology of the ameloblastic fibrosarcoma exhibits malignant transformation of the ectomesenchymal components, with high cell density and increased mitotic activity. Long-standing tumors may lack the epithelial components completely (H & E, x 160).

Right: Note a tumorous, partially ulcerated swelling; the histology revealed an ameloblastic fibrosarcoma. (from Reichart and Zobl 1978)

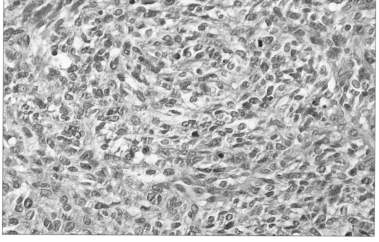

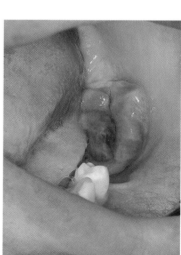

654 Odontogenic carcinoma—histology
The histologic picture reveals dentin (*) of a tooth root, with adjacent islands of malignant odontogenic epithelium (H & E, x 120).

Courtesy M. Shear

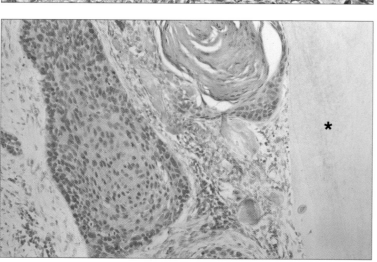

Tumors and Other Osseous Lesions

Cemento-ossifying Fibroma

The cemento-ossifying fibroma is defined as a circumscribed, seldom encapsulated neoplasia that consists of connective tissue containing varying amounts of mineralized substance. The latter may be similar to bone and/or cementum (Kramer et al 1992). In terms of differential diagnosis, this lesion is difficult to differentiate from fibrous dysplasia. In earlier classifications, the cemento-ossifying fibroma was classified as two separate entities. The lesion is detected most often in the mandibular premolar-molar region.

Patients are usually over 40 years of age when this lesion is diagnosed. The clinical growth of the cemento-ossifying fibroma is slow and painless. Radiographically, these neoplasms are well-circumscribed and contain varying amounts of radiopaque material. The lesion is usually radiolucent, with or without central opacities. Treatment consists of careful surgical removal; recurrence has occasionally been observed. In 1997, Su et al. described the characteristics of the cemento-ossifying fibroma (Su et al. 1997a, 1997b).

Osteogenic Tumors

- Cemento-ossifying fibroma

Non-neoplastic Lesions

- Fibrous dysplasia
- Cemento-osseous dysplasia
    - —Periapical cemental dysplasia
    - —Florid cemento-osseous dysplasia
    - —Other cemento-osseous dysplasias
- Cherubism
- Central giant cell granuloma
- Aneurysmae bone cyst
- Solitary bone cyst

655 Tumors and other osseous lesions—classification
The 1992 WHO classification deviated from previous classification in that it led to a combination of various pathologic entities. Particularly the cementum-containing lesions were combined.

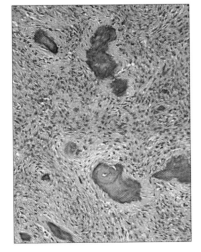
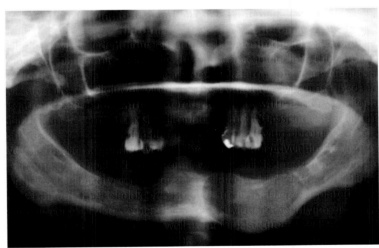

656 Cemento-ossifying fibroma
In the left side of the edentulous mandible, the panoramic radiograph clearly depicts a large, well-circumscribed radiolucency with scattered radiopaque structures, indicating a cemento-ossifying fibroma.
Left: Within the dense connective tissue stroma, which exhibits a high degree of cellularity, one observes isolated small islands of cementifying or ossifying structures as well as metaplastic bone (H & E, x 80).

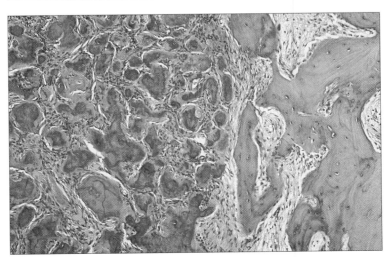

657 Cemento-ossifying fibroma
The histologic picture of cemento-ossifying fibroma exhibits multiple cementicle-like structures to the left of the existing bone within dense connective tissue; the basophilic masses resembling cementum exhibit reversal lines (H & E, x 80).

Fibrous Dysplasia

Fibrous dysplasia is a benign, self-limiting, non-encapsulated lesion most often observed in young individuals. The maxilla is often affected and the normal bone is replaced by cellular connective tissue that contains islands or trabeculae of metaplastic bone. The radiographic picture depends upon the stage of development of this lesion. During the osteolytic stage, there is a poorly demarcated radiolucency; subsequently, following the formation of dysplastic bone, milky, ground-glass structures appear (Pierce et al. 1996).

Cemento-osseous Dysplasias

The pathologic conditions known as cemento-osseous dysplasias encompass periapical cementodysplasia as well as florid cemento-osseous dysplasia (Summerlin and Tomich 1994). The cementum-containing dysplasias comprise a broad spectrum of various lesions with various clinical and histopathologic pictures. These lesions do not usually require surgical therapy.

658 Fibrous dysplasia—radiographic finding
This panoramic radiograph reveals the typical, poorly demarcated osseous structures in the region of the left mandible and the zygomatic bone of the maxilla.

Right: The skull radiograph substantiates the initial suspicion. The maxillary sinus is not discernable, and the left parietal area of the skull appears to be expanded.

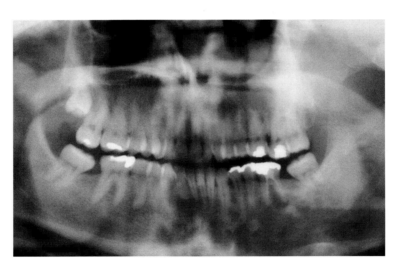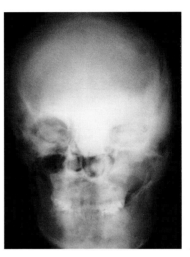

659 Fibrous dysplasia—histology/CT
Histology reveals cellular connective tissue with irregularly distributed osseous trabeculae, which are reminiscent of Chinese language characters (H & E, x 40).

Right: Computed tomography of the left maxilla. The maxillary sinuses and portions of the nasal sinuses have been compromised by fibrous-dysplastic bone. The therapy consists of conservative osteotomy, but only after the growth phase is completed.

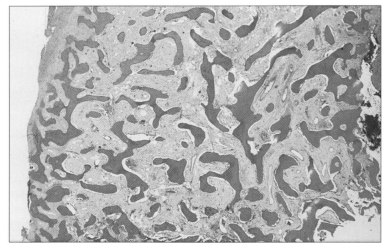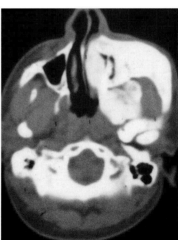

660 Periapical cementodysplasia
The panoramic radiograph depicts areas of periapical osteolysis on numerous teeth of the left mandible. Females in middle age are more often affected.

Right: Within the dense connective tissue one notes islands of metaplastic bone and cementum-like structures (H & E, x 40).

Figs. 658–660:
Courtesy B. Hoffmeister

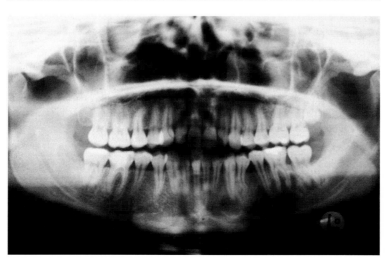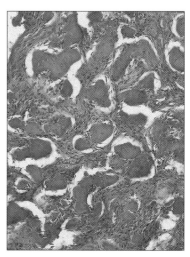

Cherubism, Central Giant Cell Granuloma

Cherubism is defined as a benign, self-limiting condition, in which the vascular connective tissue contains a varying number of multinucleated giant cells, which may be arranged diffusely or in focal groupings (Kramer et al. 1992). Children are most often affected; the lesions are recognized as familial. One or several quadrants of the jaws may be affected; the radiographic picture is one of radiolucent, multilocular regions of expanding bone. After age 12, the activity of the pathologic process increases and the histologic picture varies accordingly. The active phase is charac-terized by elevated cellularity, numerous giant cells and foci of hemorrhage.

The *central giant cell granuloma* is defined as an intraosseous lesion that consists of more or less cellular connective tissue, with multiple foci of hemorrhage, aggregations of multinucleated giant cells and occasional trabeculae of woven bone (Kramer et al. 1992). The radiographic picture is one of osseous destruction with a multilocular pattern. This lesion, therefore, is similar in radiographic

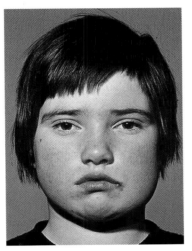 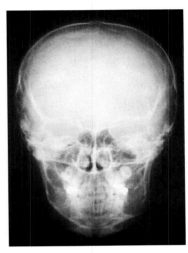

661 Cherubism
Left: Clinical picture of a young female who exhibits the typical "trumpet blower's cheeks" due to the expansion of the entire mandible. The maxilla may also be affected.

Right: The posterior–anterior skull radiograph reveals the multilocular radiolucency within the entire mandible.

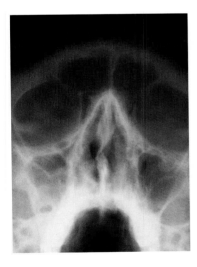 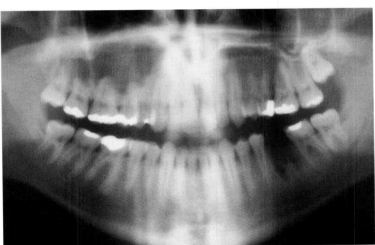

662 Central giant cell granuloma
The panoramic radiograph reveals a diffuse radiolucency in the area of the right maxilla in the region of teeth 15–18. Clinical examination revealed swelling of the alveolar process in this area.

Left: The radiograph shows a radiopacity at the floor of the right maxillary sinus.

Courtesy B. Hoffmeister

663 Central giant cell granuloma
This periapical radiograph reveals a resorptive change in the region of the mesial root of the first molar as well as the second molar. The osseous structures appear to have fused.
These radiographic findings do not permit a definitive diagnosis. This can only be achieved by means of a histologic examination.

Courtesy B. Hoffmeister

appearance to an ameloblastoma.

The central giant cell granuloma occurs in all areas of the jaws and at all ages. The most common appearance, however, is in the dentulous alveolar process of the mandible in the second and third decades of life. Females are twice as often affected as males. Perforating lesions lead to soft tissue swelling and a brownish-blue discoloration. The differential diagnosis of a peripheral giant cell granuloma can therefore be somewhat difficult (see p. 164).

The typical histologic picture exhibits focal aggregations of giant cells, but this sign is not always observed. Fresh hemorrhage and hemosiderin deposits are frequently seen. Because the interface with the surrounding healthy bone is not sharply demarcated, recurrence of the lesion may be expected following conservative surgical removal. The previous terminology, "*reparative*" giant cell granuloma, is incorrect and should no longer be employed.

Central giant cell granuloma

664 Radiographic finding
This panoramic radiograph reveals a large, multilocular lesion with expansion of the mandible in the caudal direction. Resorption of the tips of the roots of several teeth can be observed. The differentiation between giant cell granuloma and giant cell tumor is often difficult.

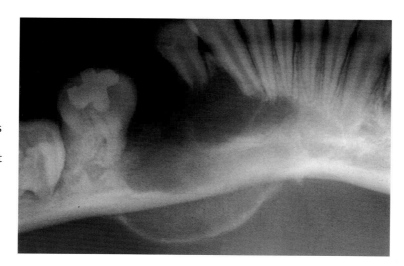

665 Radiographic finding
An area of osteolysis is observed between the maxillary canine and premolar. Following surgical excision and histologic examination, the diagnosis was central giant cell granuloma.

Right: Low-power histologic view with numerous multinucleated giant cells in a dense, cell-rich connective tissue with persisting islands of bone
(H & E, x 80).

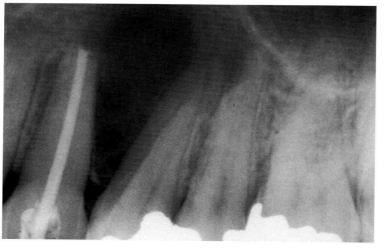
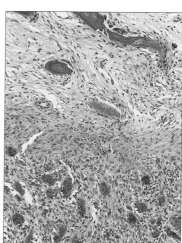

666 Histology
Higher magnification reveals the multinucleated giant cells, which derive from macrophages
(H & E, x 200). The sections often exhibit fresh hemorrhage and the deposition of fibrinoid material. Hemosiderin deposits are also frequently observed.

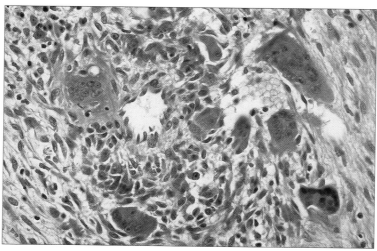

Solitary Bone Cyst, Aneurysmal Bone Cyst, Stafne's Cavity

Classified as a pseudocyst, the *solitary bone cyst* does not have an epithelial lining. It is most frequently observed in the second decade of life. The mandible is primarily affected. The radiographic picture is of a circumscribed, unilocular, radiolucent lesion that is often detected by chance. Simple surgical opening is usually therapeutically effective; regeneration of new bone occurs quickly.

The *aneurysmal bone cyst* contains blood-filled spaces associated with a fibroblastic tissue. It occurs in individuals below age 30. The mandible is more frequently affected.

Radiographically, it is a radiolucent lesion which balloons the cortex. Surgical curettage is sufficient treatment; follow-up examinations are required.

Stafne's cavity on lingual mandibular bone defect is a development defect that occurs mortly in middle-aged men at the angle of the mandible *below* the mandibular canal. This defect is caused by pressure atrophy from a lobe of the submandibular salivary gland. No treatment is necessary.

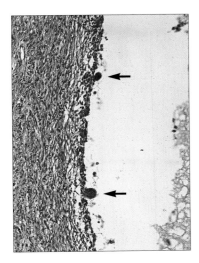
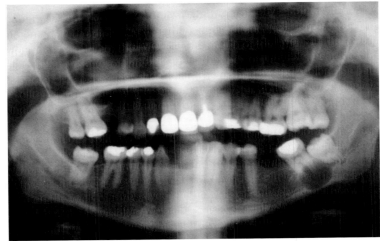
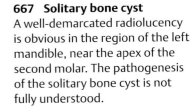

667 Solitary bone cyst
A well-demarcated radiolucency is obvious in the region of the left mandible, near the apex of the second molar. The pathogenesis of the solitary bone cyst is not fully understood.

Left: Exploration of a solitary bone cyst usually reveals that it is empty. Sometimes a thin, loose connective tissue layer is observed on the walls of the cavity. Two giant cells are visible on the surface (arrows) (H & E, x 30).

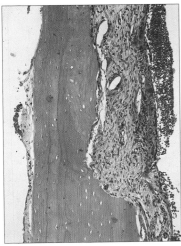
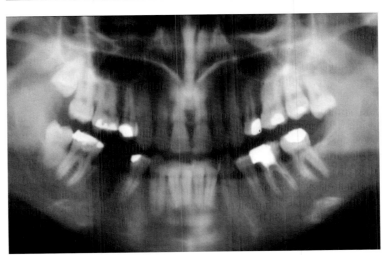

668 Aneurysmal bone cyst
The panoramic radiograph reveals a diffuse radiolucency in the anterior segment of the mandible.

Left: The histologic picture reveals normal bone with cellular connective tissue, several multinucleated giant cells, and fresh hemorrhage. This picture is in some ways similar to that of central giant cell granuloma (H & E, x 30).

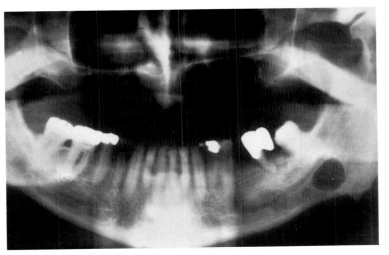

669 Stafne's cavity
The panoramic radiograph reveals a sharply demarcated radiolucency below the mandibular canal on the left side. This corresponds to a cavity in the left mandible, which is occupied by glandular tissue from the submandibular salivary gland. The close relationship between the lingual mandibular bone defect and the salivary gland lobe may be demonstrated by sialography.

Salivary Glands

Definition—Anatomy

The glands that discharge their secretions into the oral cavity are classified in two ways, anatomically and histologically. Anatomically, they are classified as the intraoral, or *minor, salivary glands* and the extraoral, or major, salivary glands. Histologically, they are characterized according to the secretion they produce—serous, mucous or mixed. The *major salivary glands,* namely the parotid gland, submandibular gland and sublingual gland, are located bilaterally. The parotid gland consists of a superficial and a deep lobe of glandular tissue. The submandibular gland is located at the posterior aspect of the mylohyoid muscle. The sublingual gland is located just subjacent to the sublingual plica in the floor of the mouth.

The oral cavity contains mixed saliva that derives from the various glands. The saliva has various functions, primarily immunological, that are expressed through the saliva's content of a variety of different immunoglobulins.

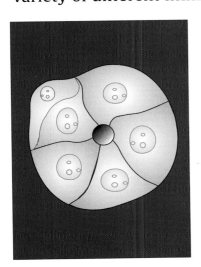

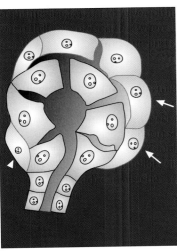

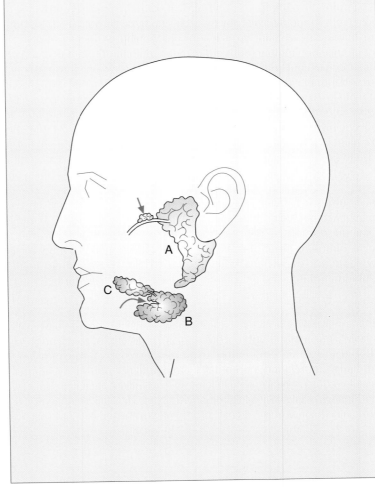

670 Anatomy of salivary glands—histology
Locations of the major salivary glands. The curved arrow indicates a notch in the submandibular gland (**B**) produced by the mylohyoid muscle. The sublingual salivary gland is labelled **C**. The straight red arrow indicates an accessory gland localized alongside the main excretory duct (Stensen's duct) of the parotid gland (**A**).

Above left: Serous acinus exhibiting pyramid-shaped gland cells and a narrow lumen. The cell nuclei are round. Myoepithelial cells are present between the basement membrane and the gland cells.

Below left: Diagram of a mixed salivary acinus. Most of the acini are purely mucous; the serous cells assume a half-moon shape (arrows). Intercellular canaliculi as well as myoepithelial cells (arrowhead) can also be observed.

Major Salivary Glands, Saliva Production

- The *parotid gland* is the largest of the three major salivary glands. It is located anterior to the ear, on the lateral surface of the masseter muscle. Saliva flow from this gland is via the parotid duct (Stensen's duct), which penetrates the buccinator muscle and the mucosa of the cheek to open opposite the maxillary first or second molars.
- The *submandibular gland* has a diameter of 4–5 cm. Secretion flows via the submandibular duct (Wharton's duct), which delivers salvia into the oral cavity via the small papillary orifices of the sublingual caruncle.

- The *sublingual gland* consists of one large and 8–20 small glands with multiple orifices into the oral cavity along the sublingual plicae.

Saliva production: Numerous factors influence the amount and composition of saliva produced. The total volume of saliva produced in an adult amounts to 600–1500 ccm/24 h. With aging, less saliva is produced and the quality of the saliva changes.

671 Saliva composition
This table shows the composition of the secretions from the various large and small glands in the oral cavity.

Gland	Serous	Mucous	Mixed
Parotid	+++		
Submandibular	++	+	+
Sublingual	+	++	+
Labial/Buccal	+	++	+
Palatal		+++	
Tongue (1)		+++	
Tongue (2)	+++		
Tongue (3)	+	++	+

672 Lingual salivary glands— localization
Three distinct groups of glands with varying localizations can be identified.

1 Posterior mucous glands (Weber)
2 Posterior serous glands in the region of the circumvalate papillae (von Ebner)
3 Anterior mixed glands (Blandin–Nuhn)

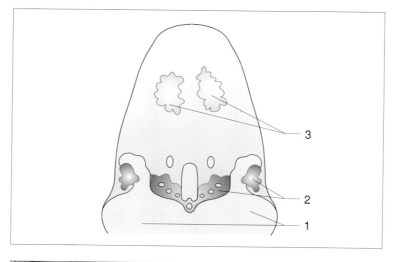

673 Histology of different types of salivary glands
Left: Biopsy of a (mixed) labial gland, which consists primarily of mucous glands. Note also the serous half-moon shaped cells (arrows) and an intercalated duct (arrowhead) (H & E, x 100).

Right: Biopsy of an accessory palatal salivary gland exhibiting typical light-staining mucous acini (Mallory, x 60).

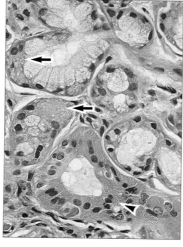
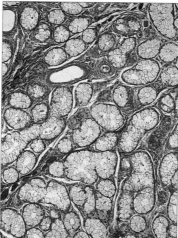

Infections—Bacterial and Viral

Parotitis, Sialadentitis

Acute epidemic sialadenitis (mumps), usually of the parotid gland, is caused by a virus from the group of paramyxoviruses. The incubation period is two to three weeks, commonly 18 days. Children are most often affected. In adults, this disease may be associated with severe symptoms such as orchitis and encephalitis. The prodromal signs are fever, anorexia and headache. In 70% of cases, both parotid glands are affected.

Suppurative parotitis is an acute, pyogenic infection that occurs most frequently in elderly patients whose general health is compromised, for example following major surgery. The infection is caused by staphylococci and streptococci, and develops through retrograde spread along Stensen's duct, from the oral cavity toward the glands.

Chronic sialadenitis commonly affects the submandibular gland, with accompanying obstruction of the ducts and orifices, and formation of sialoliths.

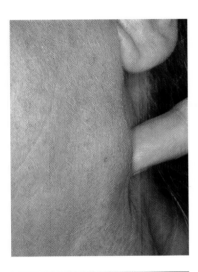
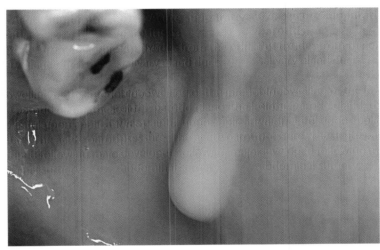

674 Acute suppurative parotitis
Pus exudes from the orifice of the salivary gland duct.

Left: Swelling of the inferior lobe of the parotid gland; the lesion was painful upon application of pressure. The acute parotitis developed following major abdominal surgery.

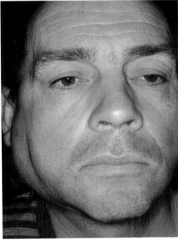
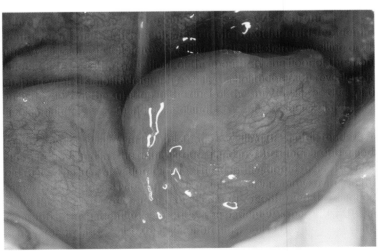

675 Chronic sialadenitis/epidemic parotitis
Note the swelling on the left side of the floor of the mouth. The radiograph revealed sialolith formation in the duct of the submandibular gland.

Left: Painful, tender swelling of the right parotid gland in a 39-year-old male. The identification of paramyxovirus in the saliva confirmed the diagnosis of epidemic parotitis. The patient was also treated for orchitis.

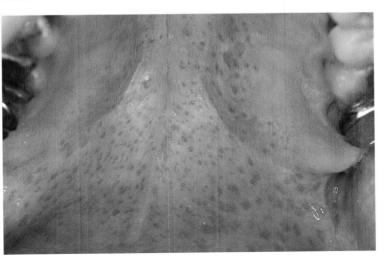

676 Chronic sialadenitis
Both hard and soft palate exhibit multiple red spots corresponding to the orifices of the palatal salivary glands. This patient's habit of consuming extremely hot beverages led to obstruction and to periductal hyperemia of the orifices of the accessory palatal salivary glands.

Mechanical and Physical Causes

Mucocele, Ranula

Mucocele, to which category the ranula also belongs, develops primarily from the minor salivary glands (see also pp. 51 and 263). Two types are distinguished:

- The more common *extravasation cyst* (no epithelial lining), in which saliva escapes into surrounding tissues following trauma to the salivary ducts, and
- The less frequently observed *retention cyst*, which is lined with epithelium from the ductal epithelium.

The mucocele of the floor of the mouth derives primarily from the sublingual glands and is larger and deeper than at other localizations. Clinically, one observes a bluish swelling that is similar to the appearance of a frog's belly (Latin: *rana* = frog), hence the term *ranula* (see p. 121). Mucoceles of the extravasation type from the sublingual gland may ramify diffusely into the neck region. This lesion has been described as a "plunging" ranula and is characterized by a high recurrence rate after surgery.

Mucocele of the floor of the mouth

677 Ranula
Typical bluish mucocele ("ranula") of the sublingual gland on the right side of the floor of the mouth. Treatment consists of broad opening of the lesion with placement of the fewest possible number of sutures; excessively tight suturing often leads to recurrence.

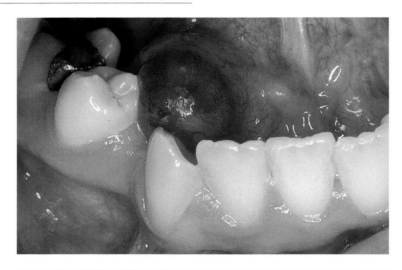

678 Recurrence
This ranula is the third recurrence. This particular type of lesion is difficult to access surgically, and frequently requires resection of the affected portion of the gland.

Right: Localization of mucosal cysts (adapted from Shear 1992).

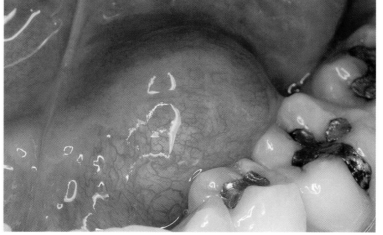

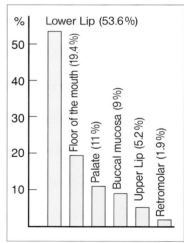

679 Histology
Histologic picture of a resected mucocele. The lining consists of a condensed layer of granulation tissue that has the appearance of an epithelial layer at this very low-power magnification (H & E, x 10).

1 Surface epithelium
2 Lining of the mucocele

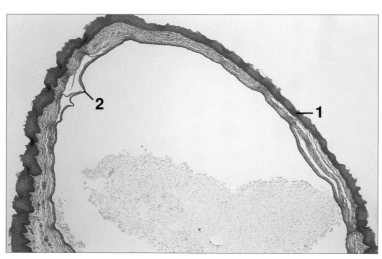

Tumor Classification

At first glance, the salivary glands appear to be relatively uncomplicated organs. However, the tumors that originate from the salivary glands exhibit a broad spectrum of clinical and microscopic appearances. For this reason, classification and diagnosis of these tumors is difficult. Two internationally accepted principles of classification are available for diagnostic purposes, the TNM system and the WHO classification.

- The *TNM system* is only applicable for carcinoma of the major salivary glands. In the TNM system, the T stands for the primary tumor and its local expansion, N for the regional lymph nodes, and the M for distant metastases (see p. 110).
- The *WHO classification* (Seifert 1991, 1997) is based upon tumor histopathology.

The diagnosis and prognosis of the salivary gland tumors was recently reviewed comprehensively (Seifert 1997).

680 Histologic classification of salivary gland tumors
Numerous types of salivary gland tumors have been described in recent years. Many of these tumors are only relatively rarely encountered clinically. This table presents a complete listing of all tumors listed in the WHO classification (1991). Only those lesions marked with a [●] are of major significance from a quantitative standpoint.

Adenomas

Pleomorphic adenoma [●]
Myoepithelioma (myoepithelial adenoma)
Basal cell adenoma
Warthin's tumor (adenolymphoma) [●]
Oncocytoma (oncocytic adenoma)
Canalicular adenoma
Sebaceous gland adenoma

Ductal adenoma
—inverted ductal papilloma
—intraductal papilloma
—sialadenoma papilliferum
Cystadenoma [●]
—papillary cystadenoma
—mucinous cystadenoma

Carcinomas

Acinus cell carcinoma
Mucoepidermoid carcinoma [●]
Adenoid cystic carcinoma [●]
Polymorphous low-grade adenocarcinoma
    (terminal duct adenocarcinoma)
Epithelial-myoepithelial carcinoma
Basal cell adenocarcinoma
Sebaceous carcinoma
Papillary cystadenocarcinoma
Mucinous adenocarcinoma

Oncocytic carcinoma
Salivary duct carcinoma
Adenocarcinoma [●]
Malignant myoepithelioma
    (myoepithelial carcinoma)
Carcinoma in pleomorphic adenoma
    (malignant mixed tumor)
Squamous cell carcinoma
Small cell carcinoma
Undifferentiated carcinoma
Other carcinomas

Non-epithelial tumors
Malignant lymphomas
Secondary tumors
Unclassified tumors

Tumor-like lesions

Sialadenosis
Oncocytosis
Necrotizing sialometaplasia
    (salivary gland infarction)
Benign lymphoepithelial lesion
Salivary gland cysts
Chronic sclerosing sialadenitis of
    submandibular gland (Küttner tumor)
Cystic lymphoid hyperplasia in AIDS

Benign Tumors

Basal Cell Adenoma

The basal cell adenoma is a benign tumor made up of basaloid cells with a prominent basal cell layer and a distinct basement membrane–like structure without mucoid stroma as seen in pleomorphic adenomas. Various cell arrangements have been described: solid, trabecular, tubular and membranous (Dardick et al. 1992).

Benign tumors of the salivary gland should be treated by means of a conservative surgical approach.

Adenolymphoma (Warthin's Tumor)

The adenolymphoma is a classic benign adenoma. This tumor consists of glandular, cystic structures, sometimes with a papillary cystic arrangement, lined with characteristic eosinophilic epithelium. The stroma contains areas of lymphoid tissue with follicles. New aspects of the pathogenesis were recently published (Aguirre et al. 1998).

681   Basal cell adenoma
In the lower half of this histologic preparation, one can observe a basal cell adenoma of the tubular type. There are many ductal structures, which are made up primarily of basaloid cells. The arrow points to normal adjacent glandular structures of the mixed, mainly mucous type (H & E, x 100).

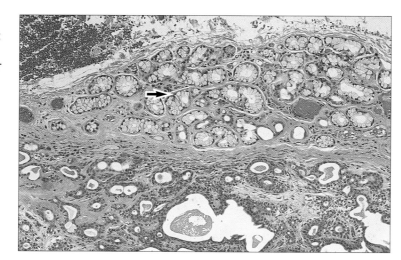

682   Adenolymphoma—histology
Adenolymphoma occurs almost exclusively in the parotid gland. This high magnification reveals a multilayered, columnar epithelium with eosinophilic cytoplasm. A lymphoid stromal tissue occupies the subepithelial area (H & E, x 200).
Right: This section reveals the papillary cystic structure of the epithelial components of the tumor. Lymphoid tissue is enclosed within various islands (arrows) (H & E, x 20).

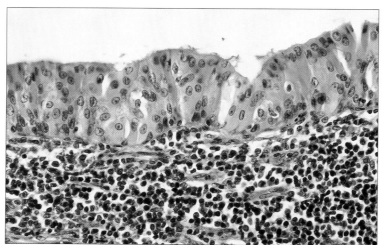
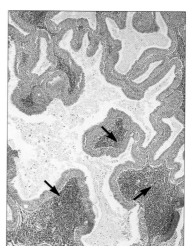

683   Age and gender data for adenolymphoma of the parotid gland
Most tumors occur in the sixth and seventh decades of life. Males are more frequently affected. The treatment for adenolymphoma is conservative surgical removal; recurrence is rare.

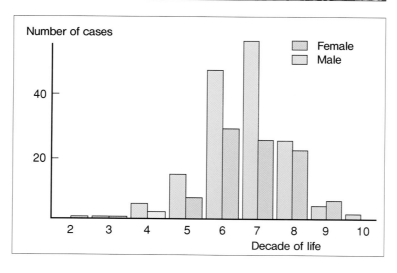

Pleomorphic Adenoma

The pleomorphic adenoma is the most common salivary gland tumor in both the major, extraoral glands as well as the minor, intraoral glands. Seventy percent of all pleomorphic adenomas occur in the parotid gland, 10% in the submandibular gland, and only very few in the sublingual gland. Twenty percent are detected in the small, intraoral accessory salivary glands. A bimodal age distribution has been described (Farina et al. 1997).

The clinical course is characterized by slow growth of a lump, which can achieve dramatic dimensions. Upon palpation, the tumor is well demarcated and may contain a variety of tissue components. The pleomorphic adenoma develops finger-like outgrowths from the main body of the tumor, which often infiltrate the capsule. If tumor tissue remnants are left *in situ* during surgical excision, recurrence can be expected. A careful, long-term follow-up is always indicated.

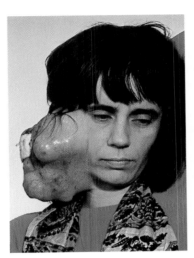 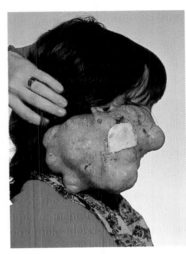

Pleomorphic adenoma

684 Clinical findings
Left: Monstrous, nodular pleomorphic adenoma in a 38-year-old woman. Being reluctant to seek medical advice, over a period of 14 years the patient changed her hairstyle in order to hide the growing tumor. The surgical specimen weighed 3.5 kilograms.
Right: Lateral view of the same patient. Carcinoma frequently develops in pleomorphic adenomas of this size.

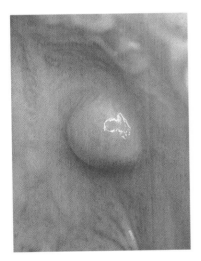 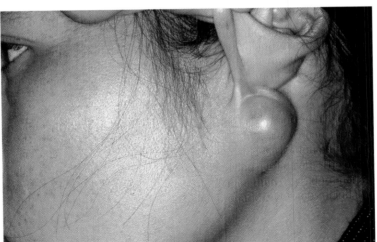

685 Clinical findings
Circumscribed pleomorphic adenoma of the left parotid gland below the elevated earlobe. This tumor developed over a 5-year period.

Left: Intraoral pleomorphic adenoma with its typical intraoral localization on the left side of the hard palate. The overlying mucosa is unremarkable; there are no signs of inflammation.

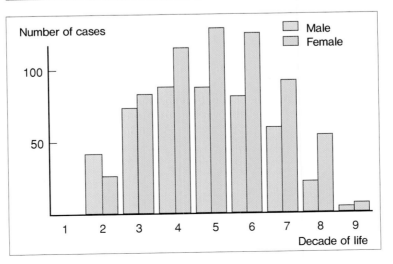

686 Age and gender distribution
The pleomorphic adenoma is more common in females than in males. For both genders, there is a broad range of onset between the fourth and seventh decades of life.

The pleomorphic adenoma is characterized *histologically* by architectural rather than cellular pleomorphism. Epithelial and modified myoepithelial elements intermingle with tissues of mucoid, myxoid or chondroid appearance. The epithelial and myoepithelial components form ducts, strands and islands. Squamous epithelial metaplasia is detected in about one-fourth of all pleomorphic adenomas. The range of histologic appearances within an individual tumor can be extreme.

No clear correlation has been found between the various histologic appearances and any given clinical behavior of the tumor. However, recurrence is more common in the stroma-rich, mucoid variant, and malignant transformation is most often associated with highly cellular tumors.

Pleomorphic adenoma

687 Histology
The histologic picture of this pleomorphic adenoma exhibits epithelial cells that have produced duct-like structures and irregular islands of tumor. The tumor stroma is loose and myxoid (H & E, x 80).

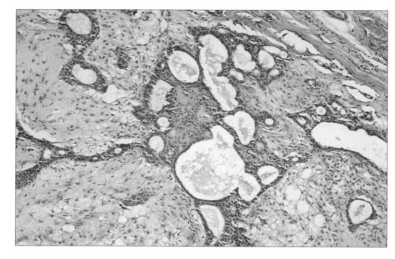

688 Histology
This pleomorphic adenoma from the palate exhibits only few epithelial tumor components. In one area (arrow) there is a proliferation of myoepithelial cells (H & E, x 80).

The connective tissue capsule around the pleomorphic adenoma is not always continuous, and may exhibit frequent tumor infiltrations. These infiltrations are responsible for the recurrences.

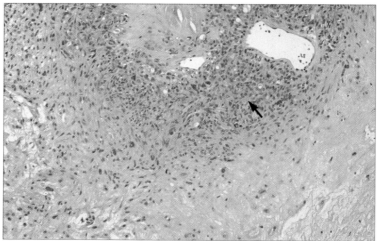

689 Histology
In this pleomorphic adenoma one notes that the epithelial component is pronounced, with the formation of duct-like structures. Some of these exhibit squamous epithelial metaplasia and the production of keratin-like material in the lumen (H & E, x 80).

Right: The tumor stroma is characterized by a myxoid and especially a chondroid appearance (H & E, x 80).

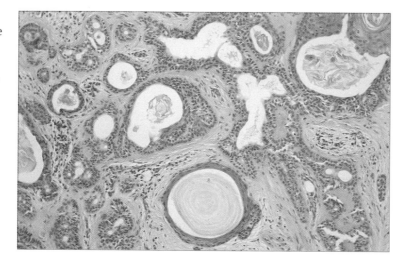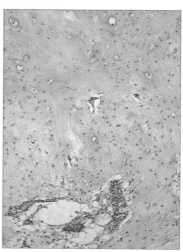

Malignant Tumors

Adenoid Cystic Carcinoma

Malignant tumors of the salivary glands are relatively common, affecting primarily the parotid gland and less often the minor, accessory glands of the oral cavity. Less aggressive tumors may produce signs and symptoms resembling those of the benign adenomas. With increasing malignancy, the growth rate increases as well as the tendency for superficial ulcerations, pain, facial paralysis and the formation of metastases to the regional lymph nodes. The adenoid cystic carcinoma is an infiltrative, malignant tumor that exhibits perineural and perivascular spread.

Mucoepidermoid Carcinoma

All mucoepidermoid carcinomas should be considered as malignant, regardless of their macroscopic or microscopic appearance; they may also metastasize.

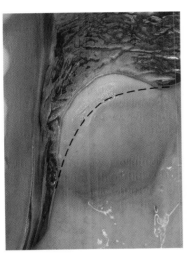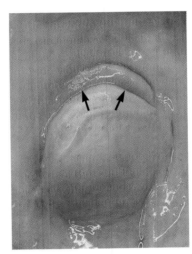

690 Adenoid cystic carcinoma
Left: Adenoid cystic carcinoma at the dorsal border of the maxillary denture. Six months previously, the border of the denture had been trimmed back (dashed line) to accommodate the growth of the tumor.

Right: The notch (arrows) resulted from continuing growth of the tumor and is visible only when the denture is removed.

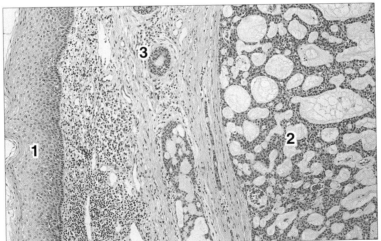

691 Adenoid cystic carcinoma—histology
The histologic picture of adenoid cystic carcinoma exhibits two patterns of growth: a glandular, or cribriform type, and a tubular type. All structural types of adenoid cystic carcinoma can occur simultaneously within the same tumor (H & E, x 80).

1 Palatal epithelium
2 Glandular/cribriform growth pattern
3 Tubular growth pattern

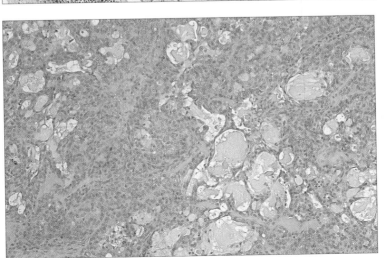

692 Mucoepidermoid carcinoma—histology
Mucoepidermoid carcinomas consist of three cell types. In addition to differentiated squamous cells, one also notes large, pale, slightly granular mucous-producing cells, and cells of intermediate type. The latter are not clearly visible in this micrograph. Microcyst formation is also often observed (H & E, x 100).

Other Lesions

Sialolithiasis ("Salivary Stone")

The term "sialolithiasis" implies the formation of stone (Greek: *lithos* = stone), either within the salivary gland ducts or within the body of the gland itself. The cause of such stone formation is not clear. Over 60% of sialoliths develop in the submandibular gland, usually in the major excretory duct (Wharton's duct). The size of sialoliths varies enormously from microscopically small to extremely large formations of 4–5 cm in diameter.

Decalcified sections of sialoliths demonstrate a structural pattern similar to that of the stones in other excretory systems (kidneys, bladder, gall bladder). A central nidus of organic debris is surrounded by laminated formations of calcified material.

The degree of obstruction determines the severity of inflammation in the gland. Small sialoliths in the duct of the submandibular gland can be removed by incising the duct. Placement of a drainage tube ensures the flow of saliva.

Sialoliths

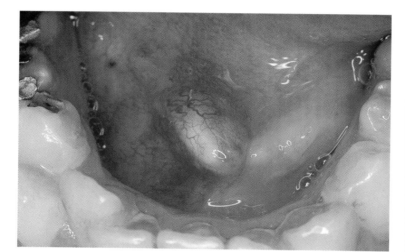

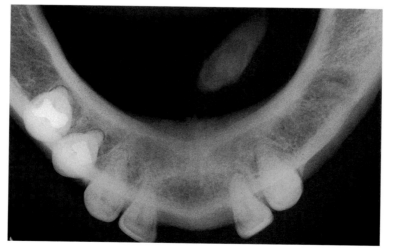

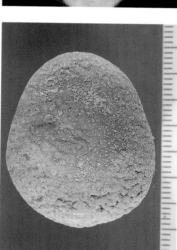

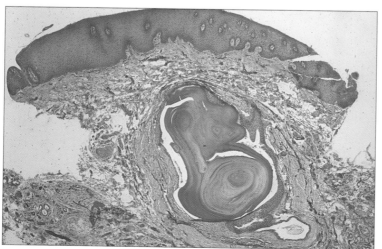

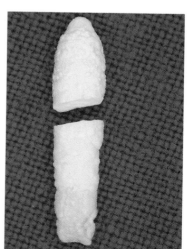

693 Clinical finding
Sialolith that developed in the right Wharton's duct. The stone can be seen through the thin mucosa of the floor of the mouth. The periductal tissue is erythematous, a sign of inflammation.

Right: A skull radiograph reveals a large, round sialolith on the left side, approaching 3 cm in diameter (see also Fig. 694, right).

694 Radiographic finding
The mandibular occlusal radiograph reveals a sialolith in the duct of the left submandibular gland.

Right: Large sialolith with a relatively smooth surface as depicted radiographically in Fig. 693, right. Stones of this size often necessitate surgical removal of the gland.

695 Histology
The histologic picture reveals sialolith formation in a labial salivary gland. Stone formation in minor salivary glands is a rare phenomenon. Note the laminated structure of the stone (H & E, x 30).

Right: Ductal sialolith (fractured during removal) from the submandibular gland (Fig. 694). This sialolith assumed an elongated form corresponding to the shape of the salivary duct.

Sjögren's Syndrome

For many years, patients exhibiting symptoms of xerostomia, keratoconjunctivitis sicca, enlarged salivary glands and rheumatoid arthritis were diagnosed as having Sjögren's syndrome. On the basis of recent research, the syndrome can be subdivided into two groups: while *primary* Sjögren's syndrome consists of symptoms in the salivary glands and the eyes without any additional connective tissue disorders, *secondary* Sjögren's syndrome is characterized by involvement of the salivary glands and/or the eyes as well as rheumatoid arthritis or other connective tissue diseases (Stiller 1997).

This syndrome occurs most frequently in post-menopausal women. Females are much more frequently affected than males, at a ratio of 9:1. In addition to dryness of the mouth, patients complain of difficulties in swallowing and also taste disturbances.

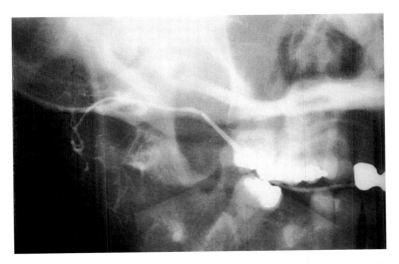

696 Sialography—normal appearance
Sialography remains the classical method for diagnosing salivary gland diseases. This picture reveals the normal duct system of the parotid gland.

Courtesy W. Golder and K. Kleim

- Dry mouth
- Burning sensation of the mucosa
- Pale or slightly reddened mucosa
- Atrophy of the lingual papillae
- Smooth surface and root caries
- Angular cheilitis

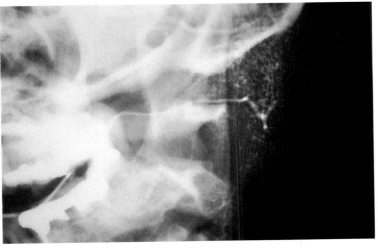

697 Sjögren's syndrome— sialography
Sialography of the parotid gland in a patient with Sjögren's syndrome reveals the appearance of "cherry tree blossoms."

Courtesy W. Golder and K. Kleim

Left: Clinical symptoms primary Sjögren's syndrome.

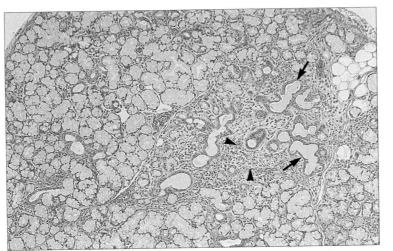

698 Sjögren's syndrome— histology
The histologic picture reveals the typical changes: widening of the ducts (arrows), lymphocytic infiltration (arrowheads), atrophy of the acini, and destruction of the lobuli. Epimyoepithelial islands are only seldom observed in the minor salivary glands (H & E, x 80).

Xerostomia

Dry mouth may be a symptom of a wide variety of disorders that have effects on the salivary glands. The term "xerostomia" encompasses a broad spectrum of patient complaints, ranging from slight reduction of saliva flow to absolute dryness of the oral cavity. Some causes of xerostomia include aplasia of the salivary glands, inflammatory conditions, radiotherapy, various types of anemia, Sjögren's syndrome, Mikulicz's syndrome or Heerfordt's syndrome, hormonal disturbances, vitamin deficiencies, inadequate nutrition and various medications.

Cystic Lymphoid Hyperplasia in AIDS

Salivary gland swelling is occasionally observed in HIV patients, particularly in children, but is also observed in adults. These salivary enlargements may mimic the clinical appearance of Sjögren's syndrome (Schmidt-Westhausen et al. 1997) with the salivary glands being enlarged bilaterally, appearing as diffuse, soft swellings. Patients may suffer from dry mouth, dry eyes, and arthralgia.

699 Xerostomia
Long-term therapy with antidepressant medication can lead to pronounced dryness of the oral cavity. This may lead to atrophy of the lingual filiform papillae and a more pronounced clinical appearance of the fungiform papillae.

Right: Medicaments that may influence saliva secretion.

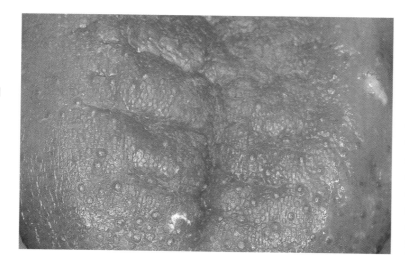

- Analgesics
- Appetite suppressants
- Antiacne preparations
- Antiarthritics
- Anticholinergics and spasmolytics
- Antidiarrhetics
- Antiemetics
- Antihistamines
- Antihypertensives
- Anti-Parkinson medication
- Diuretics
- Psychopharmacological drugs
- Antipsychotic drugs

700 Cystic lymphoid hyperplasia in AIDS
Magnetic resonance tomography of an HIV-positive patient exhibits a clear increase in size of the parotid gland on the left side, with diverse cystic cavities (from Schmidt-Westhausen et al. 1997).

Right: The left cheek is obviously swollen from the preauricular region to the angle of the mandible. No erythema of the skin is apparent. The patient complained of severe pain.

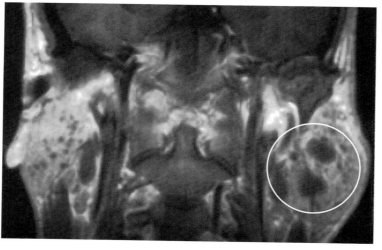

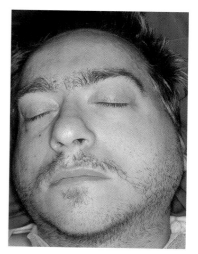

701 Cystic lymphoid hyperplasia of AIDS—histology
The histologic picture of HIV-associated salivary gland swelling is characterized mainly by a follicular, lymphatic hyperplasia in which islands of nonkeratinized squamous epithelium may appear (arrows). (H & E, x 60)

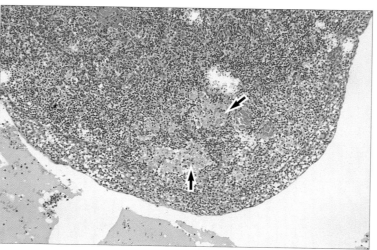

Necrotizing Sialometaplasia

Necrotizing sialometaplasia is the result of an ischemic insult, most commonly on the palate (see p. 136). The term "salivary gland infarct" derives from the similarity of the changes to that of other organs, such as the prostate gland. Males are significantly more frequently affected than females (male:female = 18:1). Most patients are heavy smokers and it has, therefore, been suspected that necrotizing sialometaplasia is actually a late stage of "smoker's palate." Histopathologically, it is important to differentiate necrotizing sialometaplasia from squamous cell carcinoma (Seifert 1998).

Mucocele

A mucocele (see pp. 51, 254) is a condition in which the secretion from a salivary gland extends into the periglandular tissue (extravasation type) or is retained in an excretory duct, resulting in enlargement (retention type). Mucoceles represent 6% of all salivary gland diseases.

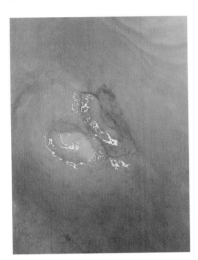
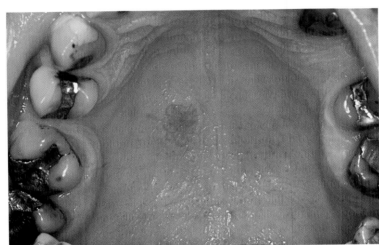
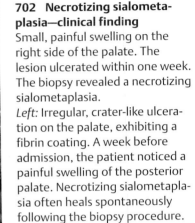

702 Necrotizing sialometaplasia—clinical finding
Small, painful swelling on the right side of the palate. The lesion ulcerated within one week. The biopsy revealed a necrotizing sialometaplasia.
Left: Irregular, crater-like ulceration on the palate, exhibiting a fibrin coating. A week before admission, the patient noticed a painful swelling of the posterior palate. Necrotizing sialometaplasia often heals spontaneously following the biopsy procedure. Surgical therapy is not necessary.

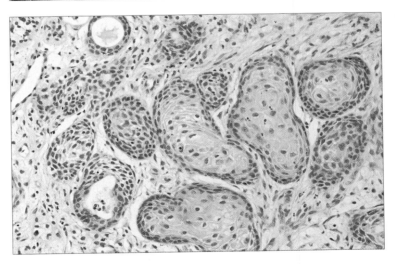

703 Necrotizing sialometaplasia—histology
The histologic picture of necrotizing sialometaplasia consists of metaplasia of the ductal epithelium into squamous epithelium as well as a diffuse inflammatory reaction. The inexperienced observer may confuse the histologic picture with that of a squamous cell carcinoma (H & E, x 160).

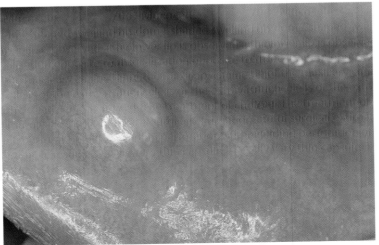

704 Mucocele
This dome-shaped swelling on the lower lip is observed at a typical localization opposite to the tip of the maxillary canine. This mucocele is of the extravasation type. The treatment of choice is careful surgical extirpation, avoiding perforation of the usually very thin capsule.

Diagnostic Key

This condensed *diagnostic key* has been included to aid readers, particularly practitioners with a patient in the chair who are seeking guidance in establishing a diagnosis. Since this *Color Atlas of Oral Pathology* deals primarily with mucosal pathology and diseases of the alveolar bone, this diagnostic key was created using straightforward basic principles. In the case of mucosal pathology, they relate to changes in tissue color and volume, and in the case of alveolar bone disorders they relate mainly to relationships to the radiographic characteristics. Within this "diagnostic pool" one can easily find the most important pathologic processes that have been described in this *Atlas*. References to the individual chapters, by means of abbreviations, should make rapid entry into the diagnostic sequence possible.

The following abbreviations have been used for the individual chapters:

Abbr.	Chapter	Pages
EC	Epithelial Cysts of the Jaw	205–219
PA	Palate	127–145
GI	Gingiva	147–175
JB	Jaw bone	189–203
LI	Lip	43– 61
FM	Floor of the Mouth	115–125
OT	Odontogenic Tumors	221–249
SG	Salivary Glands	251–263
BS	Buccal Mucosa/Sulcus	63– 87
EJ	Edentulous Jaw	177–187
TO	Tongue	89–113

White Lesions of the Oral Mucosa

Keratinizing Lesions

Condyloma acuminatum	GI
Focal epithelial hyperplasia	LI, BS, TO
Friction keratosis	EJ, GI
Leukoplakia	GI, EJ, LI, FM, BS
Lichen planus	GI, BS, TO
Discoid lupus erythematosus	BS
Oral hairy leukoplakia	TO
Papilloma	PA
Psoriasis	PA
Smoker's palate	PA
Snuff dipper's lesion	LI
Verruca vulgaris	PA, GI, TO
Verrucous hyperplasia	FM
Verrucous leukoplakia	BS
Verrucous carcinoma	PA, LI, FM
White sponge nevus	BS

Nonkeratinizing Lesions

Peripheral scar formation	TO
Scleroderma	FM
Submucous fibrosis	BS
Xanthogranuloma	GI

White/Gray Lesions of the Oral Mucosa

Pseudomembranous or Necrotic Lesions

Pseudomembranous candidiasis	TO, BS
Chemical burns	GI
Necrotizing ulcerative gingivitis	GI
Plaque accumulation	GI
Syphilis	GI
Traumatic ulceration	TO
Tuberculosis	GI, TO
Lip and cheek biting	LI, BS

Oral Ulcerations

Aphthous ulceration	LI, BS
Herpes zoster	PA
Intraoral salivary gland tumors	LI, PA, BS
Leukemia	PA, GI
Crohn's disease	FM, BS
Necrotizing sialometaplasia	PA, SG
Squamous cell carcinoma	FM, EJ, LI, TO
Syphilis (stage II and IV)	TO, GI
Traumatic ulcerations	TO
Tuberculosis	GI, TO

Oral Mucosal Fissures

Angular cheilitis	LI
Scrotal tongue	TO
Denture irritation hyperplasia	EJ

Oral Exophytic Lesions

Exophytic Anatomic Structures

Sublingual caruncule	SG
Exostoses	GI, JB
Lingual folia	TO
Palatal papilla	PA
Inferior salivary papilla	FM
Superior salivary papilla	BS
Circumvalate papillae	TO
Palatal rugae	PA

Mandibular torus	JB
Palatal torus	PA
Uvula	PA

Exophytic Lesions

Adenomatoid odontogenic tumor (peripheral type)	GI, OT
Dermoid cyst	FM
Double lip	LI
Fibrous epulis	GI
Eruption cyst	EC
Fibroma	PA, BS, TO
Gingival fibromatosis	GI
Focal epithelial hyperplasia	LI, BS
Granular cell myoblastoma	TO
Hemangioma	LI, TO
Hydantoin hyperplasia	GI
Intraoral salivary gland tumors	LI, PA, CS
Kaposi's sarcoma	PA, GI, TO
Leiomyoma	PA
Leukemic infiltrate	PA, GI
Lymphangioma	LI, TO
Medicament-induced gingival overgrowth	GI
Crohn's disease	BS
Mucocele	LI, SG
Neurilemmoma	TO
Neurofibromatosis	TO
Papilloma	PA
Peripheral ameloblastoma	OT
Squamous cell carcinoma	FM, EJ, LI, TO
Denture irritation hyperplasia	TO
Pyogenic granuloma	GI
Ranula	FM
Giant cell granuloma, peripheral	GI
Submucous abscess	PA
Verruca vulgaris	PA, GI, TO
Verrucous carcinoma	PA, FM, LI

Oral Pits and Fissures

Congenital lip pits	LI
Labial fissures	LI
Lip pits of the commissure	LI

Intraoral Brownish, Bluish or Black Lesions

Circumscribed, Demarcated

Amalgam tattoo	GI
Vascular ectasia	TO, FM, BS
Hemangioma	LI, TO
Kaposi's sarcoma	PA, GI, TO
Melanin pigmentation, physiologic	BS, GI, TO
Melanoma	PA
Melanoplakia	TO
Mucocele	LI

Nevus	PA
Oral melanotic spots	LI
Petechia and ecchymosis	PA, GI
Peutz–Jeghers syndrome	LI, BS
Giant cell granuloma, peripheral	GI
Black hairy tongue	TO

Generalized

Cyanosis (tetralogy of Fallot)	TO

Red Lesions

Solitary Red Lesions of the Oral Mucosa

Candidiasis, erythematous	PA, TO, BS
Erythroplakia	FM, BS
Vascular ectasia	TO, FM, BS
Hemangioma	PA, BS, TO, LI
Lichenoid reaction	BS
Denture stomatitis	PA
Submucous petechiae (fellatio)	PA
Ulcerations with red halo	LI, FM

Red Lesions of the Tongue

Anemic conditions	TO
Median rhomboid glossitis	TO
Geographic tongue	TO

Generalized Red Lesions of the Oral Mucosa

Benign mucous membrane pemphigoid	PA, GI
Betel chewer's mucosa	BS, TO
Candidiasis, erythematous	TO, PA, BS
Epidermolysis bullosa	LI
Erythema multiforme	LI
Herpetic gingivostomatitis	BS, GI, TO
Kaposi's sarcoma, multiple	PA, GI, TO
Lichen planus, erosive type	PA, GI, BS, TO
Discoid lupus erythematosus	BS
Crohn's disease	FM, BS
Reiter's disease	BS
Mucositis	BS
Pemphigus vulgaris	PA, GI, LI
Psoriasis	PA

Yellow Lesions of the Oral Mucosa

Epidermoid and dermoid cysts	FM	Lipoma	FM
Yellow hairy tongue	TO	Lympho-epithelial cyst	TO
Heterotopic sebaceous		Ulcerations (fibrin-coated)	TO, BS
glands (Fordyce's granules)	BS	Xanthogranuloma	GI

Radiographic Diagnostic Key

Periapical Radiolucencies of the jaws

Benign cementoblastoma (early stage)	OT
Osteomyelitis	JB
Periapical cemental dysplasia	OT
Periapical granuloma	JB
Radicular cyst	EC, JB
Cemento-ossifying fibroma	OT

Radiolucencies of the Jawbones

Adenomatoid odontogenic tumor	OT
Eosinophilic granuloma	JB
Fibrous dysplasia	JB
Follicular cyst	EC
Calcifying odontogenic cyst	OT
Calcifying epithelial odontogenic tumor	OT
Odontogenic keratocyst	JB, EC
Solid intraosseaous ameloblastoma	OT
Squamous odontogenic tumor	OT
Unicystic ameloblastoma	OT
Cemento-ossifying fibroma	JB, OT
Odontogenic myxoma	OT
Odontoma (early stage)	OT

Solitary Radiolucencies With Poorly Demarcated Borders

Chronic ostitis and osteomyelitis	JB
Bone metastasis	JB
Malignant odontogenic and non-odontogenic tumors	OT, JB
Squamous cell carcinoma, infiltrating	JB

Generalized Rarefactions of the Jaws

Hereditary hemolytic anemia	JB
Langerhans cell granulomatosis	JB
Osteoporosis	EJ

Generalized Radiopacities

Ameloblastic fibro-odontoma	OT
Florid cemento-osseous dysplasia	OT
Gardner's syndrome	JB
Calcifying epithelial odontogenic tumor	OT
Paget's disease of bone	JB
Osteogenesis imperfecta	JB

Solitary Unilocular Radiolucencies
(not associated with teeth in all cases)

Adenomatoid odontogenic tumor	OT
Aneurysmal bone cyst	JB
Langerhans cell granulomatosis	JB
Lateral periodontal cyst	EC
Metastatic carcinoma	JB
Non-odontogenic cyst	EC
Odontogenic keratocyst	JB, EC
Odontogenic fibroma	OT
Odontogenic myxoma	OT
Odontoma (early stage)	OT
Osteoblastoma	OT
Residual (radicular) cyst	EC
Giant cell granuloma, central	JB
Solid intraosseous ameloblastoma	OT
Squamous odontogenic tumor	OT
Stafne cavity	JB, OT
Traumatic cyst of bone	JB, OT
Unicystic ameloblastoma	OT
Cemento-ossifying fibroma (early stage)	OT
Central hemangioma	JB

Multilocular Radiolucencies

Aneurysmal bone cyst	JB
Cherubism	JB
Lymphoma	EJ
Metastatic tumors	JB
Odontogenic myxoma	OT
Giant cell granuloma, central	JB
Solid intraosseous ameloblastoma	OT
Unicystic ameloblastoma	OT
Central hemangioma	JB

Credits for Figures and Illustrations

Some of the illustrations in this *Atlas* were kindly provided by the colleagues listed below. Additional illustrations, primarily figures depicting rare lesions, are derived from previous publications of the authors. The illustrations and corresponding references are listed below. Partial figures are characterized by L (Left), M (Middle), and R (Right).

University Institutes

Free University of Berlin

Prof. W. Golder, Dr. K. Kliem, Radiology Clinic
Figs. 696, 697

Prof. U. Gross, Benjamin Franklin University Clinic, Institut for Pathology
Figs. 526 R, 530, 530 L, 534

Prof. Dr. B. Hoffmeister, Benjamin Franklin University Clinic, Department of Oral and Maxillofacial Surgery
Figs. 175 R, 176 L, 176 R, 417, 418, 419, 419 L, 508, 509, 509 R, 510, 511, 520, 520 R, 522, 529, 529 L, 532, 532 R, 533, 590 R, 658, 658 R, 659, 659 R, 660, 660 R

Humboldt University, Berlin

Dr. G. Bethke, Center for Dental Medicine, Department of Oral Surgery and Dental Radiolgy
Figs. 145

Dr. H.-J. Tietz, University Clinic for Dermatology
Figs. 68, 68 R, 69, 69 R, 70, 70 R

Medical University of Hannover

Dr. Dr. A. Eckardt, Clinic for Oral and Maxillofacial Surgery
Figs. 537, 537 L

Robert-Koch-Institute, Berlin

Prof. H.-R. Gelderblom
Figs. 341, 342

Free University of Amsterdam

Prof. I. van der Waal, Pathology Institute
Figs. 380, 381, 455

University of Kagoshima, Japan

Prof. K. Sugihara, Dental School, First Department of Oral and Maxillofacial Surgery
Figs. 505, 506, 507, 507 L

University of Kopenhagen

Prof. Dr. J. J. Pindborg †, Department of Oral Pathology and Medicine, School of Dentistry
Figs. 607 L

University of Oslo

Prof. T. Axéll, Department of Oral Surgery and Medicine
Figs. 118, 119, 119 R

University of Stellenbosch, Republic of South Africa

Prof. I. Thompson, Department of Oral Pathology
Figs. 514, 652

University of Witwatersrand, Republic of South Africa

Prof. M. Shear, Department of Oral Pathology
Figs. 654

Private Practitioners

Dr. K. Kalz, Berlin
Figs. 93 (L, M, R)

References

Note: Multiple entries from a single author are organized chronologically, independent of the co-authors. Family names preceded by "von" or "van" have not been acknowledged in this alphabetization.

Textbooks, Standard References and Monographs

Andersson, G.: Snuff-induced changes associated with the use of loose and portion-bag-packed Swedish moist snuff. A clinical, histological and follow-up study. Swed Dent J Suppl 75, 1991.

Bengel, W., Veltman, G.: Differentialdiagnostik der Mundschleimhauterkrankungen. Quintessenz, Berlin 1986.

Bodey, G. P.: Candidiasis. Pathogenesis, Diagnosis and Treatment. 2nd ed. Raven, New York 1993.

Burkhardt, A.: Der Mundhöhlenkrebs und seine Vorstadien. G. Fischer, Stuttgart 1980.

Cawson, R. A., Eveson, J. W.: Oral Pathology and Diagnosis. Heinemann Medical Books, London 1987.

Cawson, R. A, Binnie, W. H., Eveson, J. W.: Color Atlas of Oral Diseases. Clinical and Pathologic Correlations. Mosby-Wolfe 1994.

Cawson, R. A., Langdon, J. D., Eveson, J. W.: Surgical Pathology of the Mouth and Jaws. Butterworth-Heinemann, Oxford 1996.

Ceccotti, E. L.: Manifestaciones Orales del SIDA. Atlas Color. Editorial Médica Panamericana, Buenos Aires 1995.

Dolby, A. E.: Oral Mucosa in Health and Disease. Blackwell Scientific, Oxford 1975.

Frank, P., Rahn, R.: Zahnärztliche Anamnese und Befunderhebung. Hanser, München 1993.

Goodman, R. M., Gorlin, R. J.: Atlas of the Face in Genetic Disorders. 2nd ed. Mosby, St. Louis 1977.

Gorlin, R. J., Pindborg, J. J., Cohen, M. M.: Syndromes of the Head and Neck. McGraw-Hill, New York 1976.

Greenspan, D., Greenspan, J. S., Pindborg, J. J., Schiødt, M.: AIDS – Orale Manifestationen und Infektionsschutz. Deutscher Ärzte-Verlag, Köln 1992.

Gupta, P. C., Hamner, J. E., Murti, P. R.: Control of Tobacco-Related Cancers and Other Disease. Proceedings of an International Symposium. January 15–19, 1990, TIFR, Bombay. Oxford University Press, Bombay 1992.

Häring, R, Zilch, H.: Chirurgie. 4. Aufl. de Gruyter, Berlin 1997.

Härle, F.: Atlas der Hauttumoren im Gesicht. Hanser, München 1993.

Hausamen, J.-E., Machtens, E., Reuther, J.: Mund-, Kiefer- und Gesichtschirurgie. 3. Aufl. Springer, Berlin 1995.

Heikinheimo, K.: Cell Growth and Differentiation of Developing and Neoplastic Odontogenic Tissues. Dissertation, University of Turku, Finnland 1993.

Hornstein, O. P.: Erkrankungen des Mundes. Ein interdisziplinäres Handbuch und Atlas. Kohlhammer, Stuttgart 1996.

Husstedt, I. W.: HIV und AIDS – Fachspezifische Diagnostik und Therapie. Springer, Berlin 1998.

Jones, J. H., Mason, D.: Oral Manifestations of Systemic Disease. 2nd ed. Ballière Tindall, London 1990.

Krüger, E.: Lehrbuch der chirurgischen Zahn-, Mund- und Kieferheilkunde. Bd. 1+2. Quintessenz, Berlin 1993.

Laskaris, G.: Color Atlas of Oral Diseases. Thieme, Stuttgart 1988.

Lehnhardt, E.: HNO-Heilkunde für Zahnmediziner. 2. Aufl. Thieme, Stuttgart 1992.

Löning, T.: Immunpathologie der Mundschleimhaut. G. Fischer, Stuttgart 1984.

Lucas, R. B.: Pathology of Tumours of the Oral Tissues. 3rd ed. Churchill Livingstone, Edinburgh 1976.

de Lucas Tomás, M.: Atlas de Medicina Oral y Maxillo-Facial. Editorial cientifico-médica, Barcelona 1991.

Mackenzie, I. C, Dabelsteen, E., Squier, C. A.: Oral Premalignancy. Proceedings of the First Dows Symposium. University of Iowa Press, Iowa City 1980.

Mehta, F. S., Pindborg, J. J., Hamner, J. E., Gupta, P. C., Daftary, D. K., Sahiar, B. E., Shroff, B. C.: Report on Investigations of Oral Cancer and Precancerous Conditions in Indian Rural Populations, 1966–69. Munksgaard, Copenhagen 1971.

Mehta, F. S., Hamner, J. E.: Tobacco-related Oral Mucosal Lesions and Conditions in India. A Guide for Dental Students, Dentists, and Physicians. Tata Institute of Fundamental Research 1993.

Millard, H. D., Mason, D.: 2nd World Workshop on Oral Medicine. August 21–26, 1993, Chicago, Illinois. University of Michigan, Continuing Dental Education 1995.

Mittermayer, C.: Oralpathologie – Erkrankungen der Mundregion. Lehrbuch für Zahnmedizin, Mund- und Kieferheilkunde. Schattauer, Stuttgart 1993.

Morgenroth, K., Bremerich, A., Lange, D. E.: Pathologie der Mundhöhle. 3. Aufl. Thieme, Stuttgart 1996.

Morgenroth, K., Rühl, G.: Taschenatlas Pathohistologie der Mundhöhle. Thieme, Stuttgart 1990.

Neville, B. W., Damm, D. D., White, D. K., Waldron, C. A.: Color Atlas of Clinical Oral Pathology. Lea & Febiger, Philadelphia, London 1991.

Odds, F. C.: Candida and Candidosis. 2nd ed. Ballière Tindall, London 1988.

Pasler, F. A.: Radiologie. (Rateitschak, K. H., Wolf, H. F.: Farbatlanten der Zahnmedizin, Bd. 5.) Thieme, Stuttgart 1991.

Pindborg, J. J., Hjørting-Hansen, E.: Atlas of Diseases of the Jaws. Munksgaard, Copenhagen 1974.

Pindborg, J. J.: Atlas of Diseases of the Oral Mucosa. 5th ed. Munksgaard, Copenhagen 1992.

Pindborg, J. J., Reichart, P. A.: Atlas of Diseases of the Oral Cavity in HIV Infection. Munksgaard, Copenhagen 1995.

Pindborg, J. J., Reichart, P. A., Smith, C. J., van der Waal, I., in collaboration with L. H. Sobin and pathologists in 9 countries (WHO): Histological Typing of Cancer and Precancer of the Oral Mucosa. 2nd ed. Springer, Berlin 1997.

Porter, S. R., Scully, C.: Oral Health Care for Those with HIV Infection and Other Special Needs. Science Reviews, Northwood 1995.

Prabhu, S. R., Wilson, D. F, Daftary, D. K., Johnson, N. W.: Oral Diseases in the Tropics. Oxford University Press, 1992.

Prein, J., Remagen, W., Spiessl, B., Uehlinger, E.: Atlas der Tumoren des Gesichtsschädels. Odontogene und nicht odontogene Tumoren. Springer, Berlin 1985.

Rateitschak, K. H. & E. M., Wolf, H.: Parodontologie. 2. Aufl. (Rateitschak, K. H., Wolf, H.: Farbatlanten der Zahnmedizin, Bd. 1.) Thieme, Stuttgart 1989 (3. Aufl. in Vorbereitung).

Regezi, J. A., Sciubba, J. J.: Oral Pathology – Clinico-pathologic Correlations. Saunders 1989.

Reichart, P. A., Schulz, P., Walz, C., Beyer, D., Pape, H.-D., Hausamen, J.-E., Remagen, W., Howaldt, H.-P.: Früherkennung von Neubildungen im Kiefer-Gesichtsbereich durch den praktizierenden Zahnarzt. Deutsche Krebshilfe, Bonn 1991.

Reichart, P. A., Gelderblom, H.: AIDS-Kompendium für Zahnärzte. Hoechst Marion Roussell Deutschland 1999.

Robertson, P. B., Greenspan, J. S.: Perspectives on Oral Manifestations of AIDS. Diagnosis and Management of HIV-Associated Infections. Procter & Gamble, PSG Publishing Company, Littleton 1988.

Sailer, H. F., Pajarola, G. F.: Orale Chirurgie. (Rateitschak, K. H., Wolf, H.: Farbatlanten der Zahnmedizin, Bd. 11.) Thieme, Stuttgart 1996.

Samaranayake, L. P., MacFarlane, T. W.: Oral Candidosis. Butterworth, London 1990.

Schulten, E. A. J. M.: Oral Lesions in Human Immunodeficiency Virus (HIV) Infection. A Clinico-Pathologic Study. Academisch Proefschrift. Drukkerij Raket b. v., Pijnacker 1990.

Scully, C., Cawson, R. A.: Taschenatlas Oralpathologie. Hüthig, Heidelberg 1996.

Scully, C.: Oral pathology and medicine in periodontics. Periodontology 2000. Munksgaard, Copenhagen 1998.

Scully, C., Flint, S., Porter, S. R.: Erkrankungen der Mundhöhle. Diagnose und Therapie. 2. Aufl. Urban & Schwarzenberg 1998.

Seifert, G., Miehlke, A., Handrich, J., Chilla, R.: Diseases of the Salivary Glands. Thieme, Stuttgart 1986.

Seifert, G., in collaboration with L. H. Sobin (WHO): Histologic Typing of Salivary Gland Tumours. 2nd ed. Berlin, Springer 1991.

Seifert, G.: Oral Pathology. Actual Diagnostic and Prognostic Aspects. Springer, Berlin 1996.

Shear, M.: Cysts of the Oral Regions. 3rd ed. Wright, Oxford 1992.

Smith, C., Pindborg, J. J., Binnie, W. H.: Oral Cancer – Epidemiology, Etiology and Pathology. Hemisphere, New York 1990.

Spijkervet, F. K. L.: Irradiation mucositis. Prevention and treatment. Munksgaard, Copenhagen 1991.

Straßburg, M., Knolle, G.: Farbatlas und Lehrbuch der Mundschleimhauterkrankungen. 3. Aufl. Quintessenz, Berlin 1991.

Veltman, G.: Dermatologie für Zahnmediziner mit besonderer Berücksichtigung der Mundkrankheiten. Thieme, Stuttgart 1976.

van der Waal, I., Pindborg, J. J.: Diseases of the Tongue. Quintessenz, Chicago 1986.

van der Waal, I., van der Kwast, W. A. M.: Oralpathologie für Zahnärzte. Klinische, röntgenologische, histopathologische und therapeutische Aspekte häufiger Erkrankungen der Mundhöhle. Quintessenz, Berlin 1987.

van der Waal, I.: The Burning Mouth Syndrome. Munksgaard, Copenhagen 1990.

van der Waal, I.: Diseases of the Jaws. Diagnosis and Treatment. Textbook and Atlas. Munksgaard, Copenhagen 1991.

van der Waal, I.: Mondafwijkingen. Een atlas voor de dagelijkse praktijk. Bohn Stafleu Van Loghum, Houten/Diegem 1996.

Weismann, K., Sand Petersen, C., Søndergaard, J., Wantzin, G. L.: Skin Signs in AIDS. Textbook of AIDS/HIV. Infection-Related Dermatology. Munksgaard, Copenhagen 1988.

Wood, N. K., Goaz, P. W.: Differential Diagnosis of Oral and Maxillofacial Lesions. 5th ed. Mosby, St. Louis 1997.

World Health Organization. International Agency for Research on Cancer: IARC Monographs on the Evaluation of the Carcinogenic Risk of Chemicals to Humans. Tobacco Habit Other than Smoking, Betel-Quid and Areca-Nut Chewing; and Some Related Nitrosamines. Vol. 37. Int. Agency for Research on Cancer, Lyon 1985.

Periodicals—Continuing Education

Oral Diseases (Stockton Press, Hampshire, England)

Journal of Oral Pathology & Medicine (Munksgaard, Copenhagen)

Oral Surgery Oral Medicine Oral Pathology Oral Radiology and Endodontics (Mosby, USA)

Oral Oncology, European Journal of Cancer (Pergamon, Oxford, England)

International Journal of Oral & Maxillofacial Surgery (Munksgaard, Copenhagen)

Journal of Acquired Immunodeficiency Syndrome (Whitston)

Mund-, Kiefer-, Gesichtschirurgie (Springer)

AIDS (Current Science)

Cancer (Butterworth)

Community Dentistry and Oral Epidemiology (Munksgaard, Copenhagen)

Dento-Maxillo-Facial Radiology (Stockton, Hampshire, England)

Journal of Oral and Maxillofacial Surgery (Saunders)

Cited Literature

A

Abbey, L. M., Kaugars, G. E., Gunsolley, J. C., Burns, J. C., Page, D. G., Svirsky, J. A., Eisenberg, E., Krutchkoff, D. J.: The effect of clinical information on the histopathologic diagnosis of oral epithelial dysplasia. Oral Surg Oral Med Oral Pathol Oral Radiol Endod 85: 74–7, 1998.

Ackermann, G., Cohen, M. A., Altini, M.: The paradental cyst: A clinicopathologic study of 50 cases. Oral Surg Oral Med Oral Pathol 64: 308–12, 1987.

Aguirre, J. M., Echebarría, M. A., Martínez-Conde, R., Rodriguez, C., Burgos, J. J., Rivera, J. M.: Warthin tumor – A new hypothesis concerning its development. Oral Surg Oral Med Oral Pathol Oral Radiol Endod 85: 60–3, 1998.

Akal, Ü. K., Günhan, Ö., Güler, M.: Ameloblastic fibrodentinoma. Report of two cases. Int J Oral Maxillofac Surg 26: 455–7, 1997.

Altini, M., Shear, M.: The lateral periodontal cyst: an update. J Oral Pathol Med 21: 245–50, 1992.

Amagasa, T., Yokoo, E., Sato, K., Tanaka, N., Shioda, S., Takagi, M.: A study of the clinical characteristics and treatment of oral carcinoma in situ. Oral Surg Oral Med Oral Pathol 60: 50–5, 1985.

Andersson, G.: Snuff-induced changes associated with the use of loose and portion-bag-packed swedish moist snuff. A clinical, histological and follow-up study. Swed Dent J 75, 1991.

Antoniades, K., Eleftheriades, I., Karakis, D.: The Gardner Syndrome. Int J Maxillofac Surg 16: 480–3, 1987.

August, M., Magennis, P., Dewitt, D.: Osteogenic sarcoma of the jaws: factors influencing prognosis. Int J Oral Maxillofac Surg 26: 198–204, 1997.

Axéll, T.: A prevalence study of oral mucosal lesions in an adult Swedish population. Odontologisk Revy 27 (Suppl 36), 1976.

Axéll, T.: Occurence of leukoplakia and some other oral white lesions among 20333 adult Swedish people. Community Dent Oral Epidemiol 15: 46–51, 1987.

Axéll, T., Azul, A. M., Challacombe, S. J., Ficarra, G., Flint, S., Greenspan, D., Greenspan, J., et al.: Classification and diagnostic criteria for oral lesions in HIV infection. EC-Clearinghouse on Oral Problems Related to HIV Infections and WHO Collaborating Centre on Oral Manifestations of the Immunodeficiency Virus. J Oral Pathol Med 22: 289–91, 1993.

Axéll, T., Pindborg, J. J., Smith, C. J., van der Waal, I., and an International Collaborative Group on Oral White Lesions: Oral white lesions with special reference to precancerous and tobacco-related lesions: conclusions of an international symposium held in Uppsala, Sweden, May 18–21, 1994. J Oral Pathol Med 25: 49–54, 1996.

Axéll, T., Samaranayake, L. P., Reichart, P. A., Olsen, I.: Guest Editorial – A proposal for reclassification of oral candidosis. Oral Surg Oral Med Oral Pathol Oral Radiol Endod; 84: 111–2, 1997.

B

Badaracco, G., Venuti, A., Di Lonardo, A., Scambia, G., Mozzetti, S., Panici, P. B., Mancuso, S., Marcante, M. L.: Concurrent HPV infection in oral and genital mucosa. J Oral Pathol Med 27: 130–4, 1998.

Baden, E., Jones, J. R., Khedekar, R., Burns, W. A.: Neurofibromatosis of the tongue: a light and electronmicroscopic study with review of the literature from 1849 to 1981, J Oral Med 39, 157-64, 1984.

Baer, U., Boese-Landgraf, J.: Hämostase, Thrombose, Embolie. In Häring, R., Zilch, H.: Chirurgie, 4. Aufl. de Gruyter, Berlin 1997, (S. 163–73).

Bánóczy, J., Szabó, L., Frithiof, L.: White sponge nevus: leukoedema exfoliativum mucosae oris. A report on 45 cases. Swed Dent J 66: 481–93, 1973.

Bánóczy, J.: Follow-up studies in oral leukoplakia. J Maxillofac Surg 5: 69–75, 1977.

Bánóczy, J., Rigo, O.: Prevalence study of oral precancerous lesions with a complex screening system in Hungary. Community Dent Oral Epidemiol 19: 265–7, 1991.

Barasch, A., Gofa, A., Krutchkoff, D. J., Eisenberg, E.: Squamous cell carcinoma of the gingiva – A case series analysis. Oral Surg Oral Med Oral Pathol Oral Radiol Endod 80: 183–7, 1995.

Barrett, A. P.: Gingival lesions in leukemia – a classification. J Periodontol 55: 585–8, 1984.

Barrett, A. P., Bilous, M.: Oral patterns of acute and chronic graft-v-host disease. Arch Dermatol 120: 1461–5, 1984.

Becker, J., Gross, U., Reichart, P. A.: Klinische und histologische Nachuntersuchung nach absoluter Alveolarfortsatzerhöhung mit Hydroxylapatitgranulat. Dtsch Zahnärztl Z 43: 71–3, 1988.

Becker, J., Leser, U., Marschall, M., Langford, A., Jilg, W. S., Gelderblom, H., Reichart, P., Wolf, H.: Expression of proteins encoded by Epstein-Barr virus trans-activator genes depends on the differentiation of epithelial cells in oral hairy leukoplakia. Proc Natl Acad Sci USA 88: 8332–6, 1991.

Becker, J.: Neue Aspekte zur Immunpathogenese des oralen Lichen planus. Dtsch Zahnärztl Z 47: 872–4, 1992.

Becker, J., Schuppan, D., Philipsen, H. P., Reichart, P. A.: Ectomesenchyme of ameloblastic fibroma reveals a characteristic distribution of extracellular matrix proteins. J Oral Pathol Med 21: 156–9, 1992.

Beck-Mannagetta, J., Necek, D., Grasserbauer, M.: Zahnärztliche Aspekte der solitären Kieferhöhlen-Aspergillose. Z Stomatol 83: 283–315, 1986.

Bhonsle, R. B., Murti, P. R., Gupta, P. C., Mehta, F. S.: Reverse dhumti smoking in Goa: an epidemiologic study of 5449 villagers for oral precancerous lesions. Ind J Cancer 13: 301–5, 1976.

Bouquot, J. E., Gorlin R. J.: Leukoplakia, lichen planus and other oral keratoses in 23616 white Americans over the age of 35 years. Oral Surg 61: 373–81, 1986.

Brown, R. S., Beaver, W. T., Bootomley, W. K.: On the mechanism of drug-induced gingival hyperplasia. J Oral Pathol Med 20: 201–9, 1991.

Buchner, A., Merrell, P. W., Carpenter, W. M., Leider, A. S.: Central (intraosseous) calcifying odontogenic cyst. Int J Oral Maxillofac Surg 19: 260–2, 1990.

C

Carter, L. C, Carney, Y., Perez-Pudiewski, D.: Lateral periodontal cyst. Multifactorial analysis of a previously unreported series. Oral Surg Oral Med Oral Pathol Oral Radiol Endod 81: 210–6, 1996.

Carvalho, Y. R., Loyola, A. M., Gomez, R. S., Araújo, V. C.: Peripheral giant cell granuloma. An immunohistochemical and ultrastructural study. Oral Dis 1: 20–5, 1995.

Cawson, R. A., Langdon, I. D, Eveson, J. W.: Surgical pathology of the mouth and jaws. Wright; Oxford 1996.

Challacombe, S. J.: Immunologic aspects of oral candidiasis. Oral Surg Oral Med Oral Pathol 78: 202–10, 1994.

Chambers, M. S., Lyzak, W. A., Martin, J. W., Lyzak, J. S., Toth, B. B.: Oral complications associated in patients with a hematologic malignancy. Oral Surg Oral Med Oral Pathol Oral Radiol Endod 79: 559–63, 1995.

Chang, Y.: Identification of herpesvirus-like DNA sequences in AIDS-associated Kaposi's sarcoma. Science 266: 1865–9, 1994.

Chaudhry, A. P., Yamane, G. M, Sharlock, S. E., Raj, M. S., Jain, R.: A clinicopathological study of intraoral lymphoepithelial cysts. J Oral Med 39: 79–84, 1984.

Cohen Jr, M. M.: Perspectives on craniofacial asymmetry. VI. The hamartoses. Int J Oral Maxillofac Surg 24: 195–200, 1995.

Cruchley, A. T., Williams, D. M., Niedobitek, G., Young, L. S.: Epstein-Barr-virus: biology and disease. Oral Dis 3, Suppl. 1: 156–63, 1997.

Chrysomali, E., Papanicolaou, S. I, Dekker, N. P., Regezi, J. A.: Benign neural tumors of the oral cavity: A comparative immunhistochemical study. Oral Surg Oral Med Oral Pathol Oral Radiol Endod 84: 81–90, 1997.

D

Dagenais, M., Pharoah, M. J., Sikorski, P. A.: The radiographic characteristics of histiocytosis X. A study of 29 cases that involve the jaws. Oral Surg Oral Med Oral Pathol 74: 230–6, 1992.

Dardick, I., Lytwyn, A., Bourne, A. J., Byard, R. W.: Trabecular and solid-cribriform types of basal cell adenoma. A morphologic study of two cases of an unusual variant of monomorphic adenoma. Oral Surg Oral Med Oral Pathol 73: 75–83, 1992.

Delecluse, H. J., Anagnostopoulos, I., Dallenbach, F., Hummel, M., Marafioti, T., Schneider, U., Huhn, D., et al.: Plasmablastic lymphomas of the oral cavity: A new entity associated with the immunodeficiency virus infection. Blood 89: 1413–20, 1997.

E

EC-Clearinghouse on oral problems related to HIV infection and WHO collaborating centre on oral manifestations of the immunodeficiency virus. Classification and diagnostic criteria for oral lesions in HIV infection. J Oral Pathol Med 22: 289–91, 1993.

El-Kabir, M., Samaranayake, L.: Candidosis. In Millard, H. D., Mason, D. K.: Perspectives on 2nd World Workshop on Oral Medicine, August 21–26, 1993. University of Michigan, Michigan 1995 (pp 27–50).

Eng, H.-L., Lu, S. Y., Yang, C.-H., Chen, W. J.: Oral tuberculosis. Oral Surg Oral Med Oral Pathol Oral Radiol Endod 81: 415–20, 1996.

Epstein, J. B., Silverman, S.: Head and neck malignancies associated with HIV infection. Oral Surg Oral Med Oral Pathol 73: 193–200, 1992.

van Es, R. J. J., Keus, R. B., van der Waal, I., Koole, R., Vermey, A.: Osteosarcoma of the jaw bones. Long-term follow up of 48 cases. Int J Oral Maxillofac Surg 26: 191–7, 1997.

Esposito, M., Hirsch, J.-M., Lekholm, U., Thomsen, P.: Biological factors contributing to failures of osseointegrated oral implants. I. Success criteria and epidemiology. Eur J Oral Sci 106: 527–51, 1998.

Esser, E.: Mundhöhlen-Oropharynxkarzinom. Prognose und Radikalität. Disputation anläßlich des 48. Kongresses der Deutschen Gesellschaft für Mund-, Kiefer- und Gesichtschirurgie am 03.06.1998, Osnabrück 1998.

Ettinger, R. L., Manderson, R. D.: A clinical study of sublingual varices. Oral Surg Oral Med Oral Pathol 38: 540–5, 1974.

Eufinger, H., Machtens, E., Akuamoa-Boateng, E.: Oral manifestations of Wegener's granulomatosis. Review of the literature and report of a case. Int J Oral Maxillofac Surg 21: 50–3, 1992.

Eversole, L. R., Tomich, C. E., Cherrick, H. M.: Histogenesis of odontogenic tumours. Oral Surg 32: 569–581, 1971.

Eversole, L. R., Jacobsen, P. L., Stone, C. E.: Oral and gingival changes in systemic sclerosis (scleroderma). J Periodontol 175–8, 1984.

Eversole, L. R.: Immunopathogenic Diseases of the Oral Mucosa. In Millard, H. D., Mason, D. K.: Perspectives on 2nd World Workshop on Oral Medicine, August 21–26, 1993. University of Michigan, Michigan 1995 (pp. 129–35).

F

Fardal, Ø., Perio, D., Johannessen, A. C.: Rare case of keratin-producing multiple gingival cysts. Oral Surg Oral Med Oral Pathol 77: 498–500, 1994.

Farina, A., Pelucchi, S., Carinci, F.: Evidence of bimodal distribution of age in patients affected by pleomorphic adenoma of the parotid gland. Oral Oncol 33: 288–9, 1997.

Farthing, P. M., Maragou, P., Coates, M., Tatnall, F., Leigh, I. M., Williams, D. M.: Characteristics of the oral lesions in patients with cutaneous recurrent erythema multiforme. J Oral Pathol Med 24: 9–13, 1995.

Feifel, H., Friebel, S., Riediger, D.: Verlauf und Therapie der Osteomyelitis des Gesichtsschädels. Dtsch Zahnärztl Z 52: 691–3, 1997.

Ficarra, G., Gaglioti, D.: Facial molluscum contagiosum in HIV-infected patients. Int J Oral Maxillofac Surg 18: 200–1, 1989.

Field, E. A., Speechley, J. A., Rugman, F. R., Varga, E., Tyldesley, W. R.: Oral signs and symptoms in patients with undiagnosed vitamin B12 deficiency. J Oral Pathol Med 24: 468–70, 1995.

Flaitz, C. M., Nichols, C. M., Adler-Storthz, K., Hicks, M. J.: Intraoral squamos cell carcinoma in human immunodeficiency virus infection, Oral Surg Oral Med Oral Pathol Oral Radiol Endod 80: 55–62, 1995.

Flaitz, C. M., Nichols, M., Hicks, M. J.: Herpesviridae-associated persistent mucocutaneous ulcers in acquired immunodeficiency syndrome. A clinicopathologic study. Oral Surg Oral Med Oral Pathol Oral Radiol Endod 81: 433–41, 1996.

Fowler, C. B., Hartman, K. S., Brannon, R. B.: Fibromatosis of the oral and paraoral region. Oral Surg Oral Med Oral Pathol 77: 373–86, 1994.

Fröschl, T., Kerscher, A.: The optimal vestibuloplasty in preprosthetic surgery of the mandible. J Craniomaxillofac Surg 25: 85–90, 1997.

G

Gagari, E., Kabani, S.: Adverse effects of mouthwash use. A review. Oral Surg Oral Med Oral Pathol Oral Radiol Endod 80: 432–9, 1995.

Gardner, D. G.: Oral and maxillofacial pathology. Some current concepts on the pathology of ameloblastomas. Oral Surg Oral Med Oral Pathol Oral Radiol Endond 82: 660–9, 1996.

Gardner, D. G.: Central odontogenic fibroma-current concepts. J Oral Pathol Med 25: 556–61,1996.

Gopalakrishnan, R., Weghorst, C. M., Lehman, T. A., Calvert, R. J., Bijur, G., Sabourin, C. L. K., Mallery, S. R., et al.: Mutated and wild-type p53 expression and HPV integration in proliferative verrucous leukoplakia and oral squamous cell carcinoma. Oral Surg Oral Med Oral Pathol Oral Radiol Endod 83: 471–7, 1997.

Gorlin, R. J., Goltz, R. W.: Multiple nevoid basal cell epithelioma, jaw cysts and bifid rib: a syndrome. New Engl J Med 262: 908–12, 1960.

Gorlin, R., Pindborg, J. J., Cohen, M. M.: Tuberous Sclerosis. In: Syndromes of the Head and Neck. 2nd ed. McGraw-Hill, 1976 (pp. 704–8).

Gorlin, R. J.: Nevoid basal cell carcinoma syndrome. Dermatol Clin 13: 113–25, 1995.

Greenspan, D., de Villiers, E. M., Greenspan, J. S., de Souza, Y. G., zur Hausen, H.: Unusual HPV types in oral warts in association with HIV infection. J Oral Pathol 17: 482–7, 1988.

Greenspan, D.: Treatment of oral candidiasis in HIV infection. Oral Surg Oral Med Oral Pathol 78: 211–5, 1994.

Groot, R. H., van Merkesteyn, J. P. R., Bras, J.: Diffuse sclerosing osteomyelitis and florid osseous dysplasia. Oral Surg Oral Med Oral Pathol Oral Radiol Endod 81: 333–42, 1996.

Gupta, P. C., Murti, P. R., Bhonsle, R. B., Mehta, F. S., Pindborg, J. J.: Effect of cessation of tobacco use on the incidence of oral mucosal lesions in a 10-year follow-up study of 12212 users. Oral Dis 1: 54–8, 1995.

H

Halme, L., Meurman, J. H.; Laine, P., von Smitten, K., Syrjänen, S., Lindqvist, C., Strand-Pettingen, I.: Oral findings in patients with active or inactive Crohn's disease. Oral Surg Oral Med Oral Pathol 76: 175–81, 1993.

Hansen, L. S., Olson, J. A., Silverman, S.: Proliferative verrucous leukoplakia. A long-term study of thirty patients. Oral Surg Oral Med Oral Pathol 60: 285–98, 1985.

Härle, F.: Atlas der Hauttumoren im Gesicht. Hanser, München 1993.

Hata, T., Aikoh, T., Hirokawa, M., Hosoda, M.: Mycosis fungoides with involvement of the oral mucosa. Int J Oral Maxillofac Surg 27: 127–8, 1998.

Heikinheimo, K.: Cell Growth and Differentiation of Developing and Neoplastic Odontogenic Tissues. Academic Dissertation. Institute of Dentistry, University of Turku, and the Department of Pathology, Helsinki, Finland, 1993.

Hell, B.: Zur Schwierigkeit bei der Differentialdiagnose zwischen chronisch-sklerosierender Osteomyelitis und fibröser Dysplasie bzw. ossifizierendem/zementifizierendem Fibrom. In Pfeifer, G., Schwenzer, N.: Fortschritte der Kiefer- und Gesichtschirurgie, Bd. 31. Thieme, Stuttgart 1986 (S. 31).

Herrmann, D.: Karzinomentstehung bei oralem Lichen planus – Langzeituntersuchung an 919 Patienten. Dtsch Zahnärztl Z 47: 877–9, 1992.

Hiraga, T., Tanaka, S., Ikegame, M., Koizumi, M., Iguchi, H., Nakajima, T., Ozawa, H.: Morphology of bone metastasis. Eur J Cancer 34: 230–9, 1998.

Hiroki, A., Nakamura, S., Shinohara, M., Oka, M.: Significance of oral examination in chronic graft-versus-host disease. J Oral Pathol Med 23: 209–15, 1994.

Hirshberg, A., Leibovich, P., Buchner, A.: Metastatic tumors to the jawbones: analysis of 390 cases. J Oral Pathol Med 23: 337–41, 1994.

Hogewind, W. F. C., van der Waal, I.: Prevalence study of oral leukoplakia in a selected population of 1000 patients from the Netherlands. Community Dent Oral Epidemiol 16: 302–5, 1988.

Hogewind, W. F. C.: Oral Leukoplakia in a Dutch Population. A Clinical Study. Dissertation. Vrije Universiteit, Amsterdam, 1990.

Holland-Moritz, R.; Rimpler, M., Rudolph, P.-O.: Allergie gegenüber Gold in der Mundhöhle. Dtsch Zahnärztl Z 35: 963–67, 1980.

Hornstein, O.P.: Erkrankungen des Mundes – Ein interdisziplinäres Handbuch und Atlas. Kohlhammer, Stuttgart, 1996.

Houston, G. D., Fowler, C. B.: Extraosseous calcifying epithelial odontogenic tumor. Report of two cases and review of the literature. Oral Surg Oral Med Oral Pathol Oral Radiol Endod 83: 577–83,1997.

I

Ishigami, T., Schmidt-Westhausen, A., Philipsen, H.-P., Baiborodin, S.-I., Gelderblom, H., Reichart, P. A.: Oral manifestation of alpha-mannosidosis: report of a case with ultrastructural findings. J Oral Pathol Med 24: 85–88, 1995.

Ivanyi, L., Kirby, A., Zakrzewska, J. M.: Antibodies to mycobacterial stress protein in patients with orofacial granulomatosis. J Oral Pathol Med 22: 320–2, 1993.

J

Johnson, N. W., Ranasinghe, A. W., Warnakulasuriya, K. A. A. S.: Potentially malignant lesions and conditions of the mouth and oropharynx: natural history – cellular and molecular markers of risk. Eur J Cancer Prev 2: 31–51, 1993.

Johnson, N. W., Warnakulasuriya, S., Tavassoli, M.: Hereditary and environmental risk factors, clinical and laboratory risk markers for head and neck, especially oral, cancer and precancer. Eur J Cancer Prev 5: 5–17, 1996.

Johnson, N. W.: Essential questions concerning periodontal diseases in HIV infection. Oral Dis 3: 138–40, 1997.

Johnson, N. W.: Ursachen für Mundhöhlenkrebs. FDI World 6: 7–11, 1998.

Jonsson, R.: Oral Manifestations of Systemic Lupus Erythematosus. Dissertation. University of Göteborg, Faculty of Odontology, Göteborg, 1983.

Jordan, R. C. K., Speight, P. M.: Extranodal Non-Hodgkin's Lymphomas of the Oral Cavity. In Seifert, G.: Oral Pathology – Actual Diagnostic and Prognostic Aspects. 1st ed. Springer, Berlin 1996 (pp. 125–146).

Jorgenson, R. J., Levin S.: White sponge nevus. Arch Dermatol 117: 73–6, 1981.

Jovanovic, A.: Squamous cell carcinoma of the lip and the oral cavity – an epidemiological study. Dissertation. Academisch Ziekenhuis, Amsterdam, 1994.

Jungell, P.: Oral lichen planus. A review. Int J Oral Maxillofac Surg 20: 129–35, 1991.

Jungell, P., Malmström, M.: Cyclosporin A mouthwash in the treatment of oral lichen planus. Int J Oral Maxillofac Surg 25: 60–2, 1996.

K

Kaugars, G. E., Heise, A. P., Riley, W. T., Abbey, L. M., Svirsky, J. A.: Oral melanotic macules. A review of 353 cases. Oral Surg Oral Med Oral Pathol 76: 59–61, 1993.

Kaugars, G. E., Silverman, S., Lovas, J. G. L., Thompson, J. S., Brandt, R. B., Singh, V. N.: Use of antioxidant supplements in the treatment of human oral leukoplakia. A review of the literature and current studies. Oral Surg Oral Med Oral Pathol 81: 5–14, 1996.

Keutel, C., Vees, B., Krimmel, M., Cornelius, C. P., Schwenzer, N.: Orale, faziale und kraniale Manifestationen der Neurofibromatose von Recklinghausen (NF). Mund Kiefer Gesichts Chir 1: 268–71, 1997.

King, R. C., Smith, B. R., Burk, J. L.: Dermoid cyst in the floor of the mouth. Review of the literature and case reports. Oral Surg Oral Med Oral Pathol 78: 567–76, 1994.

Könsberg, R., Axéll, T.: Treatment of Candida-infected denture stomatitis with a miconazole lacquer. Oral Surg Oral Med Oral Pathol 78: 306–11, 1994.

Kosmehl, H., Berndt, A., Katenkamp, D., Hyckel, P., Stiller, K.-J., Gabler, U., Langbein, L., Reh, T.: Integrin receptors and their relationship to cellular proliferation and differentiation of oral squamous cell carcinoma. A quantitative immunhistochemical study. J Oral Pathol Med 24: 343–8, 1995.

Kowitz, G., Lucatorto, F., Bennett, W.: Effects of dentifrices on soft tissues of the oral cavity. J Oral Med 28: 105–9, 1973.

Kramer, J. R., Pindborg, J. J., Bezroukov, V., Infirri, J. S.: Guide to epidemiology and diagnosis of oral mucosal diseases and conditions. Community Dent Oral Epidemiol 8: 1–26, 1980.

Kramer, I. R. H., Pindborg, J. J., Shear, M.: Histologic Typing of Odontogenic Tumours. World Health Organization. 2nd ed. Springer, Berlin 1992.

Kuntz, A., Reichart, P. A.: Adenomatoid odontogenic tumour mimicking a globulo-maxillary cyst. Int J Oral Surg 15, 632-6, 1986.

L

Lamey, P. J., McNab, L., Lewis, M. A. O., Gibb, R.: Orofacial artefactual disease. Oral Surg Oral Med Oral Pathol 77: 131–4, 1994.

Lamey, P. J.: Burning mouth syndrome. Dermatol Clin 14: 339–354, 1996.

Lamster, I. B., Grbic, J. T., Bucklan, R. S., Mitchell-Lewis, D., Reynolds, H. S., Zambon, J. J.: Epidemiology and diagnosis of HIV-associated periodontal diseases. Oral Dis 3: 141–8, 1997.

Lang, N. P., Mombelli, A., Tonetti, S. M.; Brägger, U., Hämmerle, C. H. F.: Clinical trials on therapies for peri-implant infections. Ann Periodontol 2: 343–56, 1997.

Langford, A., Groth, A., Kunze, R., Gelderblom, H., Reichart, P. A.: Oral hyperpigmentation associated with HIV infection. J Dent Res 68: 189, 1989.

Langford, A., Kunze, R., Timm, H., Ruf, B., Reichart, P. A.: Cytomegalovirus-associated oral ulcerations in HIV-infected patients. J Oral Pathol Med; 19: 71–6, 1990.

Langford, A., Dienemann, D., Schürmann, D., Pohle, H.-D., Pauli, G., Stein, H., Reichart, P. A.: Oral manifestations of AIDS-associated non-Hodgkin's lymphomas. Int J Oral Maxillofac Surg 20: 136–41, 1991.

Langford, A., Langer, R., Lobeck, H., Stolpmann, H.-J., Pohle, H.-D., Reichart, P. A., Bier, J.: Human immunodeficiency virus-associated squamous cell carcinomas of the head and neck presenting as oral and primary intraosseous squamous cell carcinomas. Quintessence Int 9: 635–54, 1995.

Langstädtler, L., Reichart, P. A., Schmidt-Westhausen, A., Gross, U.: Orale Ulzerationen bei HIV1-seropositiven Patienten. Dtsch Z Mund Kiefer Gesichts Chir 20: 278–80, 1996.

Lau, K. S., Tideman, H., Wu, P. C.: Ameloblastic carcinoma of the jaws. A report of two cases. Oral Surg Oral Med Oral Pathol Oral Radiol Endod 85: 78–81, 1998.

Lay, K. M., Sein, K., Hyint, A., Ko, S. K., Pindborg J. J.: Epidemiologic study of 6000 villagers of oral precancerous lesions in Bilugyun: preliminary report. Community Dent Oral Epidemiol 10: 152–5, 1982.

Lehner, T.: Oral candidosis. Dent Pract 91: 209–16, 1967.

Lilly, J., Juhlin, T., Lew, D., Vincent, S., Lilly, G.: Wegener's granulomatosis presenting as oral lesions – A case report. Oral Surg Oral Med Oral Pathol Oral Radiol Endod 85: 153–7, 1998.

Loff, S., Wessel, L., Wirth, H., Manegold, B. C., Pilcher, H., Waag, K.-L.: Peutz-Jeghers-Syndrom – Beobachtungen am Klinikum Mannheim über 25 Jahre. Langenbecks Arch Chir 380: 43–52, 1995.

M

Machtens, E., Bremerich, A.: Infektionen. In Hausamen, J.-E., Machtens, E., Reuther, J.: Kirschnersche allgemeine und spezielle Operationslehre. Mund-, Kiefer- und Gesichtschirurgie. 3. Aufl. Springer, Berlin 1995 (S. 91–127).

MacPhail, L. A., Greenspan, D., Feigal, D. W., Lennette, E. T., Greenspan, J. S.: Recurrent aphthous ulcers in association with HIV infection. Description of ulcer types and analysis of T-lymphocyte subsets. Oral Surg Oral Med Oral Pathol 71: 678–83, 1991.

Maerker, R., Burkhardt, A.: Klinik oraler Leukoplakien und Präkanzerosen. Retrospektive Studie an 200 Patienten. Dtsch Z Mund Kiefer Gesichts Chir. 2: 206–220, 1978.

Makek, M. S., Sailer, H. F.: Endothelialer Pseudotumor (sog. pyogenes Granulom). Bericht über 140 Fälle. Schweiz Monatsschr Zahnheilkd 95: 248–60, 1985.

Markopoulos, A. K., Antoniades, D., Papanayotou, P., Trigonidis, G.: Malignant potential of oral lichen planus: a follow-up study of 326 patients. Oral Oncol 33: 263–9, 1997.

McCartan, B. E.: Psychological factors associated with oral lichen planus. J Oral Pathol Med 24: 273–5, 1995.

McCartan, B. E., McCreary, C. E.: Oral lichenoid drug eruptions. Oral Dis 3: 58–63, 1997.

McCullough, M. J., Ross, B. C., Reade, P. C.: Candida albicans: a review of its history, taxonomy, epidemiology, virulence attributes, and methods of strain differentiation. Int J Oral Maxillofac Surg 25: 136–44, 1996.

Mehta, F. S, Gupta, P. C., Daftary, D. K., Pindborg J. J., Chokso, S. K.: An epidemiologic study of oral cancer and precancerous conditions among 101761 villagers in Maharashtra, India. Int J Cancer 10: 134–41, 1972.

Mehta, F. S., Pindborg, J. J.: Spontaneous regression of oral leukoplakias among Indian villagers in 15-year-follow-up study. Community Dent Oral Epidemiol 2: 80–84, 1974.

van Merkesteyn, J. P. R., Groot, R. H., van den Akker, H. P., Bakker, D. J., Borgmeijer-Hoelen, A. M. M. J.: Treatment of chronic suppurative osteomyelitis of the mandible. Int J Oral Maxillofac Surg 26: 450–4, 1997.

Meyer, T., Hart, I. R.: Mechanisms of tumour metastasis. Eur J Cancer 34: 214–21, 1998.

Meyer, U., Kleinheinz, J., Gaubitz, M., Schulz, M., Weingart, D., Joos, U.: Orale Manifestationen bei Patienten mit systemischem Lupus erythematodes. Mund Kiefer Gesichts Chir 1: 90–4, 1997.

Mighell, A. J., Robinson, P. A., Hume, W. J.: Peripheral giant cell granuloma: a clinical study of 77 cases from 62 patients, and literature review. Oral Dis 1: 12–9, 1995.

Mobini, N., Nagarwalla, N., Ahmed, R. A.: Oral pemphigoid – Subset of cicatricial pemphigoid? Oral Surg Oral Med Oral Pathol Oral Radiol Endod 85: 37–43, 1998.

Mohammadi, H., Said-Al-Naief, N. A. H., Heffez, L. B.: Arteriovenous malformation of the mandible. Report of a case with a note on the differential diagnosis. Oral Surg Oral Med Oral Pathol Oral Radiol Endod 84: 286–9, 1997.

Muller, S., Parker, D. C., Kapadia, S. B., Budnick, S. D., Barnes, E. L.: Ameloblastic fibrosarcoma of the jaws. A clinicopathologic and DNA analysis of five cases and review of the literature with discussion of its relationship to ameloblastic fibroma. Oral Surg Oral Med Oral Pathol Oral Radiol Endod 79: 469–77, 1995.

N

Nagler, R., Peled, M., Laufer, D.: Cervicofacial actinomycosis: a diagnostic challenge. Oral Surg Oral Med Oral Pathol Oral Radiol Endod 83: 652–6, 1997.

Nakamura, S., Hiroki, A., Shinohara, M., Gondo, H., Ohyama, Y., Mouri, T., Sasaki, M., et al.: Oral involvement in chronic graft-versus-host disease after allogeneic bone marrow transplantation. Oral Surg Oral Med Oral Pathol Oral Radiol Endod 82: 556–63, 1996.

Newton, A. V.: Denture sore mouth. Brit Dent J 112: 357–60, 1962.

Ng, H. K., Siar, C. H., Ganesapillai, T.: Sarcoid-like foreign body reaction in body piercing – A report of two cases. Oral Surg Oral Med Oral Pathol Oral Radiol Endod 84: 28–31, 1997.

Nxumalo, T. N., Shear, M.: Gingival cysts in adults. J Oral Pathol Med 21: 309–13, 1992.

O

Oehlers, F. A. C.: Periapical lesions and residual dental cysts. Brit J Oral Surg 8: 103–13, 1970.

Ogden, R. G., Cowpe, J. G., Wight, A. J.: Oral exfoliative cytology: review of methods of assessment. J Oral Pathol Med 26: 201–5, 1997.

P

Parkin, D. M., Muir, C. S., Whelan S. C.: Cancer Incidence in Five Continents. Vol. 6. Int. Agency for Research on Cancer, Lyon. IARC Scientific Publication No. 120, 1992.

Pedersen, A.: Recurrent aphthous ulceration: Virological and immunological aspects. APMIS 101, suppl. 37, 1993.

Pheiffer, K. F., Ould, G., Hoffmeister, B., Sterry, W., Kunstmann, P., Kirch, W.: Syndrome vulvo-vagino-gingival non spécifique. Rev Stomatol Chir Maxillofac 89: 109–11, 1988.

Phelan, J. A., Freedman, P. D., Newsome, N., Klein, R. S.: Major aphthous-like ulcers in patients with AIDS. Oral Surg Oral Med Oral Pathol 71: 68–72, 1991.

Philipsen, H. P.: Om Keratocyster i Kæberne. Tandlægebladet 60: 963–80, 1956.

Philipsen, H. P., Birn, H.: The adenomatoid odontogenic tumor. Acta Pathol Microbiol Scand 75: 375–98, 1969.

Philipsen, H. P., Reichart, P. A., Zhang, K. H., Nikai, H., Yu, Y. X.: Adenomatoid odontogenic tumor: biologic profile based on 499 cases. J Oral Pathol Med 20: 149–58, 1991.

Philipsen, H. P., Ormiston, I. W., Reichart, P. A.: The desmo- and osteoplastic ameloblastoma. Histologic variant or clinicopathologic entity? Case reports. J Oral Maxillofac Surg 21: 352–7, 1992.

Philipsen, H. P., Samman, N., Ormiston, I. W., Wu, P. C., Reichart, PA.: Variants of the adenomatoid odontogenic tumor with a note on tumor origin. J Oral Pathol Med 21: 348–52, 1992.

Philipsen, H. P., Reichart, P. A.: Squamous odontogenic tumor (SOT): a benign neoplasm of the periodontium. A review of 36 reported cases. J Clin Periodontol 23: 922–6, 1996.

Philipsen, H. P., Reichart, P. A.: The adenomatoid odontogenic tumour: ultrastructure of tumour cells and non-calcified amorphous masses. J Oral Pathol Med 25: 491–6, 1996.

Philipsen, H. P., Reichart, P. A., Prætorius, F.: Mixed odontogenic tumours and odontomas. Considerations on interrelationship. Review of the literature and presentation of 134 new cases of odontomas. Oral Oncol 33: 86–99, 1997.

Philipsen, H. P., Reichart, P. A.: The unicystic ameloblastoma – a review of 193 cases from the literature. Oral Oncol 34: 317–25, 1998.

Philipsen, H. P., Reichart, P. A.: The adenomatoid odontogenic tumor. Facts and figures. Oral Oncol 35: 125–131, 1999

Pierce, A. M., Sampson, W. J., Wilson, D. F., Goss, A. N.: Fifteen-year follow-up of a family with inherited craniofacial fibrous dysplasia. J Oral Maxillofac Surg 54: 780–8, 1996.

Piffkó, J., Bánkfalvi, A., Öfner, D., Berens, A., Tkotz, T., Joos, U., Böcker, W., Schmid, K. W.: Expression of p53 protein in oral squamous cell carcinomas and adjacent non-tumorous mucosa of the floor of the mouth: an archival immunohistochemical study using wet autoclave pretreatment for antigen retrieval. J Oral Pathol Med 24: 337–42, 1995.

Pindborg, J. J.: Calcifying epithelial odontogenic tumors. Acta Pathol Microbiol Scand 3: 71–6, 1955.

Pindborg, J. J.: Krebs und Vorkrebs der Mundhöhle. Quintessenz, Berlin 1982.

Pindborg, J. J., Reichart, P. A.: Atlas of Diseases of the Oral Cavity in HIV Infection. Munksgaard, Copenhagen 1995.

Pindborg, J. J., Reichart, P. A., Smith, C. J., van der Waal, I.: Histological Typing of Cancer and Precancer of the Oral Mucosa. 2nd ed. Springer, Berlin 1997.

Pisano, J. J., Coupland, R., Chen, S.-Y., Miller, A. S.: Plasmocytoma of the oral cavity and jaws. A clinicopathologic study of 13 cases. Oral Surg Oral Med Oral Pathol Oral Radiol Endod 83: 265–71, 1997.

Porter, S. R., Scully, C.: Orofacial manifestations in the primary immunodeficiency disorders. Oral Surg Oral Med Oral Pathol 78: 4–13, 1994.

Prabhu, S. R.: Protozoal infections. In Prabhu, S. R., Wilson, D. F., Daftary, D. K., Johnson, N. W.: Oral Diseases in the Tropics. Oxford University Press 1992 (pp. 145–9).

Prabhu, S. R., Prætorius, F.: Mixed Bacterial Infections of Oral Tissues: Fusospirochaetal Diseases. In Prabhu, S. R., Wilson, D. F., Daftary, D. K., Johnson N. W.: Oral Diseases in the Tropics. Oxford University Press 1992 (pp. 264–9).

Prabhu, S. R., Ramanathan, K., Guimaraes, S. A. C., Yip, W. K.: Fungal infections. In Prabhu, S. R., Wilson, D. F., Daftary, D. K., Johnson, N. W.: Oral Diseases in the Tropics. Oxford University Press 1992 (pp. 154–79).

Prætorius-Clausen, F.: Rare oral viral disorders. (Molluscum contagiousum, localized keratoacanthoma, verrucae, condyloma acuminatum and focal epithelial hyperplasia). Oral Surg Oral Med Oral Pathol 34: 604–18, 1972.

R

Raab-Traub, N., Webster-Cyriaque, J.: Epstein-Barr virus infection and expression in oral lesions. Oral Dis 3: 164–70, 1997.

Ramirez-Amador, V., Silverman S., Mayer, P., Tyler, M., Quivey, J.: Candidal colonization and oral candidiasis in patients undergoing oral and pharyngeal radiation therapy. Oral Surg Oral Med Oral Pathol Oral Radiol Endod 84: 149–53, 1997.

Rateitschak, K. H., & E. M., Wolf, H. and Hassell, T. M.: *Color Atlas of Periodontology,* Third Edition. Thieme Medical Publishers, Stuttgart & New York, 2001.

Reich, R. H., Reichart, P. A., Ostertag, H.: Ameloblastic fibro-odontome. J Maxillofac Surg 12: 230–4, 1984.

Reichart, P. A.: The clinical picture: Cancrum oris. Quintessence Int 5: 77–8, 1974.

Reichart, P. A.: Pathologic changes in the soft palate in lepromatous leprosy. Oral Surg Oral Med Oral Pathol 38: 898–904, 1974.

Reichart, P. A.: Facial and oral manifestations in leprosy. An evaluation of seventy cases. Oral Surg Oral Med Oral Pathol 41: 385–99, 1976.

Reichart, P. A.: Infektionen der Mundschleimhaut (Teil I). Mund Kiefer Gesichtschir 3: 236–41, 1999a.

Reichart, P. A.: Infektionen der Mundschleimhaut (Teil II). Mund Kiefer Gesichtschir 3: 298–308, 1999b.

Reichart, P. A.: Clinical management of selected oral fungal and viral infections during HIV- disease. Int Dent J 49: 251–9, 1999c.

Reichart, P. A., Ananatasan, T., Reznik, G.: Gingiva and periodontium in lepromatous leprosy – a clinical, radiological and microscopical study. J Periodontol 47: 455–60, 1976.

Reichart, P. A., Dornow, H.: Gingivo-periodontal manifestations in chronic benign neutropenia. J Clin Periodontol 5: 74–80, 1978.

Reichart, P. A., Köster, J.: Selbstinduzierte Gingivamutilationen – ein diagnostisches und therapeutisches Problem. Dtsch Zahnärztl Z 33: 93–5, 1978.

Reichart, P. A., Zobl, H.: Transformation of ameloblastic fibroma to fibrosarcoma. Int J Oral Surg 7: 503–7, 1978.

Reichart, P. A., Lubach, D., Vonnahme F.-J.: Zur Klinik und Morphologie der fokalen epithelialen Hyperplasie. Dtsch Z Mund Kiefer Gesichts Chir 6: 249–52, 1982.

Reichart, P. A., Srisuwan, S., Metah, D.: Lesions of the facial and trigeminal nerve in leprosy: an evaluation of 43 cases. Int J Oral Surg 11: 14–20, 1982.

Reichart, P. A., Lubach, D., Becker, J.: Gingival manifestation in linear nevus sebaceous syndrome. Int J Oral Surg 12: 437–43, 1983.

Reichart, P. A., Ries, P.: Considerations on the classification of odontogenic tumours. Int J Oral Surg 12: 323–33, 1983.

Reichart, P. A., Mohr, U., Srisuwan, S., Geerlings, H., Theetranont, C., Kangwanpong, T.: Precancerous and other oral mucosal lesions related to chewing, smoking and drinking habits in Thailand. Community Dent Oral Epidemiol 15: 152–60, 1987.

Reichart, P. A., Neuhaus, F., Sookasem, M.: Prevalence of torus palatinus and torus mandibularis in Germans and Thai. Community Dent Oral Epidemiol 16: 61–4, 1988.

Reichart, P. A., Langford, A., Gelderblom, H. R., Pohle, H. D., Becker, J., Wolf, H.: Oral hairy leukoplakia: observations in 95 cases and review of the literature. J Oral Pathol Med 18: 410–5, 1989.

Reichart, P. A., Philipsen, H. P., Dürr, U.: Epulides in dogs. J Oral Pathol Med 18: 92–6, 1989.

Reichart, P. A., Schiødt, M.: Non-pigmented oral Kaposi's sarcoma (AIDS). Int J Oral Maxillofac Surg 18: 197–9, 1989.

Reichart, P. A., Roy, R. G., Prabhu S. R.: B. Leprosy (Hansen's disease). In Prabhu, S. R., Wilson, D. F., Daftary, D. K., Johnson N. W.: Oral Diseases in the Tropics. Oxford University Press 1992 (pp. 202–14).

Reichart, P. A., Langford, A., Pohle, H. D.: Epidemic oro-facial Kaposi's sarcoma (eKS) – report on 124 cases. Oral Oncol, Eur J Cancer 29B: 187–9, 1993.

Reichart, P. A., van Wyk, C. W., Becker, J., Schuppan, D.: Distribution of procollagen type III, collagen type VI and tenascin in oral submucous fibrosis (OSF). J Oral Pathol Med 23: 394–8, 1994.

Reichart, P. A., Philipsen, H. P., Sonner, S.: Ameloblastoma: biological profile of 3677 cases. Oral Oncol, Eur J Cancer 2: 86–99, 1995.

Reichart, P. A.: Oral Pathology of Acquired Immunodeficiency Syndrome and Orofacial Kaposi's Sarcoma. In Seifert, G.: Oral Pathology – Actual Diagnostic and Prognostic Aspects. Springer Berlin 1996 (pp. 97–124).

Reichart, P. A., Kohn, H.: Prevalence of oral leukoplakia in 1000 Berliners. Oral Dis 2: 291–4, 1996.

Reichart, P. A., Philipsen, H.P.: Betel and Miang – Vanishing Thai Habits. White Lotus, Bangkok 1996.

Reichart, P. A., Weigel, D., Schmidt-Westhausen, A., Pohle, H.D.: Exfoliative cheilitis (EC) in AIDS – association with Candida infection. J Oral Pathol Med 26: 290–3, 1997.

Reichart, P. A., Philipsen, H. P.: Betel chewer's mucosa – a review. J Oral Pathol Med 27: 239–42, 1998.

Reichart, P. A.: Surgical Management of Non-malignant Lesions of the Mouth. In Booth, P. W., Hausamen, J. E.: Maxillofacial Surgery. Churchill Livingstone 1999.

Reichart, P. A., Gelderblom, H. R.: AIDS-Kompendium für Zahnärzte. Hoechst Marion Roussell Deutschland 1999.

Reinish, E. I., Raviv, M., Srolovitz, H., Gornitsky, M.: Tongue, primary amyloidosis, and multiple myeloma. Oral Surg Oral Med Oral Pathol 77: 121–5, 1994.

Riethdorf, S., Friedrich, R. E., Ostwald, C., Barten, M., Gogacz, P., Gundlach, K. K. H., Schlechte, H., et al.: p53 gene mutations and HPV infection in primary head and neck squamous cell carcinomas do not correlate with overall survival: a long term follow-up study. J Oral Pathol Med 26: 315–21, 1997.

Robert-Koch-Institut: AIDS/HIV Halbjahresbericht I / 1999. Bericht des AIDS-Zentrums im Robert Koch-Institut über aktuelle epidemiologische Daten, S. 1–20, 1999.

Robinson, J. C., Lozada-Nur, F., Frieden, I.: Oral pemphigus vulgaris – A review of the literature and a report on the management of 12 cases. Oral Surg Oral Med Oral Pathol Oral Radiol Endod 84: 349–55, 1997.

Roed-Petersen, B., Bánóczy, J., Pindborg, J. J.: Smoking habits and histological characteristics of oral leukoplakias in Denmark and Hungary. Br J Cancer 28: 575–9, 1973.

Roed-Petersen, B., Renstrup, G.: A topographical classification of the oral mucosa suitable for electronic data processing. Its application to 560 leukoplakias. Acta Odontol Scand 27: 681–95, 1969.

Romagnoli, P., Pimpinelli, N., Mori, M., Reichart, P. A., Eversole, L. R., Ficarra, G.: Immunocompetent cells in oral candidiasis of HIV-infected patients: an immunohistochemical and electron microscopical study. Oral Dis 3: 99–105, 1997.

Rossie, K. M., Guggenheimer, J.: Thermally induced „nicotine" stomatitis. Oral Surg Oral Med Oral Pathol 70: 597–9, 1990.

Rubens, R. D.: Bone metastases – The clinical problem. Eur J Cancer 34: 210–3, 1998.

Rubright, W. C., Walker J. A., Karlsson U. L., Diehl D. L.: Oral slough caused by dentifrice detergents and aggravated by drugs with antisialic activity. J Am Dent Assoc 97: 215–220, 1978.

Rutkauskas, J. S., Davis, J. W.: Effects of chlorhexidine during immunosuppressive chemotherapy. A preliminary report. Oral Surg Oral Med Oral Pathol 76: 441 –8, 1993.

S

Safrin, S.: Herpes Simplex Virus Infections in HIV-Infected Patients: Clinical Course and Management. DAAC Forum, 1996 (S. 12–17).

Sailer, H. F., Pajarola, G. F.: *Oral Surgery for the General Dentist.* Thieme Medical Publishers, Stuttgart & New York, 1999.

Sakki, T., Knuuttila, M. L. E., Läärä, E., Antilla, S. S.: The association of yeasts and denture stomatitis with behavioral and biologic factors. Oral Surg Oral Med Oral Pathol Oral Radiol Endod 84: 624–9, 1997.

Sankaranarayanan, R., Mathew, B., Varghese, C., Sudhakaran, P. R., Menon, V., Jayadeep, A., Nair, M. K., et al.: Chemoprevention of oral leukoplakia with vitamin A and beta carotene: an assessment. Oral Oncol 33: 231–6, 1997.

Savage, N. W.: Oral lichenoid drug eruptions. Oral Dis 3: 55–7, 1997.

Saxon, M. A., Ambrosius, W. T., Rehemtula, A.-K. F., Russell, A. L., Eckert, G. J.: Sustained relief of oral aphthous ulcer pain from topical diclofenac in hyaluronan. A randomized, double-blind clinical trial. Oral Surg Oral Med Oral Pathol Oral Radiol Endod 84: 356–61, 1997.

Scheifele, C., Reichart, P. A.: Orale Leukoplakien bei manifestem Plattenepithelkarzinom – eine prospektive Studie an 101 Patienten. Mund Kiefer Gesichts Chir, 1998, im Druck.

Schell, H. Schönberger, A.: Zur Lokalisationshäufigkeit von benignen und präkanzerosen Leukoplakien und von Karzinomen in der Mundhöhle. Z Hautkr 62: 798–804, 1987.

Schenk, R. K.: Bone Regeneration: Biologic Basis. In Buser, D., Dahlin, C., Schenk, R. K.: Guided Bone Regeneration in Implant Dentistry. Quintessence, Chicago 1994 (pp. 49–100).

Schepman, K. P., van der Waal, I.: A proposal for a classification and staging system for oral leukoplakia: a preliminary study. Oral Oncol, Eur J Cancer, 31: 396–8, 1995.

Schliephake, H., Eckardt, A., Gaida-Martin, C., Pytlik, C.: PCNA/Cyclin-Antikörper als Proliferationsmarker bei Mundschleimhauterkrankungen. Dtsch Zahnärztl Z 47: 845–8, 1992.

Schmidt-Westhausen, A., Gelderblom, H. R., Reichart, P. A.: Oral hairy leukoplakia in an HIV-seronegative heart transplant patient. J Oral Pathol Med 19: 192–4, 1990.

Schmidt-Westhausen, A., Philipsen, H. P., Reichart, P. A.: Das ameloblastische Fibrom – ein odontogener Tumor im Wachstumsalter. Dtsch Zahnärztl Z 46: 66–8, 1991.

Schmidt-Westhausen, A., Gelderblom, H. R., Neuhaus, P., Reichart, P. A.: Epstein-Barr virus in lingual epithelium of liver transplant patients. J Oral Pathol Med 22: 274–6, 1993.

Schmidt-Westhausen, A., Becker, J., Schuppan, D., Burkhardt, A., Reichart, P. A.: Odontogenic myxoma-characterisation of the extracellular matrix (ecm) of the tumour stroma. Oral Oncol, Eur J Cancer 18:377–80, 1994.

Schmidt-Westhausen, A., Grünewald, T., Reichart, P. A., Pohle, H. D.: Oral manifestations in 70 German HIV-infected women. Oral Dis 3: 28–30, 1997.

Schmidt-Westhausen, A., Pohle, H. D., Lobeck, H, Reichart, P. A.: HIV-assoziierte Speicheldrüsenerkrankungen. Literaturübersicht und drei Fallbeschreibungen. Mund Kiefer Gesichts Chir 1: 82 –85, 1997.

Schmidt-Westhausen, A., Grünewald, T., Reichart, P. A., Pohle, H. D.: Oral manifestations of toxic epidermal necrolysis (TEN) in patients with AIDS – Report of five cases. Oral Dis 4: 90–4, 1998.

Schmidt-Westhausen, A., Reichart, P. A.: Orofaziale Manifestation der HIV-Infektion. In Husstedt, I. W.. HIV und AIDS – Fachspezifische Diagnostik und Therapie. Springer, Berlin 1998 (S. 96–125).

Scully, C., El-Kabir, M., Samaranayake, L. P.: Candida and Oral Candidosis: A Review. Critical Rev Oral Biol Med. 5: 125–57, 1994.

Scully, C.: New Aspects of Oral Viral Diseases. In G. Seifert: Oral Pathology – Actual Diagnostic and Prognostic Aspects. Springer, Berlin 1996 (S. 29–96).

Seifert, G.: Histologic Typing of Salivary Gland Tumours. 2nd ed. Springer, Berlin 1991.

Seifert, G.: Diagnose und Prognose der Speicheldrüsentumoren. Eine Interpretation der neuen revidierten WHO-Klassifikation. Mund Kiefer Gesichts Chir 1: 252–67, 1997.

Seifert, G.: Diagnostische „Fallstricke" („pitfalls") bei benignen und malignen Speicheldrüsenkrankheiten. Ihre Bedeutung für Prognose und Therapie. Mund Kiefer Gesichts Chir 2: 62–9, 1998.

Sewerin, J.: The sebaceous glands in the vermilion border of the lips and the oral mucosa of man. Acta Odontol Scand 33, suppl 68, 1975.

Seymour, R. A., Thomason, J. M., Nolan, A.: Oral lesions in organ transplant patients. J Oral Pathol Med 26: 297–304, 1997.

Shear, M.: Cysts of the Oral Regions. 3rd ed. Wright, Oxford 1992.

Silverman, S., Gorsky, M.: Proliferative verrucous leukoplakia. A follow-up study of 54 cases. Oral Surg Oral Med Oral Pathol Oral Radiol Endod 84: 154–7, 1997.

Slootweg, P. J., Müller, H.: Verrucous hyperplasia or verrucous carcinoma. J. Maxillofac Surg 11: 13–9, 1983.

Smith, L. W., Bhargava, K., Mani, N. J., Malaowalla, A. M., Silverman Jr., S.: Oral cancer and precancerous lesions in 57518 industrial workers of Gujarat, India. Ind J Cancer 12: 118–23, 1975.

Soll, D. R., Morrow, B., Srikantha, T., Vargas, K., Wertz, P.: Developmental and molecular biology of switching in Candida albicans. Oral Surg Oral Med Oral Pathol 78: 194–201, 1994.

Sonner, S.: Das Ameloblastom. 1. Erstellung eines Tumorbioprofils, 2. Immunhistochemische Studie über die extrazelluläre Bindegewebsmatrix. Dissertation. Fachbereich Zahn-, Mund- und Kieferheilkunde der Freien Universität, Berlin 1993.

Sonner, S., Reichart, P. A.: Orale Metastasen maligner Melanome. Dtsch Z Mund Kiefer Gesichtschir 18: 131–5, 1994.

Stiller, M.: Orale Manifestationen autoimmunologischer Erkrankungen mit einer Sicca-Symptomatik. Vergleichende Untersuchungen von Patienten mit einem primären und sekundären Sjögren-Syndrom. Mund Kiefer Gesichts Chir 1: 78–81, 1997.

Straßburg, M., Schneider, W.: Orale Frühmanifestationen akuter Leukämien. Dtsch Zahnärztl Z 48: 10–17, 1993.

Su, L., Weathers, D. R., Waldron, C. A.: Distinguishing features of focal cemento-osseous dysplasias and cemento-ossifying fibromas. I. A pathologic spectrum of 316 cases. Oral Surg Oral Med Oral Pathol Oral Radiol Endod 84: 301–309, 1997a.

Su, L., Weathers, D. R., Waldron, C. A.: Distinguishing features of focal cemento-osseous dysplasia and cemento-ossifying fibromas. II. A clinical and radiologic spectrum of 316 cases. Oral Surg Oral Med Oral Pathol Oral Radiol Endod 84: 540–9, 1997b.

Sugihara, K., Reichart, P. A., Gelderblom, H. R.: Molluscum contagiosum associated with AIDS: a case report with ultrastructural study. J Oral Pathol Med 19: 235–9, 1990.

Sugihara, K., Reupke, H., Schmidt-Westhausen, A., Pohle, H.-D., Gelderblom, H., Reichart, P. A.: Negative staining EM for the detection of Epstein-Bar virus in oral hairy leukoplakia. J Oral Pathol Med 19: 367–70, 1990.

Summerlin, D.-J., Tomich, C. E.: Focal cemento-osseous dysplasia: A clinicopathologic study of 221 cases. Oral Surg Oral Med Oral Pathol 78: 611–620, 1994.

Sun, A., Chang, J. G., Chu, C. T., Liu, B. Y., Yuan, J. H., Chiang, C. P.: Preliminary evidence for an association of Epstein-Barr virus with preulcerative oral lesions in patients with recurrent aphthous ulcers or Behçet's disease. J Oral Pathol Med 27: 168–75, 1998.

Syrjänen, S.: Viral infections of the oral mucosa. Dtsch Zahnärztl Z 52: 657–67, 1997.

T

Takeda, Y.: So-called "immature dentinoma": a case presentation and histological comparison with ameloblastic fibrodentinoma. J Oral Pathol Med 23: 92–6, 1994.

Tanaka, N., Amagasa, T., Iwaki, H., Shioda, S., Takeda, M., Ohashi, K., Reck, S. F.: Oral malignant melanoma in Japan. Oral Surg Oral Med Oral Pathol 78: 81–90, 1994.

Tanaka, N., Nagai, I., Hiratsuka, H., Kohama, G.-I.: Oral malignant melanoma: long-term follow up in three patients. Int J Oral Maxillofac Surg 27: 111–4, 1998.

Thomason, I. M., Ellis, J. S., Kelly, P. J, Seymour, R. A.: Nifedipine pharmacological variables as risk factors for gingival overgrowth in organtransplant patients. Clin Oral Invest 1: 35–9, 1997.

Thorn, J. J., Holmstrup, P. Rindum, J., Pindborg, J. J.: Course of various clinical forms of oral lichen planus. A prospective follow-up study of 611 patients. J Oral Pathol 17: 213–8, 1988.

Toida, M.: So-called calcifying odontogenic cyst: review and discussion on the terminology and classification. J Oral Pathol Oral Med 27: 49–52, 1998.

Tourne, L. P. M., Fricton, J. R.: Burning mouth syndrome. Critical review and proposed clinical management. Oral Surg Oral Med Oral Pathol 74: 158–67, 1992.

Tsuji, T. Mimura, Y., Wen, S., Li, X., Kanekawa, A., Sasaki, K., Shinozaki, F.: The significance of PCNA and p53 protein in some oral tumors. Int J Oral Maxillofac Surg 24: 221–5, 1995.

Tyler, M. T., Bentley, K. C., Cameron, J. M.: Atypical migratory stomatitis and Münchhausen syndrome presenting as periorbital ecchymosis and mandibular subluxation. Oral Surg Oral Med Oral Pathol Oral Radiol Endod 80: 414–9, 1995.

U

Ulmansky, M., Hjørting-Hansen, E., Prætorius, F., Haque, M. F.: Benign cementoblastoma. A review and five new cases. Oral Surg Oral Med Oral Pathol 77: 48–55, 1994.

V

Vedtofte, P., Holmstrup, P., Hjørting-Hansen, E., Pindborg, J. J.: Surgical treatment of premalignant lesions of the oral mucosa. Int J Oral Maxillofac Surg 16: 656–64, 1987.

Vettin, L., Rohrer, M. D., Young, S. K., Reichart, P. A.: Orale Manifestationen bei Morbus Crohn. Dtsch Z Mund Kiefer Gesichtschir 12: 473–6, 1988.

Vicente, M., Soria, A., Mosquera, A., Pérez, J. Lamas, A., Castellano, T., Ramos, A.: Immunoglobulin G subclass measurements in recurrent aphthous stomatitis. J Oral Pathol Med 25: 538–40, 1996.

de Visscher, J. G. A. M., Bouwes Bavinck, J. N., van der Waal, I.: Squamous cell carcinoma of the lower lip in renal-transplant recipients – Report of six cases. Int J Oral Maxillofac Surg 26: 120–3, 1997.

Voorsmit, R. A. C. A.: The Incredible Keratocyst. MD Dissertation, University of Nijmegen. Los Printers, Naarden 1984.

Voûte, A. B. E.: Oral Lichen Planus. A Clinical Study. Dissertation, Vrije Universiteit, Amsterdam, 1994.

W

van der Waal, I.: Diseases of the jaws. Diagnosis and treatment. Munksgaard, Copenhagen 1991 (pp. 113–6).

van der Waal, I., Schepman, K. P., van der Mei, E. H., Smeele, L. E.: Oral leukoplakia: a clinicopathological review. Oral Oncol 33: 291–301, 1997.

Wahi, P. N., Mital, V. P., Lahiri, B., Luthra, U. K., Seth, R. K., Arora, G. D.: Epidemiological study of precancerous lesions of the oral cavity. A preliminary report. Ind J Med Res 58: 1361–91, 1970.

Waldron, C. A., Shafer, W. G.: Leukoplakia revisited. A clinicopathologic study of 3256 oral leukoplakias. Cancer 36: 1386–1392, 1975.

Ward, K. A., Napier, S. S., Winter, P. C., Maw, R. D., Dinsmore, W. W.: Detection of human papilloma virus DNA sequences in oral squamous cell papillomas by the polymerase chain reaction. Oral Surg Oral Med Oral Pathol Oral Radiol Endod 80: 63–6, 1995.

Warnakulasuriya, K. A. A. S., Johnson, N. W.: Sensitivity and specificity of OraScan toluidine blue mouthrinse in the detection of oral cancer and precancer. J Oral Pathol Med 25: 97- 103, 1996.

Weinberg, M. A., Insler, M. S., Campen, R. B.: Mucocutaneous features of autoimmune blistering diseases. Oral Surg Oral Med Oral Pathol Oral Radiol Endod 84: 517–34, 1997.

Williams, D. M.: Vesiculobullous mucocutaneous disease: pemphigus vulgaris. J Oral Pathol Med 18: 544–553, 1989.

Williams, H. K., Williams, D. M.: Oral granular cell tumours: a histological and immunocytochemical study. J Oral Pathol Med 26: 164–9, 1997.

Willinger, B., Beck-Mannagetta, J., Hirschl, A. M., Makristathis, A., Rotter, M. L.: Wirkung von Zinkoxid auf Aspergillus-Arten: Eine mögliche Ursache der lokalen nichtinvasiven Kieferhöhlen-Aspergillose. Mycoses 39: 20–5, 1996.

Wilsch, L, Hornstein, O. P., Bruning, H. et al.: Oral leukoplakia II. Dtsch Zahnärztl Z 33: 132–42, 1978.

Winnie, R., deLuke, D. M.: Melkersson-Rosenthal syndrome. Review of literature and case report. Int J Oral Maxillofac Surg 21: 115–7, 1992.

Woo, S. B., Lee, S. F.-K.: Oral recrudescent herpes simplex virus infection. Oral Surg Oral Med Oral Pathol Oral Radiol Endod 83: 239–43, 1997.

World Health Organisation, Geneva: HIV/AIDS: Global AIDS surveillance. Wkly Epidemiol Rec 47: 401–8, 1999; 48; 406–14, 1999.

Y

Yadav, M., Arivanathan, M., Chandrashekran, A., Tan, B. S, Hashim, B. Y.: Human herpesvirus-6 (HHV-6) DNA and virus-encoded antigen in oral lesions: J Oral Pathol Med 26: 393–401, 1997.

Z

Zakrzewska, J. M., Lopes, V., Speight, P., Hopper, C.: Proliferative verrucous leukoplakia. A report of ten cases. Oral Surg Oral Med Oral Pathol Oral Radiol Endod 82: 396–401, 1996.

Zaridze, D. G.: The effect of nass use and smoking on the risk of oral leukoplakia. Cancer Detect Prev 9: 435–40, 1986.

Zhang, X., Langford, A., Gelderblom, H., Reichart, P.: Ultrastructural findings in oral hyperpigmentation of HIV-infected patients. J Oral Pathol Med 18: 471–4, 1989.

Zheng, T., Holford, T., Chen, Y., Jiang, P., Zhang, B., Boyle, P.: Risk of tongue cancer associated with tobacco smoking and alcohol consumption: a case-control study. Oral Oncol 33: 82–5, 1997.

Zimmer, W. M., Rogers, R. S., Reeve, C. M., Sheridan, P. J.: Orofacial manifestations of Melkersson-Rosenthal syndrome. A study of 42 patients and review of 220 cases from the literature. Oral Surg Oral Med Oral Pathol 74: 610–9, 1992.

Index